Acupuncture: A Clinical Guide

Edited by Ophelia Burnett

hayle
medical

New York

Hayle Medical,
750 Third Avenue, 9ᵗʰ Floor,
New York, NY 10017, USA

Visit us on the World Wide Web at:
www.haylemedical.com

ISBN: 978-1-63241-815-9

Cataloging-in-Publication Data

Acupuncture : a clinical guide / edited by Ophelia Burnett.
     p. cm.
Includes bibliographical references and index.
ISBN 978-1-63241-815-9
1. Acupuncture. 2. Acupuncture points. 3. Alternative medicine. I. Burnett, Ophelia.
RM184 .A28 2019
615.892--dc23

Table of Contents

Permissions

List of Contributors

Index

Preface

The practice of alternative medicine in which thin needles are inserted into the skin for the purpose of curing diseases or relieving the pain is known as acupuncture. It is an integral part of traditional Chinese medicine. It is mostly used in conjunction with other treatment modalities. Filiform needles, nine ancient needles and three-edged needles are the common types of needles used in acupuncture. Some of the common procedures involved in it include needle insertion, cupping therapy and moxibustion. It is most commonly used to treat lower back pain, headache, migraine, arthritis pain and postoperative pain. This book unfolds the innovative aspects of acupuncture, which will be crucial for the progress of this field in the future. It presents researches and studies performed by experts across the globe. This book is a vital tool for all researching or studying acupuncture as it gives incredible insights into emerging trends and concepts.

This book is the end result of constructive efforts and intensive research done by experts in this field. The aim of this book is to enlighten the readers with recent information in this area of research. The information provided in this profound book would serve as a valuable reference to students and researchers in this field.

At the end, I would like to thank all the authors for devoting their precious time and providing their valuable contribution to this book. I would also like to express my gratitude to my fellow colleagues who encouraged me throughout the process.

Editor

Bee venom acupuncture alleviates trimellitic anhydride-induced atopic dermatitis-like skin lesions in mice

Bongjun Sur[1†], Bombi Lee[1†], Mijung Yeom[1], Ju-Hee Hong[1], Sunoh Kwon[1], Seung-Tae Kim[2], Hyang Sook Lee[1,3], Hi-Joon Park[1,3], Hyejung Lee[1,3] and Dae-Hyun Hahm[1,3*]

Abstract

Background: Bee venom acupuncture (BVA), a novel type of acupuncture therapy in which purified bee venom is injected into the specific acupuncture point on the diseased part of the body, is used primarily for relieving pain and other musculoskeletal symptoms. In the present study, therapeutic potential of BVA to improve atopic dermatitis, a representative allergic dysfunction, was evaluated in the mouse model of trimellitic anhydride (TMA)-induced skin impairment.

Methods: Mice were treated with 5 % TMA on the dorsal flank for sensitization and subsequently treated with 2 % TMA on the dorsum of both ears for an additional 12 days after a 3-day interval. From the 7th day of 2 % TMA treatment, bilateral subcutaneous injection of BV (BV, 0.3 mg/kg) was performed daily at BL40 acupuncture points (located behind the knee) 1 h before 2 % TMA treatment for 5 days.

Results: BVA treatment markedly inhibited the expression levels of both T helper cell type 1 (Th1) and Th2 cytokines in ear skin and lymph nodes of TMA-treated mice. Clinical features of AD-like symptoms such as ear skin symptom severity and thickness, inflammation, and lymph node weight were significantly alleviated by BV treatment. BV treatment also inhibited the proliferation and infiltration of T cells, the production of Th1 and Th2 cytokines, and the synthesis of interleukin (IL)-4 and immunoglobulin E (IgE)—typical allergic Th2 responses in blood. The inhibitory effect of BVA was more pronounced at BL40 acupoint than non-acupuncture point located at the base of the tail.

Conclusions: These results indicate that BV injection at specific acupuncture points effectively alleviates AD-like skin lesions by inhibiting inflammatory and allergic responses in a TMA-induced contact hypersensitivity mouse model.

Keywords: Atopic dermatitis, Bee venom, Acupuncture, BL40, Trimellitic anhydride

Background

In traditional Oriental medicine, bee venom acupuncture (BVA), a peculiar type of acupuncture, has been used to relieve pain and to treat various chronic inflammatory diseases in humans. It exerts not only pharmacological effects due to its various bioactive components, but also exerts an acupuncture effect by mechanical stimulation of acupuncture points [1].

BV seems to be much like a double-edged sword. In traditional Oriental medicine, BV therapy relieves pain and inflammation in various acute or chronic diseases [2]. On the other hand, it also induces a systemic or local allergic response, with fever, pain, and itching, sometimes leading to anaphylaxis [3]. According to clinical reports of BVA therapy, subcutaneous or intramuscular injection of BV often causes instant pain and inflammation around the injection site, as well as relieving pain and inflammation [4]. It has even been argued by Oriental physicians treating some musculoskeletal and

* Correspondence: dhhahm@khu.ac.kr
†Equal contributors
[1]Acupuncture and Meridian Science Research Center, College of Korean Medicine, Kyung Hee University, Hoegi-ding, Dongdaemoon-gu, Seoul 130-701, Republic of Korea
[3]The Graduate School of Basic Science of Korean Medicine, College of Korean Medicine, Kyung Hee University, Seoul 130-701, Republic of Korea
Full list of author information is available at the end of the article

immunological diseases using BV therapy that the greater the allergic response the better therapeutic effect is [5].

A growing number of studies provide compelling evidence for the anti-inflammatory effects of BVA in several animal pain models. For example, BVA can inhibit formalin-induced pain and carrageenan-induced inflammation in rat models [6, 7]. Recently, BV and its constituent, melittin, were reported to possess anti-inflammatory, antinociceptive, and anticancer effects, and also have a therapeutic effect against bacterial diarrhea in piglets [8–11]. BVA has also been used to relieve arthritic pain and edema in Korean traditional medicine [12]. Despite the many clinical and animal studies elucidating the medicinal effects of BVA in various pain and inflammatory diseases, there have been few studies of BVA as an alternative therapy for atopic diseases. Because BV sometimes induces systemic anaphylactic responses when injected in excessive amounts, it is reasonable to expect that diseases caused by immunological hypersensitivity, including atopic dermatitis, can be treated by honey bee venom, which is well known to be an inflammatory agent as well as an allergen. To the best of our knowledge, this is the first study to elucidate the medicinal effect of BV on atopic dermatitis-like skin disease in mice.

In this study, an atopic mouse model of allergen-induced contact hypersensitivity was used to assess BVA therapy for human atopic dermatitis. In contrast to other spontaneous (NC/Nga) transgenic and knockout mouse models, this model is simple to develop and its atopic symptoms are highly reproducible. Trimellitic anhydride (TMA), used in this study as an allergen, is a known respiratory sensitizer that induces T cell-dependent contact hypersensitivity in mice, eliciting eosinophil and T cell infiltration, T helper cell type 2 (Th2) cytokine production, and IgE release [13]. In the TMA-induced atopic model, mice are first sensitized on flank skin with TMA, and then T cell-dependent skin inflammation is induced by topical challenge with TMA on the dorsal surfaces of the ears 1 week after sensitization. The severity of atopic inflammation can easily be evaluated by observing ear appearance and measuring ear thickness. The effects of TMA-induced skin inflammation on the cutaneous cytokine profile, infiltration of immune cells, and serum IgE levels have been previously studied [14–16].

Although anti-inflammatory steroids are a conventional therapy for atopic dermatitis, there are however several concerns with this therapy, especially with long-term use. Mid- to high-potency steroids are contraindicated for use on the body and in intertriginous areas because of their side effects, including skin atrophy, hypopigmentation, striae, secondary infection, and acne [17]. Alternative treatments using BV are of particular interest, because BV seems to be effective without causing severe adverse effects like those that are often observed with steroid therapy.

For this purpose, we investigated the medicinal effect of BVA on atopic dermatitis using a TMA-induced contact hypersensitivity dermatitis mouse model. BVA injection was performed at the BL40 acupoint, which is known to cool down the body in Korean traditional medicine [18]. In addition to clinical observation, we also investigated the infiltration of immune cells in ear tissue by histological staining, serum IgE levels by enzyme-linked immunosorbent assay (ELISA), and T cell cytokine profiles in ears and lymph nodes using the Bio-Plex® suspension array system.

Methods
Animals
Male BALB/c mice weighing 28–30 g (10 weeks old) were purchased from Samtaco Co. (Osan, Korea). The mice were housed in a limited-access rodent facility with up to five mice per polycarbonate cage. They were housed in an air-conditioned animal room with a 12 h light/dark cycle (08:00–20:00 h light, 20:00–08:00 h dark) at 23 ± 2 °C and with 50 ± 10 % humidity. Mice were provided with a standard laboratory diet and water *ad libitum*. The animal experiments were conducted in accordance with the *Guide for the Care and Use of Laboratory Animals* (NIH Publication No. 80–23, revised in 1996), and were approved by the Kyung Hee University Institutional Animal Care and Use Committee. All animal experiments began at least 7 days after the animals arrived.

Chemicals and drugs
All chemicals including TMA (98 %), bee venom, prednisolone, isopropyl myristate (98 %), dimethylsulfoxide, ethanol and corn oil were purchased from Sigma-Aldrich Co. (St. Louis, MO, USA). TMA was dissolved in a mixed solvent of acetone (Merck, Darmstadt, Germany) and isopropyl myristate (4:1, v/v) immediately before use. Bee venom was dissolved in saline, and prednisolone was dissolved in a mixed solvent of dimethylsulfoxide, ethanol and corn oil (5:3:92, v/v/v).

Development of atopic dermatitis
A modified version of a protocol described by Schneider et al. was used to induce atopy-like skin dermatitis in mice [19]. Mice were first sensitized with 50 μL of 5 % TMA on the shaved dorsal flank skin on day 0. After an interval for 3 days, the animals received 10 μL of 2 % TMA once a day from days 3 to 14 on both sides of both ears. The mice were sacrificed under anesthesia with pentobarbital on the last day of the experiment. At autopsy, blood was collected from the retro-orbital

plexus, and both ears and auricular lymph nodes were excised.

Experimental groups

The mice were randomly divided into five experimental groups of ten animals each as follows: non-treated naive group (NOR, $n = 10$), vehicle-treated & TMA-treated atopic group (AD, $n = 10$), BV-treated at BL40 acupoint & TMA-treated atopic group (AD + BVA, $n = 10$), BV-treated at non-acupoint & TMA-treated atopic group (AD + BVNA, $n = 10$), and prednisolone-treated & TMA-treated atopic group (AD + PRE, $n = 10$). Prednisolone (30 mg/kg, p.o.) was used as a positive control.

BVA and drug treatments

To determine the optimum conditions for BV injection, changes in skin temperature at the injection site were analyzed under conditions of subcutaneous, intradermal, and intramuscular injection of BV. BV (0.3 mg BV/kg body weight) was injected into the mid-back after hair removal, and the temperature at the injection site was measured using an infrared thermometer (HuBDIC Thermofinder (FS-300), Beauty Korea World Co., Ltd., Seoul, Korea). Each type of BV injection was performed in at least three mice, and temperature measurement was repeated three times per injection site per time point.

Daily treatment with BV and prednisolone was performed 1 h before TMA challenge on days 9 to 14 (a total of six times) (Fig. 1). For BVA treatment, the mice were gently immobilized with hands, and 20 μL BV solution (0.3 mg/kg) was injected bilaterally at a depth of 1 mm at the BL40 acupoints, located in the center of the popliteal crease between the tendons of the biceps femoris and semitendinosus muscles on both legs, using a 1 mL insulin syringe (needle gauge 26; BD Biosciences Co., CA, USA). A non-acupuncture point at the base of the tail was used as a control. The needles were removed from the acupoints immediately after BV injection. As a positive control, prednisolone, a glucocorticoid prodrug, was administered orally to mice at a dose of 30 mg/kg body weight.

Scoring of ear skin manifestations

The ear skin of mice in each experimental group was photographed using a digital camera (Canon 20D; Canon Inc., Tokyo, Japan) to analyze changes in atopic symptoms and clinical appearance of the ear skin and tissues. The severity of atopic dermatitis was macroscopically assessed, and scored in a blinded fashion every 2 days starting from the day after the first 5 % TMA challenge, according to the protocol of Shin HK et al. [20]. Atopic symptoms of ear skins were evaluated by scoring scaling and dryness, hemorrhage and excoriation, and edema and redness, and by then calculating the sum of the individual symptom scores for both ears, graded as 0 (no symptoms), 1 (mild), 2 (moderate), or 3 (severe). The total score for each animal ranges from 0 to 9.

Measurements of ear thickness and auricular lymph node weight

Ear thickness and auricular lymph node weights of all 10 mice in each experimental group was measured. Ear thickness was measured with a dial thickness gauge (Ozaki Seisakusho Co., Tokyo, Japan), and the weight of the auricular lymph node was measured with a digital balance (Mettler-Toledo Inc., Columbus, OH, USA).

ELISA of immune mediators

After scoring of ear skin manifestation, blood samples were rapidly collected from all 10 mice in each experimental group under anesthesia on the day of killing via the retro-orbital plexus using a capillary pipette. Serum was obtained from the blood samples by centrifugation at 6500 rpm for 20 min, and was stored at −70 °C until use. Serum IL-4 and IgE levels were measured using an ELISA kit (R&D Systems Inc., MN, USA and Bethyl Laboratories Inc., TX, USA, respectively). After coating the inner surfaces of microplate wells with each antibody at 4 °C overnight, serum samples (50 μL, 3-fold dilution) were dispensed into the wells and incubated for 1 h. After washing the plate twice, 100 μL avidin-horseradish peroxidase (HRP)-conjugated antibody was added. After another wash, tetramethylbenzidine (TMB) solution was added, and the plate was incubated for 30 min in the dark. After stopping the reaction with 50 μL stop solution, the absorbance at 450 nm was measured using an ELISA reader (Multi-Read 400; Authos Co., Austria).

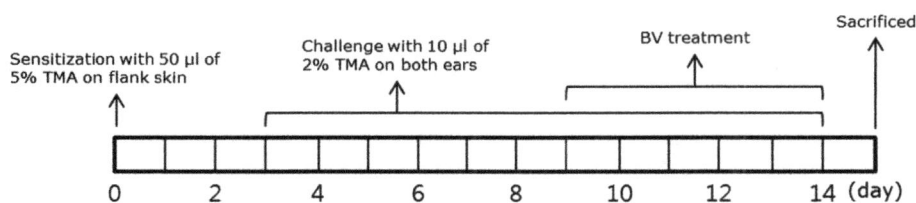

Fig. 1 Experimental schedules for developing TMA-induced atopic dermatitis and treating with BV in mice. TMA, trimellitic anhydride; BV, bee venom

RT-PCR analysis of immune mediators

For this, 5 mice from each group ($n = 10$) were deeply anesthetized with sodium pentobarbital (50 mg/kg, i.p.), and their ear tissues and auricular lymph nodes were quickly collected. Total RNA was isolated from each tissue sample of ear or lymph node. After excision, tissue samples were quickly stored at −80 °C until use. Total RNA was isolated using TRIzol® reagent (Gibco BRL Co., MD, USA). Complementary DNA (cDNA) was synthesized from total RNA with reverse transcriptase (Takara Co., Shiga, Japan). The expression levels of mRNAs were determined by PCR analysis using cDNA as the template. PCR was performed using a PTC-100 programmable thermal controller (MJ Research Co., MA, USA). Primers were designed based on published mRNA sequences using Primer3 primer selection software (Whitehead institute for Biomedical Research, Cambridge, MA: http://biotools.umassmed.edu/bioapps/primer3_www.cgi). Glyceraldehyde 3-phosphate dehydrogenase (GAPDH) was used as a housekeeping gene. PCR products were separated on 1.2 % agarose gels and stained with ethidium bromide. Subsequently, band densities were analyzed using an image analysis system (i-Max™; Core Bio System Co., Ltd., Seoul, Korea). Relative gene expression was determined by calculating the relative band intensity for each gene compared to GAPDH. Table 1 provides the primer sequences and annealing conditions for PCR.

Histology and immunohistochemistry

Five mice from each group ($n = 10$) were deeply anesthetized with sodium pentobarbital (50 mg/kg, i.p.), and their ear tissues were quickly collected. Each ear tissue was embedded in paraffin, and cut into 6 μm-thick sections using a rotatory microtome (Finesse 325; Thermo Shandon Co., UK). The sections were deparaffinized before staining. To demonstrate morphologic changes and eosinophil infiltration, sections were stained with hematoxylin (Merck, Darmstadt, Germany) and 1 % eosin (Sigma-Aldrich Co.) [21]. Staining with toluidine blue (Merck) was performed for mast cell detection. For immunohistochemistry, the other half of each ear was embedded in paraffin and cut into 6 μm-thick sections. The sections were deparaffinized before immunohistochemistry. Slides were incubated overnight at 4 °C in a primary antibody solution containing anti-mouse cluster of differentiation (CD)4 and anti-mouse CD8 rabbit antibodies (1:200 dilution; Novus Biologicals Co., Littleton, USA), after which they were incubated with anti-rabbit secondary antibody (1:500 dilution; Vector Laboratories Inc., CA, USA). Next, the slides were treated with a Vectastain™ Elite ABC kit (Vector Laboratories Inc.). Immunopositive spots on the slides were developed using diaminobenzidine (DAB) as a colorimetric substrate. A cover slip was then placed over the tissue. All slides were examined at 100× magnification using a microscope equipped with a digital camera (BX51; Olympus Co., Tokyo, Japan) and DP2-BSW analysis software (Olympus Co).

Bio-Plex analysis of Th1 and Th2 cytokines in auricular lymph node tissue

Five mice from each group ($n = 10$) were deeply anesthetized with sodium pentobarbital (50 mg/kg, i.p.), and their auricular lymph nodes were quickly collected. Cytokine assay of each auricular lymph node was performed using the Bio-Plex Mouse Cytokine 8-Plex Panel (one 96-well plate) (Bio-Rad Laboratories, Inc., CA, USA) according to the manufacturer's instructions. This is a multiplex bead-based assay (xMAP Technology) involving diverse matrices that are designed to simultaneously quantitate many cytokines in a small amount of tissue. The assay was performed as follows. The wells of a 96-well filter plate were pre-wetted with 100 μL Bio-Plex assay buffer. Multiplex bead working solution was vortexed for 15–20 s at medium speed, and 50 μL solution was added to each well. The buffer was removed by vacuum filtration and 100 μL fresh Bio-Plex wash buffer was added to each well. The buffer was again removed by vacuum filtration. This step was repeated once again and 50 μL diluted standard or sample was added to each well. The plate was covered with aluminum foil and shaken at 1100 rpm for 30 s, and then shaken at

Table 1 Nucleotide sequences of primers and operating condition for PCR analysis

Gene		Nucleotide sequence	Operating condition
GAPDH	sense	5′-AACTTTGGCATTGTGGAAGG-3′	94 °C, 30s
	antisense	5′-ACACATTGGGGGTAGGAACA-3′	
IL-1β	sense	5′-GGCTGTGGAGAAGCTGTGGC-3′	58 °C, 30s
	antisense	5′-GGGTGGGTGTGCCGTCTTTC-3′	
TNF-α	sense	5′-GCAGAAGAGGCACTCCCCCA-3′	72 °C, 30s, 30 cycles
	antisense	5′-GATCCATGCCGTTGGCCAGG-3′	
IL-4	sense	5′-TCAACCCCCAGCTAGTTGTC-3′	
	antisense	5′-TGTTCTTCGTTGCTGTGAGG-3′	

T thymine, *A* adenine, *C* cytosine, *G* guanine, *GAPDH* glyceraldehyde-3-phosphate dehydrogenase, *IL* interleukin, *TNF* tumor necrosis factor

300 rpm for 90 min at room temperature. Next, the plate was washed three times with 100 µL Bio-Plex wash buffer. After vacuum filtration, vortexed working solution of Bio-Plex Detection Antibody (25 µL) was gently added to each well, and the plate was shaken as described above and washed three times with Bio-Plex washing buffer. Vigorously vortexed 1× streptavidin-peroxidase solution (50 µL) was added to each well, and the plate was shaken at 1100 rpm for 30 s, and subsequently at 300 rpm for 10 min. After three washes, the beads in each well were resuspended with 125 µL Bio-Plex assay buffer, and the plate was shaken at 1100 rpm for 30 s. Beads were read using Bio-Plex Manager® software.

Statistical analysis

All measurements were performed by an independent investigator blinded to the experimental conditions. Results in figures are expressed as mean ± standard error of means (SEM). Experimental data were analyzed by one-way ANOVA using SPSS version 13.0 (IBM, Chicago, USA). Statistical differences among groups were further analyzed using Tukey's post hoc test. All p values less than 0.05 were considered statistically significant.

Results

Clinical manifestation of TMA-treated atopy-like ear skin lesions

Repeated application of TMA to mouse ear skins induced atopy-like skin lesions with typical atopic symptoms such as erythema, excoriation, erosion, scaling, and dryness (Fig. 2a). The severity of atopic disease was evaluated by individually scoring the symptoms (skin dryness, hemorrhage and excoriation, and edema and redness). The atopic dermatitis-like skin symptoms began to be observed on day 3 during the 5 % TMA challenge period, and showed maximum exacerbation on day 9 during the 5 % TMA challenge period, as shown in Fig. 2b. BV treatment was started on day 9, when atopy-like symptoms reached their peak. Daily BV treatment at the BL40 acupoint markedly alleviated the symptoms without apparent initial signs of acute inflammation or hypersensitivity due to BV injection. There were also no inflammation responses in the skin tissues around the BL40 acupoint after BV injection (data not shown). The therapeutic efficacy of BVA at BL40 was similar to that of prednisolone, a steroid drug, which was used as a positive control in the present study. Acupuncture stimulation at a non-acupuncture point (AD+ BVNA) showed no therapeutic effect on atopic dermatitis-like symptoms in mice.

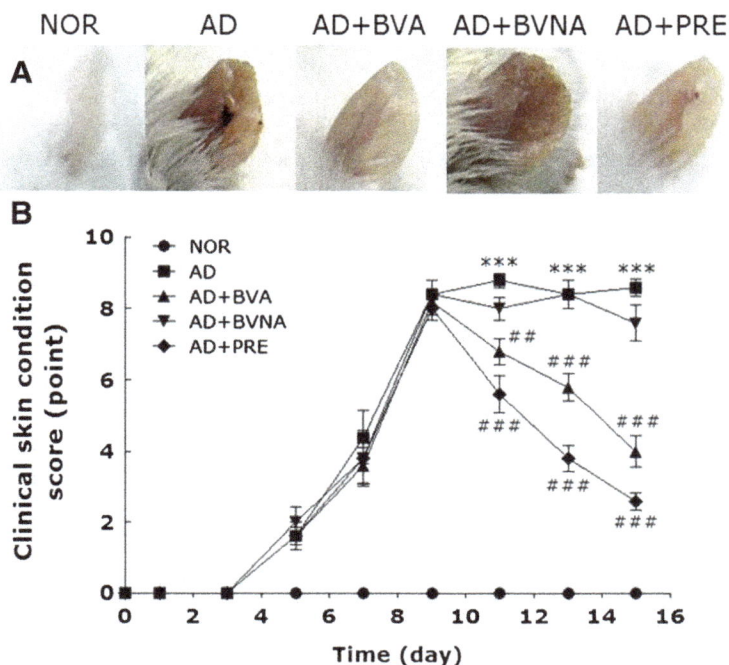

Fig. 2 Representative images (**a**) of mouse ears and scoring graph (**b**) in the NOR, AD, AD + BVA, AD + BVNA and AD + PRE groups. The graph indicates time-course severities of atopic dermatitis by scoring each image between 0 and 9 points depending on the following skin symptoms: scaling and dryness, hemorrhage and excoriation, and edema and redness. The arrow indicates the initiation of BV or prednisolon treatment. [***]$p < 0.001$ vs. the NOR group; [##]$p < 0.01$, [###]$p < 0.001$ vs. the AD group

Changes in ear thickness and auricular lymph node weight

In addition to morphological changes in inflamed ear skin, repeated application of TMA to the ear skin also induced a significant increase in ear thickness in mice (Fig. 3a). Mouse ear thickness increased about 3-fold by TMA treatment, and BV injection at acupoint BL40 significantly suppressed the increase in ear thickness on day 14 ($p < 0.001$). The medicinal efficacy of BVA treatment on reducing ear thickness in the AD + BVA group was similar to that of prednisolone in the AD + PRE group. Although BVA stimulation at a non-acupuncture point also reduced ear thickness, the effect was negligible, as compared to that of acupuncture stimulation at BL40. As shown in Fig. 3b, repeated treatments of TMA in the AD group induced a significant increase in auricular lymph node weight.

Auricular lymph node weight on day 14 after TMA treatment increased about 13-fold. Whereas BV injection at a non-acupuncture point on the tail had no effect on the increase in auricular lymph node weight, the same treatment at acupoint BL40 significantly reduced auricular lymph node weights ($p < 0.001$). Moreover, the decrease in auricular lymph node weight in the AD + BVA group was similar to that in the AD + PRE group, a positive control group.

Changes of serum IL-4 and IgE levels

Serum levels of IgE and IL-4, which are increased in most patients with atopic dermatitis, were determined in the TMA-induced mouse model as a parameter for humoral (Th2) responses [22, 23]. In the present study, as shown in Fig. 4, serum levels of IL-4 and IgE were elevated about 3.7-fold and 6.5-fold, respectively, in the AD group on day 14 after TMA treatment. The secretion profiles of these factors are very similar to the profile for eosinophil activation, which plays a crucial role in aggravating atopic dermatitis symptoms [24]. BV

injection at acupoint BL40 significantly suppressed the elevation of IL-4 and IgE levels ($p < 0.001$) on day 14. Notably, the suppressive effect of BV treatment at acupoint BL40 on serum IL-4 level in the AD + BVA group was comparable to that in the AD + PRE group. BV injection at a non-acupuncture point on the tail did not reduce serum IgE and IL-4 levels.

Histological changes of ear skin tissues

Morphological changes in inflamed skin layers and cutaneous infiltration of immune cells were characterized by histochemical techniques (Fig. 5). Inflammatory responses such as thickening of ear skin including dermis and epidermis, edema and epidermal hyperplasia, which leads to massive infiltration of various immune cells from the blood vessels into the dermis layers, were observed in coronal sections of ear skin tissues stained with hematoxylin and eosin in the AD group (Fig. 5a1-a5). BV treatment at acupoint BL40 significantly inhibited these inflammatory changes in both the epidermis and dermis, although its suppressive efficacy was lower than that of prednisolone. BVA therapy at a non-acupuncture point had no significant effect on histochemical changes in inflammation.

Of the pathogenic features of blood in atopic dermatitis patients, such as IgE, eosinophils, and mast cells, the role of mast cells is demonstrated by increases in cell numbers and mast cell activation in atopic dermatitis lesions [25]. In the present study, mast cells in the dermis in mice with TMA-induced atopy-like dermatitis were analyzed by toluidine blue staining (Fig. 5b1-b5). Topical application of TMA markedly increased mast cell infiltration in the epidermis and dermis of ear skin in the AD group. BV treatment at acupoint BL40 significantly alleviated the TMA-induced infiltration of mast cells. Its therapeutic efficacy was similar to that of prednisolone. BV stimulation at a non-acupuncture point had no such effect.

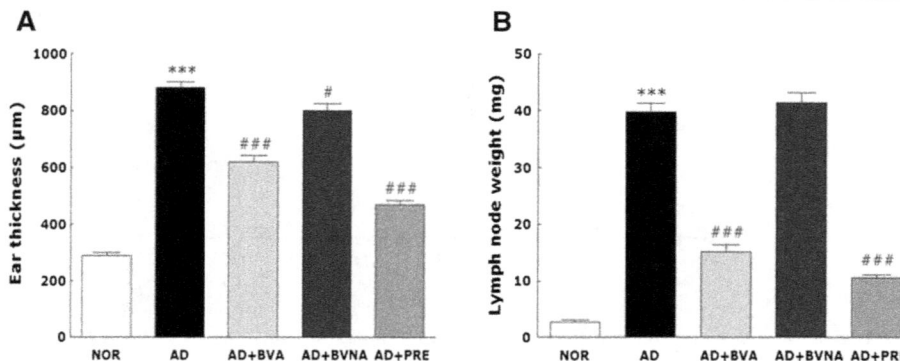

Fig. 3 Ear thickness (**a**) and lymph node weights (**b**) of the mice in the NOR, AD, AD + BVA, AD + BVNA and AD + PRE groups. $^{***}p < 0.001$ vs. the NOR group; $^{#}p < 0.05$, $^{###}p < 0.001$ vs. the AD group

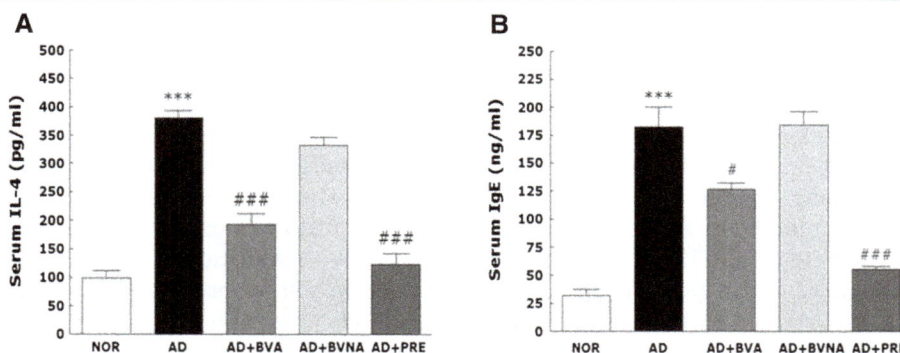

Fig. 4 Serum levels of IL-4 (**a**) and IgE (**b**) in the NOR, AD, AD + BVA, AD + BVNA and AD + PRE groups using an ELISA. IL, interleukin; IgE, immunoglobulin E; ELISA, enzyme-linked immunosorbent assay. ***$p < 0.001$ vs. the NOR group; #$p < 0.05$, ###$p < 0.001$ vs. the AD group

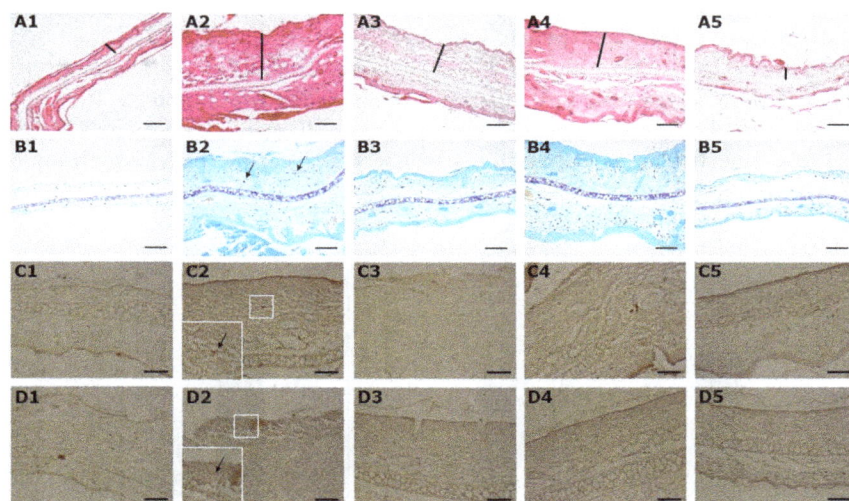

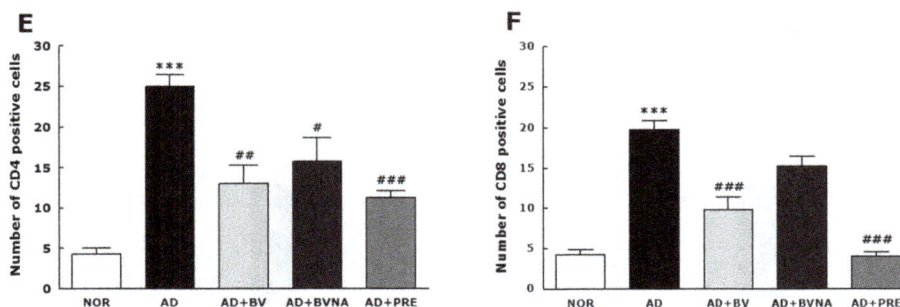

Fig. 5 Histological images and graphs indicating relative percentage of CD4- and CD8-immunopositive cells of the ear sections. Ear sections in each group were stained with hematoxylin and eosin (**a**1-**a**5), toluidine blue (**b**1-**b**5), anti-mouse CD4 IgG (**c**1-**c**5) and anti-mouse CD8 IgG (**d**1-**d**5). Black scale bar indicates 100 μm (100× magnification). Black thick lines in the images of H-E staining indicate the thickness of ear skins. Small white squares (200×) in the centers of immunohistological staining images (**c**2 & **d**2 of AD group) are magnified in the lower left corners to observe CD4- and CD8-positive cells infiltrated into the skin tissues. The representative CD4- and CD8-immunopositive cells were indicated by black arrows in indicated in small white squares in C2 and D2, respectively. The numbers of CD4- and CD8-immunopositive cells in the fixed area of the images are depicted in the bar graphs **e** and **f**, respectively, below the histological images. IgG, immunoglobulin G; CD, cluster of differentiation. ***$p < 0.001$ vs. the NOR group; #$p < 0.05$, ##$p < 0.005$ and ###$p < 0.001$ vs. the AD group

To investigate cutaneous infiltration of allergen-specific T cells, CD4[+], and CD8[+] T cells were analyzed in ear skin tissues using an immunohistochemical technique (Fig. 5c1-c5 and d1-d5). In the present study, CD4[+] T cell infiltration was predominantly observed in the dermis and CD8[+] T cells were mainly localized in the epidermis in the AD group, as shown in Fig. 5c2 and d2. BV injection at acupoint BL40 significantly inhibited the infiltration of CD4[+] and CD8[+] T cells caused by repeated application of TMA (Fig. 5e and f). Its therapeutic efficacy was similar to that of prednisolone. BV stimulation at a non-acupuncture point had no effect of suppressing the infiltration of CD8[+] T cells even though there was little effect of non-acupoint stimulation in case of CD4[+] T cells.

RT-PCR analysis of cytokine mRNA expression in ear skin and auricular lymph nodes

To investigate Th1 and Th2 cytokine gene expression, mRNA levels of cytokines such as tumor necrosis factor (TNF)-α, IL-1β, and IL-4 were determined in ear and auricular lymph node tissue homogenates using RT-PCR (Fig. 6). TNF-α and IL-1β were selected as Th1 inflammatory cytokines for the auricular lymph node and ear, respectively, and IL-4 was selected as a representative

Th2 cytokine for both tissues. In ear tissues, mRNA expression of IL-1β and IL-4 showed similar patterns: repeated application with TMA induced significant increases in the expression of IL-1β and IL-4 mRNAs, and BV treatment at acupoint BL40 significantly suppressed the TMA-induced mRNA expression of both cytokines. The suppressive effect of BV treatment at acupoint BL40 was similar to that of prednisolone. In all cases, BV stimulation at a non-acupuncture point showed weaker suppressive effects even though suppression levels were insignificant than that in the BL40 acupoint stimulation except IL-1β.

In auricular lymph node tissues, topical application of TMA induced significant increases in the expression of TNF-α and IL-4 mRNAs. BV treatment at acupoint BL40 significantly suppressed TMA-induced mRNA expression of both cytokines in the lymph node. In the case of TNF-α, application of BVA to a non-acupuncture point had a non-significant suppressive effect on mRNA expression of the cytokines.

Bio-Plex analysis of Th1 and Th2 cytokine production in the auricular lymph node

When allergens including TMA activate naïve anti-allergen T cells in mice, lymph node IL-4 concentrations

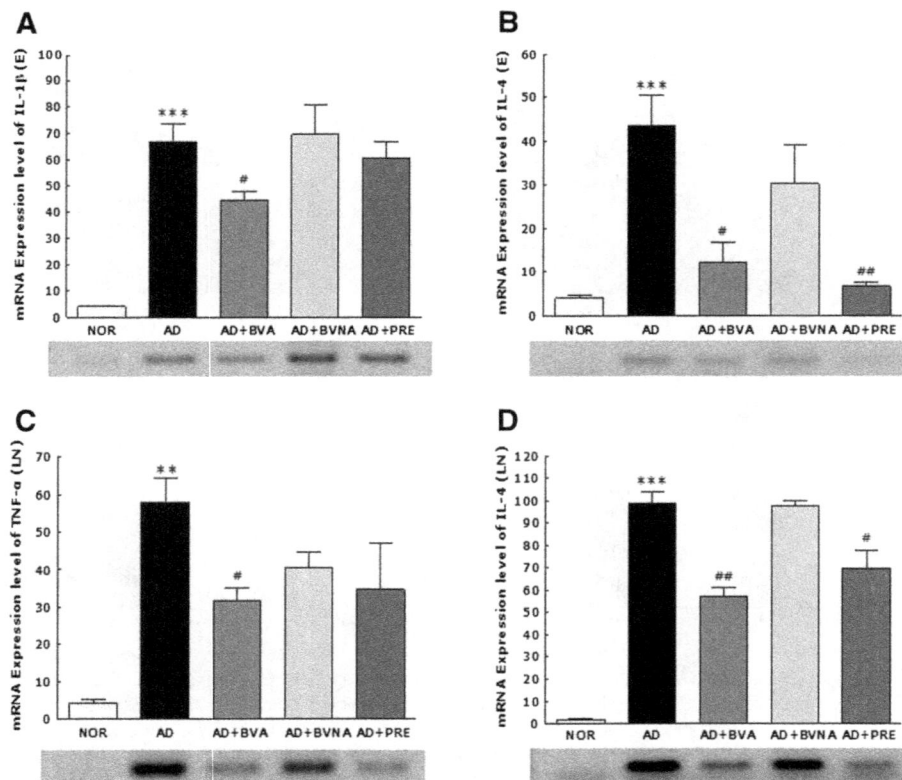

Fig. 6 The mRNA expression levels of IL-1β (**a**) and IL-4 (**b**) in ear tissue (E), and TNF-α (**c**), and IL-4 (**d**) in auricular lymph node (LN) in mice. IL, interleukin; TNF, tissue necrosis factor. [**]$p < 0.01$, [***]$p < 0.001$ vs. the NOR group; [#]$p < 0.05$, [##]$p < 0.01$, [###]$p < 0.001$ vs. the AD group

are abruptly increased, and subsequently induce naïve T cells to differentiate into Th2 effector cells. These Th2 cells then secrete Th2 cytokines to promote isotype switching to IgE in activated B cells, and to influence other immune cells responding to the allergen [26, 27]. In the present study, the secretion profiles of cutaneous

cytokines in auricular lymph node tissues were measured at the protein level using the Bio-Plex suspension array system (Fig. 7). IL-2 (a), IL-12 (b), interferon (IFN)-γ (c) and TNF-α (d) were quantified as Th1 inflammatory cytokines, and IL-5 (e), IL-10 (f), granulocyte-macrophage colony-stimulating factor (GM-CSF) (g) and IL-4 (h) as

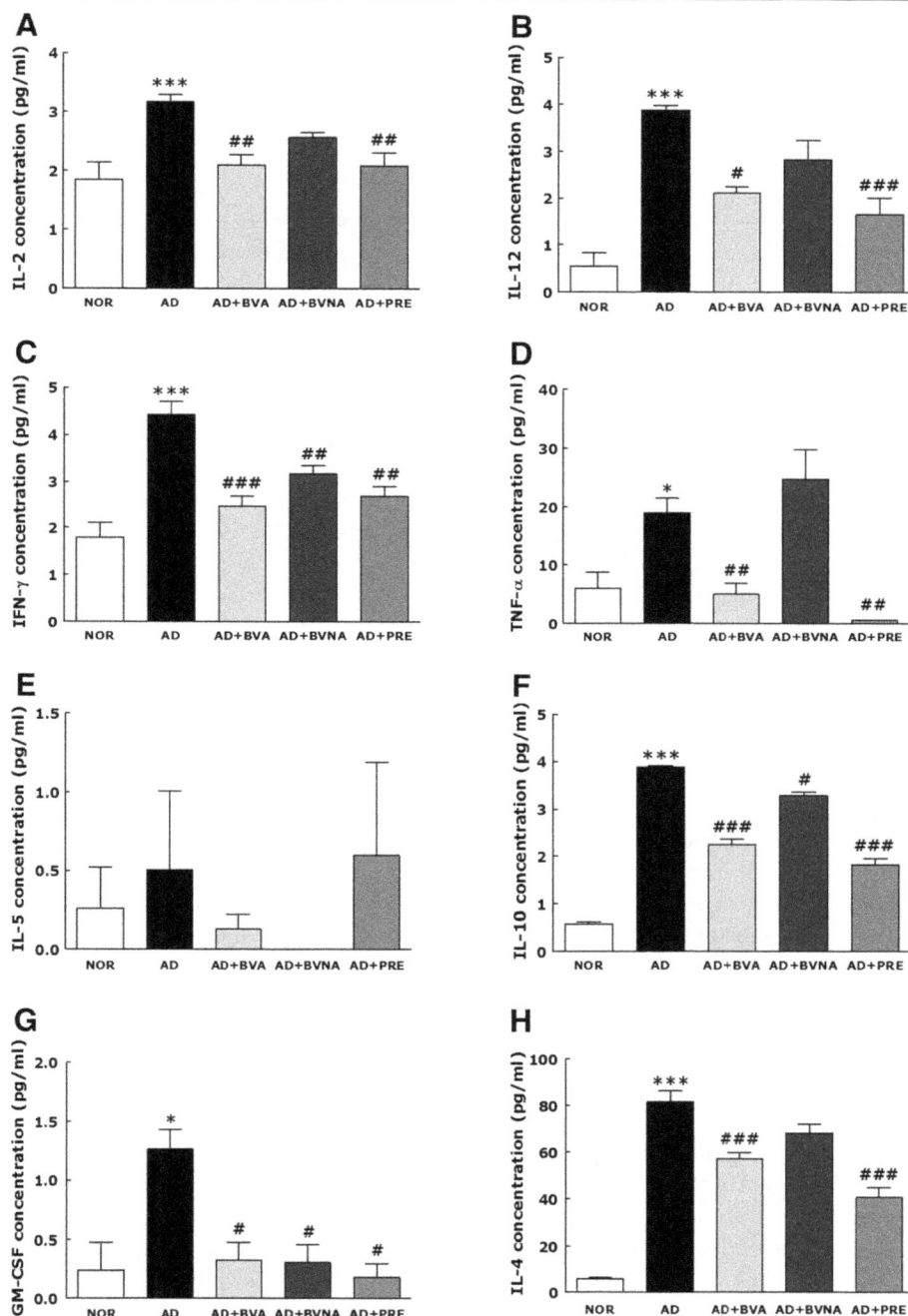

Fig. 7 Analysis of the levels of cytokines such as IL-2(**a**), IL-12(**b**), IFN-γ(**c**), IL-5(**d**), IL-10(**e**), GM-CSF(**f**), TNF-α(**g**) and IL-4(**h**). The analysis was performed using the Bio-Plex® suspension array system, in the auricular lymph node in mice. GM-CSF, granulocyte macrophage colony-stimulating factor; IFN, interferon; IL, interleukin; TNF, tissue necrosis factor. $^{*}p < 0.05$, $^{***}p < 0.001$ vs. the NOR group; $^{#}p < 0.05$, $^{##}p < 0.01$, $^{###}p < 0.001$ vs. the AD group

Th2 cytokines in auricular lymph node tissues. Repeated challenge with TMA caused significant increases in the secretion of all cytokines, regardless of Th1/Th2 phenotype. Among the cytokines examined, IL-5 showed the weakest induction after repeated topical application of TMA, and IL-4 showed the strongest. BV treatment at acupoint BL40 significantly suppressed the TMA-induced increases in the secretion of these cytokines. BV treatment at a non-acupuncture point had a little significant suppressive effect on protein expression of the cytokines such as IFN-γ, IL-10 and GM-CSF while there were also non-significant effects of suppression in cases of IL-2, IL-4, IL-5 and IL-12 expression. In the AD + BVA group, the protein expression levels of the Th1 cytokines IL-2, IL-12, IFN-γ, and TNF-α decreased to 2.1 ± 0.17 ($p < 0.01$, AD group vs. AD + BVA group), 2.12 ± 0.13 ($p < 0.05$, AD group vs. AD + BVA group), 2.48 ± 0.21 ($p < 0.001$, AD group vs. AD + BVA group), and 5.04 ± 1.76 ($p < 0.01$, AD group vs. AD + BVA group), respectively, from 3.17 ± 0.12, 3.88 ± 0.1, 4.43 ± 0.27, and 19.0 ± 2.5 in the AD group. In the AD + BVA group, the protein expression levels of the Th2 cytokines IL-5, IL-10, GM-CSF, and IL-4 decreased to 0.13 ± 0.1, 2.23 ± 0.12 ($p < 0.001$, AD group vs. AD + BVA group), 0.33 ± 0.15 ($p < 0.05$, AD group vs. AD + BVA group), and 57.23 ± 2.7 ($p < 0.001$, AD group vs. AD + BVA group), respectively, from 0.5 ± 0.5, 3.87 ± 0.03, 1.26 ± 0.17, and 81.64 ± 4.72 in the AD group. The therapeutic efficacy of BVA treatment at suppressing the secretion of TNF-α and IL-2 (Th1 cytokines), and IL-4, IL-10, and GM-CSF (Th2 cytokines), was similar to that of prednisolone.

Discussion

There have been few objective ways to determine the optimum dose of BV in clinics and animal studies. According to unpublished reports from Oriental clinics, the best outcome with BVA can be achieved with the maximum dose of BV, with substantial heat and pain around the injection site. Because the injection of excessive amounts of BV sometimes induces anaphylactic symptoms, physicians using BVA gradually increase its dose according to the patient's verbal response to treatment. One possible way to objectively optimize the injection method or daily dose is to measure the skin temperature around the BV injection site. We measured the temperature at the injection site after intradermal, subcutaneous, and intramuscular injection of BV into the backs of mice, and eventually adopted subcutaneous injection for BVA in this study (Additional file 1: Figure S1).

In the present study, BV therapy was used to treat atopic dermatitis, a typical allergic disease in which the intrinsic immune system is over-activated in response to various environmental factors. To investigate anti-inflammatory activities of BVA, we produced chronic

TMA-induced T cell-dependent skin inflammation in mouse ears using the protocol of Schneider et al. [19]. In this model, the repeated challenge of ear skin with 2 % TMA for 12 days after one-shot sensitization with 5 % TMA on day 0 caused atopic dermatitis-like skin symptoms, such as increased skin thickness, change in skin morphology, and infiltration of immune cells [28]. It is widely accepted that eosinophils, mast cells, and CD4$^+$ T cells mainly infiltrated the dermis and CD8$^+$ T cells mainly infiltrated the epidermis [29]. And our results were also coincident with the previous findings. From histological findings that the majority of skin-infiltrating T cells in active atopic dermatitis lesions in humans are CD4$^+$ T cells, CD4$^+$ T cells are considered pivotal to the development of eczema and skin eosinophilic inflammation, because they produce a mixed pattern of Th1 and Th2 cytokines in the pathological development of atopic dermatitis [26]. CD8$^+$ T cells are also dominant effector cells. They are responsible for allergen-induced skin inflammation, and thus their infiltration is required for the development of atopic dermatitis-like lesions and the initiation of mixed Th1/Th2 skin inflammation in rodent models.

Local lymph node weight is also increased by topical application of allergens including TMA or haptens such as dinitrofluorobenzene, 2,4-dinitrochlorobenzene, and trinitrochlorobenzene [30]. Hence, local lymph node weight was recently validated as a main index of allergic and immune responses in murine models. In the present study, lymph node weight also significantly increased after repeated challenge of ear skin with TMA (Fig. 3b).

Repeated topical application of allergens or haptens causes significant increases in blood IgE and IL-4 levels in a rodent allergy model [23, 31]. Topical exposure of haptens including dinitrofluorobenzene, 2,4-dinitrochlorobenzene (DNCB), and trinitrochlorobenzene (TNCB) also developed severe contact hypersensitivity in the mice. However, unlike allergens including TMA, the significant increases in eosinophil and T-cell infiltration, Th2 cytokine production and IgE levels were not observed in the serum of these hapten-induced hypersensitivity animal models, although a minor increase was reported previously [32].

In the present study, TMA treatment directly triggered a T cell-mediated contact hypersensitivity reaction and also caused distinct changes in the innate and adaptive immune systems, primarily indicated by increases in the secretion of Th1 and inflammatory cytokines, and the production of Th2 cytokines and IgE, respectively.

Serological and tissue investigations also showed an increased serum IgE level and Th2 cytokine dominance in the serum, ear skin, and auricular lymph node, despite the simultaneous dominance of Th1 cytokines such as TNF-α, IL-1β, IL-2, IL-12, and IFN-γ in ear or lymph node tissues. In ear and auricular lymph node tissues in our atopic animal model, Th1 cytokines were strongly secreted, although Th2 cytokines dominated. This might be due to a longer period of 2 % TMA challenge on both ears (3 days longer than in Schneider's protocol) to elicit an intensified immune response.

As an alternative therapy, BV was injected to stimulate a specific skin point behind the knee. The stimulation point is located far away from the ears where allergic inflammation is induced by repeated exposure to TMA, and a specific component of BV can hardly be responsible for alleviation of skin symptoms. Thus, our results demonstrate that stimulation of the specific acupoint by BV significantly inhibited TMA-induced skin inflammation in the ears, probably due to modulation of the systemic immune system. Although the detailed mechanism has not yet been elucidated, the improvement in symptoms must be attributed to certain systemic changes being able to affect every part of the body as well as being triggered by local BV stimulation.

On the other side, as reported previously, BV contains several biologically active peptides, including melittin, apamin, and adolapin [33, 34]. Many studies indicate that BVA can modulate a systemic immune response by inhibiting inflammatory mediators, similar to non-steroidal anti-inflammatory drugs (NSAIDs) [35]. Other studies reported that BV has in vitro anti-inflammatory activity which is ascribed to the transcriptional downregulation of NF-κB and MAPKs in target tissues [36]. One can speculate that Th1 cytokine-based inflammatory symptoms in atopic dermatitis were alleviated by BV components and that this pharmacological anti-inflammatory effect was exerted via modulation of NF-κB and MAPK signal transduction pathways.

Since atopic dermatitis is primarily characterized by skin symptoms such as erythema, edema, excoriation, and scaling, we first investigated the therapeutic effects of BVA on ear edema and thickness in our animal model [37]. At the maximum severity of AD-like symptoms, we started BVA treatment at a dose of 0.3 mg/kg at the BL40 acupoints on both legs and found significant reductions in ear edema and thickness 2 days after starting BVA treatment. We thereafter confirmed that BVA treatment was very effective at inhibiting activation of resident mast cells and infiltration of immune cells by histological analysis. Because mast cells play a key role in mediating allergic inflammation in asthma, atopic dermatitis, and sinusitis, we also focused on changes in mast cells in the dermis of inflamed skin. BV treatment significantly decreased mast cell infiltration in ear tissues [38]. Thus, it is likely that BV regulates the infiltration of mast cells and inhibits immune cells, thereby normalizing the inflammatory response. Aggregation of FcεRI triggers AD. After induction of AD, mast cells are activated by crosslinking of adjacent IgE molecules [39]. Notably, IgE is responsible for both acute and chronic symptoms in atopy-like skin diseases, and repeated injection of TMA increases serum IgE levels in the mice [40]. We found that total serum IgE levels in mice were significantly increased by repeated TMA treatment. BV treatment significantly reduced total serum IgE levels in TMA-treated mice.

Many studies suggest that an imbalance between Th1 and Th2 responses is closely associated with many immune disorders, including atopic dermatitis [41]. In typical allergic diseases, there are increases in the levels of Th2 cytokines and decreases in the levels of Th1 cytokines [42]. Many studies also support the assertion that restoration of the balance between Th1 and Th2 cell numbers, which can be achieved by either stimulation of Th1 cell development or inhibition of Th2 cell development, has remedial value in AD treatment [43]. However, interestingly, in our mouse model of atopy-like skin dermatitis, in which the expression levels of both Th1 and Th2 cytokines simultaneously increased, the alleviation of atopic skin symptoms by BV treatment was attributed to downregulation of both Th1 and Th2 cytokines. Th2-dominated cytokine profile plays a central role in the initiation of AD symptoms in the early stage, and in the chronic stage of human atopic dermatitis, cytokine profile shift from Th2 to Th1 is quite critical for aggravation of AD leading to severe dermal inflammation. Although our atopic model of TMA-induced hypersensitivity for 2 weeks seems to show such a mixed profile of both Th1 and Th2 dominance and thus be close to human chronic dermatitis of atopy, we do not have a confidence because we did not analyze time-course profiles of Th1- and Th-2 expression.

Local injection of BV exhibited simultaneous anti-inflammatory and anti-allergy effects for the treatment of atopic skin symptoms. This phenomenon might be caused by the double-sided character of BV, as mentioned earlier, although we did not clearly elucidate its mechanism in this study.

Unlike usual immunotherapies for immune diseases, venom therapy not only induces a rapid shift in cytokine expression from Th2 (IL-4) to Th1 (IFN-γ) cytokines, but also leads to increased production of immunosuppressive cytokine IL-10 during the initial phase of the treatment [44]. Furthermore, it was reported that although low-dose BV treatment initially upregulated Th1 cytokine expression in experimental immunotherapy, aggravating inflammation, pain, and scratching behavior, it eventually relieved those symptoms [45].

In the present study, BV stimulation at a non-acupuncture point also exhibited a significant suppressive effect on TMA-induced edema formation, T-cell activation and the levels of inflammatory cytokine mRNAs and proteins. It means that BV itself showed certain levels of anti-inflammatory and anti-allergic activities, regardless of the use of specific acupuncture point.

Although we addressed that BVA significantly inhibited the TMA-induced expression of Th2- and Th1- cytokines in the present study, the detailed mechanisms of how BVA modulated the expression levels of Th1- and Th2-cytokines together should be elucidated in the future.

Conclusion

In the atopy-like dermatitis mouse model, the expression of Th2 cytokines such as IL-4, IL-5, and IL-10 in the lymph nodes of TMA-treated mice was found to be elevated, and BVA largely abrogated TMA-induced production of Th2 cytokines. Levels of Th1 cytokines (IL-2, IL-12, IFN-γ, and TNF-α) were also increased by TMA treatment, and the increases were suppressed by BVA treatment. This means that BVA significantly suppressed the expression of both Th1 and Th2 cytokines, indicating comprehensive modulation of the Th1-Th2 balance. Although the precise mechanism by which BV inhibits Th2 cytokines and Th1 cytokines in our atopic mouse model was not explicitly elucidated in this study, the remedial value of BV therapy might be attributed to not only its widely known anti-inflammatory activity, but also its strong anti-allergic activity, which we report here for the first time.

Additional file

Additional file 1: Figure S1. Time-courses of surface temperatures at the skin sites that BV was injected in subcutaneously, intradermally or intramuscularly. BV (0.3 mg /kg body weight) was injected into the mid-back after hair removal, and the temperature at the injection site in the skin was measured using an infrared thermometer (HuBDIC Thermofinder (FS-300), Beauty Korea World Co., Ltd., Seoul, Korea). BV injections were performed in at least three mice, and temperature measurement was repeated three times per injection per time point.

Abbreviations

AD: atopic dermatitis; BV: bee venom; BVA: bee venom acupuncture; CD: cluster of differentiation; cDNA: complementary DNA; DAB: diaminobenzidine; ELISA: enzyme-linked immunosorbent assay; GAPDH: glyceraldehyde 3-phosphate dehydrogenase; GM-CSF: granulocyte-macrophage colony-stimulating factor; HRP: avidin-horseradish peroxidase; IFN: interferon; IgE: immunoglobulin E; IL: interleukin; Th1: T helper cell type 1; Th2: T helper cell type 2; TMA: trimellitic anhydride; TMB: tetramethylbenzidine; TNF: tumor necrosis factor.

Competing interests

The authors declare that they have no competing interests.

Authors' contributions

Author contributions to the study and manuscript preparation are as follows. Conception and design: BS, BL and DH. Carried out the experiments: BS, BL and JH. Acquisition of data: BS, BL, MY and SK. Analysis and interpretation: BL, JH, STK, HSL and DH. Drafting the article: BL, HP and DH. Statistical analysis: BS and BL. Study supervision: HL and DH. All authors read and approved the final manuscript.

Acknowledgements

This research was supported by grants from the National Research Foundation of Korea funded by the Korean government (NRF-2013R1A1A2008487 & NRF-2015M3A9E3052338).

Author details

[1]Acupuncture and Meridian Science Research Center, College of Korean Medicine, Kyung Hee University, Hoegi-ding, Dongdaemoon-gu, Seoul 130-701, Republic of Korea. [2]Division of Meridian and Structural Medicine, School of Korean Medicine, Pusan National University, Yangsan 628-870, Republic of Korea. [3]The Graduate School of Basic Science of Korean Medicine, College of Korean Medicine, Kyung Hee University, Seoul 130-701, Republic of Korea.

References

1. Jung TW, Lee JY, Shim WS, Kang ES, Kim JS, Ahn CW, et al. Adiponectin protects human neuroblastoma SH-SY5Y cells against MPP + −induced cytotoxicity. Biochem Biophys Res Commun. 2006;343(2):564–70.
2. Kwon YB, Yoon SY, Kim HW, Roh DH, Kang SY, Ryu YH, et al. Substantial role of locus coeruleus-noradrenergic activation and capsaicin-insensitive primary afferent fibers in bee venom's anti-inflammatory effect. Neurosci Res. 2006;55(2):197–203.
3. Lee MS, Pittler MH, Shin BC, Kong JC, Ernst E. Bee venom acupuncture for musculoskeletal pain: a review. J Pain. 2008;9(4):289–97.
4. Kwon YB, Lee JD, Lee HJ, Han HJ, Mar WC, Kang SK, et al. Bee venom pretreatment has both an antinociceptive and anti-inflammatory effect on carrageenan-induced inflammation. J Vet Med Sci. 2001;63(3):251–9.
5. Kwon YB, Kim JH, Yoon JH, Lee JD, Han HJ, Mar WC, et al. The analgesic efficacy of bee venom acupuncture for knee osteoarthritis: a comparative study with needle acupuncture. Am J Chin Med. 2001;29(2):187–99.
6. Yang CY, Park SA, Oh KJ, Yang YS. The assessment of bee venom responses in an experimental model of mono-arthritis using Tc-99m DPD bone scintigraphy. Ann Nucl Med. 2010;24(6):455–60.
7. Jeong I, Kim BS, Kim H, Lee KM, Shim I, Kang SK, et al. Prolonged analgesic effect of PLGA-encapsulated bee venom on formalin-induced pain in rats. Int J Pharm. 2009;380(1–2):62–6.
8. Nam KW, Je KH, Lee JH, Han HJ, Lee HJ, Kang SK, et al. Inhibition of COX-2 activity and proinflammatory cytokines (TNF-alpha and IL-1beta) production by water-soluble sub-fractionated parts from bee (Apis mellifera) venom. Arch Pharm Res. 2003;26(5):383–8.
9. Kim HW, Kwon YB, Ham TW, Roh DH, Yoon SY, Lee HJ, et al. Acupoint stimulation using bee venom attenuates formalin-induced pain behavior and spinal cord fos expression in rats. J Vet Med Sci. 2003;65(3):349–55.
10. Orsolic N, Sver L, Verstovsek S, Terzic S, Basic I. Inhibition of mammary carcinoma cell proliferation in vitro and tumor growth in vivo by bee venom. Toxicon. 2003;41(7):861–70.
11. Choi SH, Cho SK, Kang SS, Bae CS, Bai YH, Lee SH, et al. Effect of apitherapy in piglets with preweaning diarrhea. Am J Chin Med. 2003;31(2):321–6.
12. Kwon YB, Lee JD, Lee HJ, Han HJ, Mar WC, Kang SK, et al. Bee venom injection into an acupuncture point reduces arthritis associated edema and nociceptive responses. Pain. 2001;90(3):271–80.
13. Bernstein DI, Patterson R, Zeiss CR. Clinical and immunologic evaluation of trimellitic anhydride- and phthalic anhydride-exposed workers using a questionnaire with comparative analysis of enzyme linked immunosorbent and radioimmunoassay studies. J Allergy Clin Immunol. 1982;69(3):311–8.
14. Dearman RJ, Warbrick EV, Skinner T, Kimber I. Cytokine fingerprinting of chemical allergens: species comparison and statistical analyses. Food Chem Toxicol. 2002;40(12):1881–91.
15. Dearman RJ, Smith S, Basketter DA, Kimber I. Classification of chemical allergens according to cytokine secretion profiles of murine lymph node cells. J Appl Toxicol. 1997;17(1):53–62.
16. Sailstad DM, Ward MDW, Boykin EH, Selgrade MK. A murine model for low molecular weight chemicals: differentiation of respiratory sensitizers (TMA) from contact sensitizers (DNFB). Toxicology. 2003;194(1–2):147–61.

17. Furue M, Terao H, Rikihisa W, Urabe K, Kinukawa N, Nose Y, et al. Clinical dose and adverse effects of topical steroids in daily management of atopic dermatitis. Br J Dermatol. 2003;148(1):128–33.

18. Ahn AC, Park M, Shaw JR, McManus CA, Kaptchuk TJ, Langevin HM. Electrical impedance of acupuncture meridians: the relevance of subcutaneous collagenous bands. PLoS One. 2010;5(7), e11907.

19. Schneider C, Döcke WD, Zollner TM, Röse L. Chronic mouse model of TMA-induced contact hypersensitivity. J Invest Dermatol. 2009;129(4):899–907.

20. Lee H, Lee JK, Ha H, Lee MY, Seo CS, Shin HK. Angelicae Dahuricae Radix inhibits dust mite extract-induced atopic dermatitis-like skin lesions in NC/Nga mice. Evid Based Complement Alternat Med. 2012;2012:743075.

21. Yan HX, Wang Y, Yang XN, Fu LX, Tang DM. A new selective vascular endothelial growth factor receptor 2 inhibitor ablates disease in a mouse model of psoriasis. Mol Med Rep. 2013;8(2):434–8.

22. Hoffmann MK, Weiss O, Koenig S, Hirst JA, Oettgen HF. Suppression and enhancement of the T cell-dependent production of antibody to SRBC in vitro by bacterial lipopolysaccharide. J Immunol. 1975;114(2 pt 2):738–41.

23. Secrist H, Chelen CJ, Wen Y, Marshall JD, Umetsu DT. Allergen immunotherapy decreases interleukin 4 production in CD4+ T cells from allergic individuals. J Exp Med. 1993;178(6):2123–30.

24. Cheung PF, Wong CK, Ho AW, Hu S, Chen DP, Lam CW. Activation of human eosinophils and epidermal keratinocytes by Th2 cytokine IL-31: implication for the immunopathogenesis of atopic dermatitis. Int Immunol. 2010;22(6):453–67.

25. Liu FT, Goodarzi H, Chen HY. IgE, mast cells and eosinophils in atopic dermatitis. Clin Rev Allergy Immunol. 2011;41(3):298–310.

26. Hennino A, Vocanson M, Toussaint Y, Rodet K, Benetière J, Schmitt AM, et al. Skin-infiltrating CD8+ T cells initiate atopic dermatitis lesions. J Immunol. 2007;178(9):5571–7.

27. Hamid Q, Tulic M. Immunobiology of asthma. Annu Rev Physiol. 2009;71:489–507.

28. Sung YY, Yang WK, Lee AY, Kim DS, Nho KJ, Kim YS, et al. Topical application of an ethanol extract prepared from Illicium verum suppresses atopic dermatitis in NC/Nga mice. J Ethnopharmacol. 2012;144(1):151–9.

29. Akdis M, Simon HU, Weigl L, Kreyden O, Blaser K, Akdis CA. Skin homing (cutaneous lymphocyte-associated antigen-positive) CD8+ T cells respond to superantigen and contribute to eosinophilia and IgE production in atopic dermatitis. J Immunol. 1999;163(1):466–75.

30. Stahlmann R, Wegner M, Riecke K, Kruse M, Platzek T. Sensitising potential of four textile dyes and some of their metabolitesin a modified local lymph node assay. Toxicology. 2006;219(1–3):113–23.

31. Lee K-S, Jeong E-S, Heo S-H, Seo J-H, Jeong D-G, Choi Y-K. A novel model for human atopic dermatitis: application of repeated DNCB patch in Balb/c mice, in comparison with NC/Nga mice. Lab Anim Res. 2010;26(1):95–102.

32. Farraj AK, Harkema JR, Kaminski NE. Allergic rhinitis induced by intranasal sensitization and challenge with trimellitic anhydride but not with dinitrochlorobenzene or oxazolone in A/J mice. Toxicol Sci. 2006;92(1):321–8.

33. Moon DO, Park SY, Lee KJ, Heo MS, Kim KC, Kim MO, et al. Bee venom and melittin reduce proinflammatory mediators in lipopolysaccharide-stimulated BV2 microglia. Int Immunopharmacol. 2007;7(8):1092–101.

34. Lariviere WR, Melzack R. The bee venom test: a new tonic-pain test. Pain. 1996;66(2–3):271–7.

35. Kwon YB, Kang MS, Kim HW, Ham TW, Yim YK, Jeong SH, et al. Antinociceptive effects of bee venom acupuncture (apipuncture) in rodent animal models: a comparative study of acupoint versus non-acupoint stimulation. Acupunct Electrother Res. 2001;26(1–2):59–68.

36. Wang C, Chen T, Zhang N, Yang M, Li B, Lü X, et al. Melittin, a major component of bee venom, sensitizes human hepatocellular carcinoma cells to tumor necrosis factor-related apoptosis-inducing ligand (TRAIL)-induced apoptosis by activating CaMKII-TAK1-JNK/p38 and inhibiting IkappaBalpha kinase-NFkappaB. J Biol Chem. 2009;284(6):3804–13.

37. Kim TH, Jung JA, Kim GD, Jang AH, Cho JJ, Park YS, et al. The histone deacetylase inhibitor, trichostatin A, inhibits the development of 2,4-dinitrofluorobenzene-induced dermatitis in NC/Nga mice. Int Immunopharmacol. 2010;10(10):1310–5.

38. Bae Y, Lee S, Kim SH. Chrysin suppresses mast cell-mediated allergic inflammation: involvement of calcium, caspase-1 and nuclear factor-Kb. Toxicol Appl Pharmacol. 2011;254(1):56–64.

39. Lee CH, Chuang HY, Shih CC, Jong SB, Chang CH, Yu HS. Transepidermal water loss, serum IgE and beta-endorphin as important and independent

biological markers for development of itch intensity in atopic dermatitis. Br J Dermatol. 2006;154(6):1100–7.

40. Jang AH, Kim TH, Kim GD, Kim JE, Kim HJ, Kim SS, et al. Rosmarinic acid attenuates 2,4-dinitrofluorobenzene-induced atopic dermatitis in NC/Nga mice. Int Immunopharmacol. 2011;11(9):1271–7.

41. Grewe M, Bruijnzeel-Koomen CA, Schöpf E, Thepen T, Langeveld-Wildschut AG, Ruzicka T, et al. A role for Th1 and Th2 cells in the immunopathogenesis of atopic dermatitis. Immunol Today. 1998;19(8):359–61.

42. Packard KA, Khan MM. Effects of histamine on Th1/Th2 cytokine balance. Int Immunopharmacol. 2003;3(7):909–20.

43. Wakugawa M, Hayashi K, Nakamura K, Tamaki K. Evaluation of mite allergen-induced Th1 and Th2 cytokine secretion of peripheral blood mononuclear cells from atopic dermatitis patients: association between IL-13 and mite-specific IgE levels. J Dermatol Sci. 2001;25(2):116–26.

44. Bellinghausen I, Metz G, Enk AH, Christmann S, Knop J, Saloga J. Insect venom immunotherapy induces interleukin-10 production and a Th2-to-Th1 shift, and changes surface marker expression in venom-allergic subjects. Eur J Immunol. 1997;27(5):1131–9.

45. McHugh SM, Deighton J, Stewart AG, Lachmann PJ, Ewan PW. Bee venom immunotherapy induces a shift in cytokine responses from a TH-2 to a TH-1 dominant pattern: comparison of rush and conventional immunotherapy. Clin Exp Allergy. 1995;25(9):828–38.

2

Case report: fainting during acupuncture stimulation at acupuncture point LI4

O sang Kwon, Kwang-Ho Choi, Junbeom Kim, Seong Jin Cho, Suk-Yun Kang, Ji-Young Moon and Yeon Hee Ryu[*]

Abstract

Background: Fainting is one of the major adverse events that can occur as a result of acupuncture treatment. However, the observation of changes in biological parameters is rarely available when fainting occurs. In this case report, we could observe changes in the electroencephalogram (EEG) in a participant who fainted while participating in a clinical trial aiming to observe a relationship between acupuncture stimulation at LI4 acupuncture point and EEG in healthy adults.

Case presentation: The EEG pattern of participant changed twice. The first change was in response to the acupuncture needle insertion, and the second change occurred during fainting. Both changes consisted of a burst in EEG amplitude, but the pattern of details was different. Multiple areas of the cortex were activated, and the increased ratio of the γ wave was not observed during fainting. While acupuncture needle insertion, only the sensory cortex were activated and increased the ratio of the γ wave.

Conclusions: This single case is presented to improve the understanding of fainting during acupuncture as an adverse event and to explore the mechanism of acupuncture treatment, despite the absence of statistics and repeatability. This information can provide a new viewpoint about the mechanism of acupuncture treatment and the possibility of new techniques based on acupuncture.

Keyword: Fainting during acupuncture, Acupuncture, Fainting, EEG, sLoreta

Background

The efficacy, economical feasibility and safety of acupuncture treatment have been demonstrated in thousands of clinical studies. Acupuncture treatment can replace or reduce the dosage of the drugs such as amitriptyline [1], taxane [2] or morphine [3] to prevent adverse event that are prescribed to patients to treat various disease including chronic pain. This replacement reduces the adverse effects of drugs, however, acupuncture treatment may also be associated with minor and less critical adverse effects.

Pain and bleeding are reviewed as the most common adverse events (AEs) of acupuncture treatment from 73 case reports and 14 case series [4]. In addition to these mild AEs, fainting, stroke, haemorrhage or traumatic injuries were reported as serious AEs and led to death in some cases [4]. However, a more recent survey indicated that acupuncture clinics and the potential of severe AEs are rare [5].

Fainting is a common AE which contains dizziness, perspiration and syncope as a symptom [6], during acupuncture treatment and has not been classified as a critical AE because fainting does not kill the patient or have long-term effects, although it does cause some patients to avoid future acupuncture treatments because of the traumatic experience. However, some researchers have proposed that fainting can be used to access the mechanism of acupuncture treatment in the brain. The mechanism and cause of fainting during acupuncture treatment have not been closely examined because researchers cannot induce participants to faint.

This case occurred as an adverse event during a clinical trial designed to observe changes in EEG patterns affected by acupuncture treatment. EEG signals were recorded in the pre-stage before acupuncture needle insertion, and recording was discontinued when the participant fell down. The EEG pattern during fainting was collected until the participant fall down, and we present the data of this single case herein.

* Correspondence: yhryu@kiom.re.kr
KM Fundamental Research Division, Korea Institute of Oriental Medicine, Daejeon, Korea

Case presentation

Participant information

Age: 20

    Gender: female

    Height: 160.0 cm

    Weight: 41.0 kg

    Body temperature: 37.4 °C

    Average blood pressure: 106/61 mmHg

    Marriage: none

    Job: student (college)

    Diet: regular

    Exercise: none

    Smoking: none

    Drinking: 0.5 bottle (beer)/week

    Specific disease: none

    Medical history: no specific medical history

Adverse event

Participant were participated in the clinical trial to observe the effect of acupuncture stimulation at the electroencephalogram (EEG) and peripheral nerve system in male and female adults at the Daejeon Korean medicine hospital of Daejeon university (KCT0001871). The adverse event occurred during visit 2 (2015.05.20). The participant arrived at 10 am, and her behaviour and language were normal. The participant was prepared for measurements with a multichannel EEG (ActiveTwo, BIOSEMI, Netherland) and was placed in a seated position on a chair. Electrodes were attached, and the strength of the electrical stimulation was calibrated. A sterilised single-use acupuncture needle (0.3 × 30 mm, Dongbang medical, Korea) was inserted into the acupuncture point large intestine 4 (LI4, Hapgok) of right hand of participant approximately in depth of 1.8 cm by licensed KMD who has a 10 year's career and 4 year of the career was as a assistant teacher of acupuncture practice at the university, after 30 min of rest. The EEG data were recorded for approximately 5 min before the acupuncture needle was inserted, and researchers noticed the fainting approximately 4 min after needle insertion. The participant did not report any symptoms or uncomfortable feelings. The researchers heard the sound of some objects falling down and saw participant falling at that time. The EEG electrodes were separated from the participant's body due to the impact of falling down.

Subsequent observations

We placed the participant on the bed in a supine position. The participant recovered before 1 min had passed. The participant drank a cup of warm water and rested for 30 min while lying on the bed.

The participant's condition was observed at both 7 and 30 days after fainting. The participant did not report any uncomfortable feeling or poor condition. She also did not show any traumatic reaction or negative opinion about acupuncture treatment and was willing to receive acupuncture treatment again.

During the first interview, the participant admitted that she had been on a diet while participating in the test.

Analysis

Frequency analysis using Fourier transformation was performed to quantitatively analyse the changes in EEG activity. A window of 2 s (75% sliding window) was applied to the full-time data. The ratio was normalized as the ratio of the total power at each window after adding the absolute power of each frequency band (ϵ: 5–8 Hz, α: 9–12 Hz, β: 13–30 Hz, γ: over 30 Hz).

Standard low-resonance electromagnetic tomography analysis (sLoreta) [7, 8] was performed using a LORETA-KEY program available at: http://www.uzh.ch/keyinst/loreta.htm.

EEG wavelength amplitude

The absolute power of the EEG signal increased twice during the procedure. The first burst was observed after the acupuncture needle was inserted (300 s). The next burst was observed after the participant fainted (540 s). An increase in the γ wave was observed (Fig. 1). The ratios of the ϵ, α, β and γ wave bands showed a specific pattern at the same time of the bursts. The ratios of the ϵ and γ waves increased significantly, and the ratio of the β wave decreased significantly (Figs. 2 and 3).

EEG activity in the brain

EEG activity in the brain was analysed using the Brodmann area (BA) [9]. The orbitofrontal cortex (BA11) was activated before acupuncture treatment. The medial part of the primary sensory cortex (BA3, 1 and 2) and the somatosensory association cortex (BA5) were activated after the acupuncture needle was inserted. While the patient was fainting, the EEG signal was activated at various areas: the dorsolateral prefrontal cortex (DLPFC, BA46,9) or insula cortex (BA16); pars orbitalis (BA 47); part of the secondary visual cortex (V2, BA18) and the associative visual cortex (V3,V4,V5, BA19); and the middle temporal gyrus (BA21).

Discussion and Conclusion

Fainting during acupuncture treatment is one of the most common adverse effects that occurs at the acupuncture clinic [4] and is believed by some researchers to be related to the mechanisms of acupuncture treatment. However, studies on fainting during acupuncture have not been performed because of ethical and technical issues. Thus, fainting during acupuncture in a clinical trial, particularly a brain imaging study, can be a great opportunity to observe what happens as

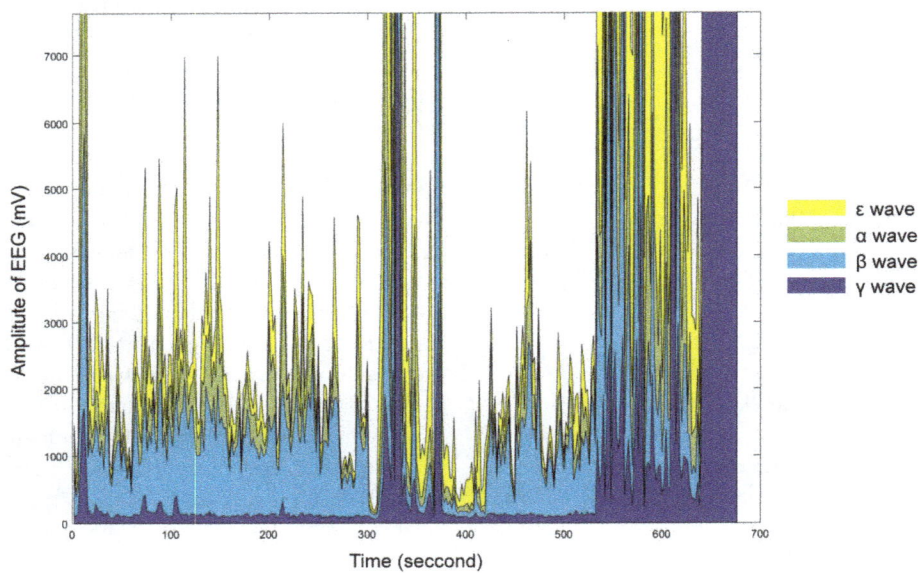

Fig. 1 Changes in the absolute power of EEG bands. The acupuncture needle was inserted at approximately 300 s (*red vertical line*), and fainting was observed at approximately 540 s. The EEG amplitude rapidly increased twice: once at the time of needle insertion and once at the time of fainting

fainting occurs. In this study, we had the opportunity to observe EEG patterns during fainting and present the data herein to enlarge our experience and understanding the relationship between the brain and acupuncture.

Before acupuncture needle injection, the amplitude of the EEG did not show a specific pattern. EEG activity was detected in the orbitofrontal cortex (BA11), which is known to be related to the reward system [10]. We hypothesized that the patient was anxious and afraid of

acupuncture following her interview; this was her first experience with acupuncture.

The absolute power of the EEG signal significantly increased twice, and the patterns of the two bursts were different. The ratio and absolute power of the γ wave, which is related to the somatosensory [11] area and perception [12], increased significantly and appeared to modulate the stimulation from the acupuncture needle insertion. This analysis was supported by sLoreta location analysis, which showed EEG activity in the medial

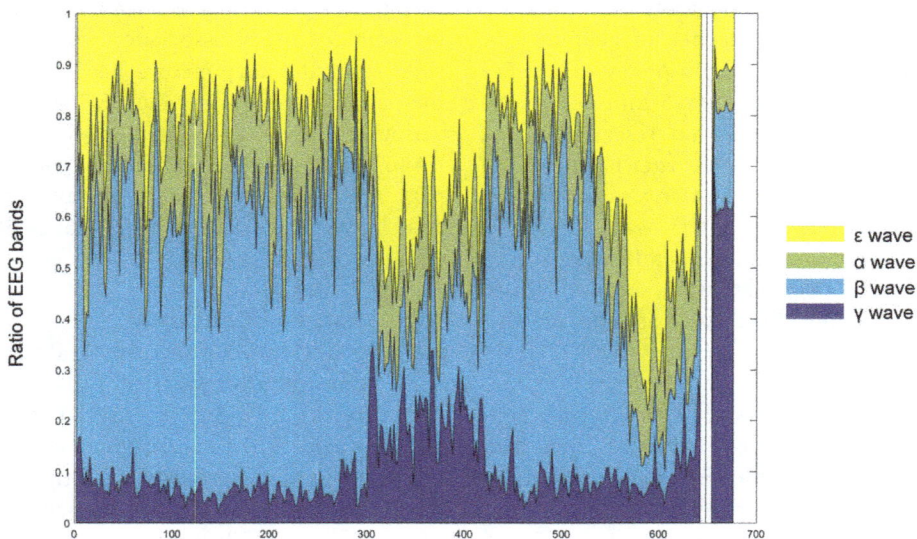

Fig. 2 Changes in ratio between each EEG band. Both activity bursts showed an increase in the ε wave ratio. The ratio of the γ wave did not significantly increase when the patient fainted, but it did increase significantly when the acupuncture needle was inserted

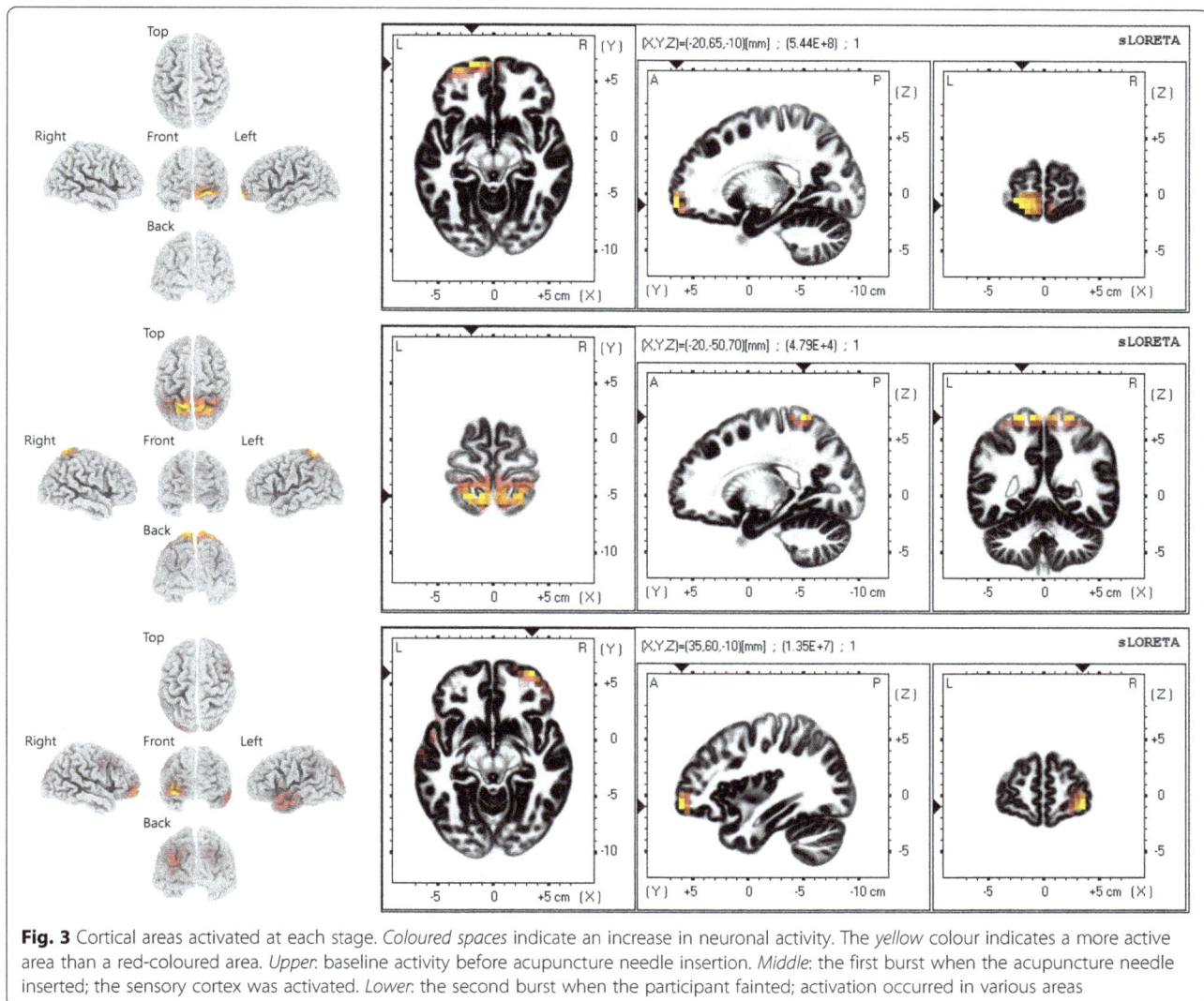

Fig. 3 Cortical areas activated at each stage. *Coloured spaces* indicate an increase in neuronal activity. The *yellow* colour indicates a more active area than a red-coloured area. *Upper*: baseline activity before acupuncture needle insertion. *Middle*: the first burst when the acupuncture needle inserted; the sensory cortex was activated. *Lower*: the second burst when the participant fainted; activation occurred in various areas

part of the primary sensory cortex (BA3, 1 and 2) and the somatosensory association cortex (BA5), thus which indicating stimulation of the forearm or hand. The increase of EEG amplitude was observed at prior studies [13, 14] and even very significantly increasing of the amplitude also observed [15], however, in some study, we could find that most of channels are not changed [1].

The second burst showed a different pattern. The ratio and absolute power of the γ wave did not increase when the burst started, whereas the first burst showed an increase in the γ wave at the start of the burst. The sLoreta analysis also indicated different locations of activation. The amplitude of the brain waves increased at various locations of cortex, such as the DLPFC, the insula cortex, the pars orbitalis, part of the secondary/associative visual cortex and the middle temporal gyrus. Activation of the DLPFC and the insula cortex during acupuncture treatment has been reported by various

researchers [16, 17]. However, the other areas were not reported to have a major role and did not have any relationship with the efficacy area of LI4. Thus, we considered that additional excitation at these areas may provoke fainting, although the mechanism and connection between these area is not clear.

In the later interview, participant reported that she had never experienced fainting or syncope. Participant's average systolic/diastolic blood pressure before the test was 106/61 and we concluded it as a normal range and not enough for fainting regarding her body mass index. She reported she was not fasted although she was trying to lose her weight. There was no patients of epilepsy, amyotrophic lateral sclerosis or other genetic neural disease in her family according herself and she had never experienced fainting before the test in accordance with her statement. We also asked the participant to contact us when she experience fainting or similar situation again and we could get any message from her for more than one and half years. We concluded that her physical statement such as blood pressure, body weight or etc. stayed at the low but normal range and may work without any problem before, however, those statement may affected her to faint when we induced acupuncture stimulation.

This case is the first reported case of EEG changes observed while fainting caused by acupuncture stimulation and comparison or statistical analysis could not performed. Thus, this one case cannot reveal the parameters or mechanisms of fainting during acupuncture treatment. However, fainting cannot be intentionally induced by acupuncture, and this accidental case is considered to be the first report about what occurs in the brain when people faint during acupuncture treatment.

Acknowledgement
This study was funded by Korea Institute of Oriental Medicine (KIOM) (grant no. K16070).

Funding
This study was funded by Korea Institute of Oriental Medicine (KIOM) (grant no. K16070).

Authors' contributions
KO mainly analysed and wrote script text, K-HC and JK analysed EEG data, CSJ edited paragraphs, KS-Y and MJ-Y analysed brain areas, RYH corrected data analysis and manuscript text. All authors read and approved the final manuscript.

Competing interest
The authors declare that they have no competing interests.

References
1. Choi K-H, Kwon OS, Cho SJ, Lee S, Kang S-Y, Ahn SH, Ryu Y. Evaluating acupuncture point and nonacupuncture point stimulation with EEG: a high-frequency power spectrum analysis. Evid Based Complement Altern Med. 2016;2016:2134364.
2. Greenlee H, Crew KD, Capodice J, Awad D, Buono D, Shi Z, Jeffres A, Wyse S, Whitman W, Trivedi MS. Randomized sham-controlled pilot trial of weekly electro-acupuncture for the prevention of taxane-induced peripheral neuropathy in women with early stage breast cancer. Breast Cancer Res Treat. 2016;156(3):453–64.
3. Gwak YS, Kim HY, Lee BH, Yang CH. Combined approaches for the relief of spinal cord injury-induced neuropathic pain. Complement Ther Med. 2016;25:27–33.
4. Zhang J, Shang H, Gao X, Ernst E. Acupuncture-related adverse events: a systematic review of the Chinese literature. Bull World Health Organ. 2010; 88(12):915–21.
5. Ernst E, White AR. Prospective studies of the safety of acupuncture: a systematic review. Am J Med. 2001;110(6):481–5.
6. Association TKAaM. The acupuncture and moxibustion. In: Jipmundang. 2008. p. 474–5.
7. Pascual-Marqui RD. Standardized low-resolution brain electromagnetic tomography (sLORETA): technical details. Methods Find Exp Clin Pharmacol. 2002;24(Suppl D):5–12.
8. Pascual-Marqui RD. Discrete, 3D distributed, linear imaging methods of electric neuronal activity. Part 1: exact, zero error localization. arXiv preprint arXiv:07103341 2007.
9. Brodmann K. Brodmann's: Localisation in the cerebral cortex. Springer Science & Business Media 2007.
10. Rogers RD, Owen AM, Middleton HC, Williams EJ, Pickard JD, Sahakian BJ, Robbins TW. Choosing between small, likely rewards and large, unlikely rewards activates inferior and orbital prefrontal cortex. J Neurosci. 1999; 19(20):9029–38.
11. Cardin JA, Carlen M, Meletis K, Knoblich U, Zhang F, Deisseroth K, Tsai L-H, Moore CI. Driving fast-spiking cells induces gamma rhythm and controls sensory responses. Nature. 2009;459(7247):663–7.
12. Fries P. Neuronal gamma-band synchronization as a fundamental process in cortical computation. Annu Rev Neurosci. 2009;32(1):209–24.
13. Pei X, Wang J, Deng B, Wei X, Yu H. WLPVG approach to the analysis of EEG-based functional brain network under manual acupuncture. Cogn Neurodyn. 2014;8(5):417–28.
14. Kim MS, Kim HD, Seo HD, Sawada K, Ishida M. The effect of acupuncture at PC-6 on the electroencephalogram and electrocardiogram. Am J Chin Med. 2008;36(03):481–91.
15. Sakai S, Hori E, Umeno K, Kitabayashi N, Ono T, Nishijo H. Specific acupuncture sensation correlates with EEGs and autonomic changes in human subjects. Auton Neurosci. 2007;133(2):158–69.
16. Chae Y, Lee I-S, Jung W-M, Park K, Park H-J, Wallraven C. Psychophysical and neurophysiological responses to acupuncture stimulation to incorporated rubber hand. Neurosci Lett. 2015;591:48–52.
17. Napadow V, Dhond RP, Kim J, LaCount L, Vangel M, Harris RE, Kettner N, Park K. Brain encoding of acupuncture sensation - coupling on-line rating with fMRI. Neuro Image. 2009;47(3):1055–65.

3

Sex differences in acupuncture effectiveness in animal models of Parkinson's disease

Sook-Hyun Lee[1], Maurits van den Noort[2], Peggy Bosch[3] and Sabina Lim[1,2,4*] iD

Abstract

Background: Many animal experimental studies have been performed to investigate the efficacy of acupuncture in Parkinson's disease (PD). Sex differences are a major issue in all diseases including PD. However, to our knowledge, there have been no reviews investigating sex differences on the effectiveness of acupuncture treatment for animal PD models. The current study aimed to summarize and analyze past studies in order to evaluate these possible differences.

Method: Each of 7 databases (MEDLINE, EMBASE, the Cochrane Library, 3 Korean medical databases, and the China National Knowledge Infrastructure) was searched from its inception through March 2015 without language restrictions.

Results: We included studies of the use of acupuncture treatment in animal models of PD. A total of 810 potentially relevant articles were identified, 57 of which met our inclusion criteria. C57/BL6 mice were used most frequently (42 %) in animal PD models. Most of the studies were carried out using only male animals (67 %); only 1 study (2 %) was performed using solely females. The further 31 % of the studies used a male/female mix or did not specify the sex.

Conclusions: The results of our review suggest that acupuncture is an effective treatment for animal PD models, but there is insufficient evidence to determine whether sex differences exist. Future studies of acupuncture treatment for PD should use female animal models because they reflect the physiological characteristics of both males and females to fully evaluate the effect and the safety of the treatment for each sex.

Keywords: Electro-acupuncture, Manual acupuncture, Bee-venom acupuncture, C57/BL6, Acupuncture point

Background

Parkinson's disease (PD) is a progressive neurodegenerative disease caused by the loss of dopaminergic neurons in the substantia nigra [1]. PD usually occurs in individuals over 50 years of age, and its incidence and prevalence increases among individuals approximately 60 years of age and older. PD has become more common due to the rapid aging of human populations around the world [2]. Epidemiological studies have

reported that the incidence of PD is 1.5–2 times higher in men than in women, and the onset of symptoms may occur later in women due to the neuroprotective effects of estrogen [3]. For the disease manifestations of PD, women have higher Unified Parkinson's Disease Rating Scale (UPDRS) motor scores, but present with dyskinesia, tremor, and PD-related complications more often than men [4].

Because the FDA reported that eight out of ten new drugs that had been sold on the market were discontinued because they resulted in far more detrimental side effects in women, the sex perspective began to be discussed in many other fields as well [5]. Adverse drug reactions can be caused by the physiological difference between men and women, and women can be

* Correspondence: lims@khu.ac.kr
[1]Department of Applied Korean Medicine, Graduate School, Kyung Hee University, Seoul, Republic of Korea
[2]Research Group of Pain and Neuroscience, WHO Collaborating Center for Traditional Medicine, East–west Medical Research Institute, Kyung Hee University, Seoul, Republic of Korea
Full list of author information is available at the end of the article

more vulnerable to a particular drug [6]. Because sex is often not considered an important variable in animal research with the exception of research related to features of a particular sex, such as reproduction and endocrine secretion, the overwhelming majority of experimental research uses only males and many studies do not even disclose the sex of the experimental animals. Basic research studies using cells in culture also often fail to present the sex of the organism from which the cell strain originated, but the results of such basic research has been applied generally to humans. Because medical research studies are performed primarily by male researchers [7–9], the research subjects are also mostly males [10–12], and there has been a tendency to be careless of females [13], which can aggravate treatment problems related to the physiological differences between men and women. The National Institutes of Health (NIH) requires applicants to report their cell and animal inclusion plans as part of the preclinical experimental design [14]. Therefore, studies are being performed to determine what sex differences need to be accounted for in preclinical and clinical stages, and the importance of the applying these principles is being highlighted [15].

PD treatment options include pharmacological treatment, non-pharmacological treatment, surgical therapy, and dopaminergic cell transplantation [15]. Acupuncture has long been employed for numerous disorders, and it has been traditionally used to relieve PD-related symptoms and to delay the clinical progression of PD symptoms [16]. We have reported that acupuncture exerts increased neuroprotective effects in regions including the substantia nigra, caudate, thalamus, and putamen in animal models of PD [17–20]. Acupuncture was also found to inhibit microglial activation, inflammation, and iron-related oxidative damage in PD [21].

Sex differences have emerged recently as an important issue, but sufficient efficacy tests for sex differences in acupuncture, as in preclinical studies for drug development, have not yet been performed. It is necessary to clarify efficacy differences according to sex in order to more effectively utilize acupuncture in clinical practice. Therefore, we carried out the present study to identify whether adequate research has been conducted so far to determine the sex differences in the efficacy of acupuncture. Specifically, we analyzed past studies of acupuncture treatment conducted in animal PD models, and determined whether the body of data was sufficient to determine the effects of sex differences on the effectiveness of acupuncture treatment. This review provides the basis for establishing whether future animal model studies are necessary to determine possible sex-related differences in the efficacy of acupuncture for PD.

Methods

Search methods for the identification of studies

The search was performed without restrictions on language or year of publication. We searched Medline, EMBASE, and the Cochrane Central Register of Controlled Trials from the inception of each database through March 2015. For Korean publications, we searched three Korean medical databases (Research Information Service System, National Discovery for Science Leaders, and OASIS). For Chinese articles, we searched the China National Knowledge Infrastructure. The keywords used for the search were the following: "Parkinson's disease" OR "Parkinson" AND "acupuncture" OR "acupoints" OR "electroacupuncture" OR "electro-acupuncture" OR "auriculotherapy" OR "auriculoacupuncture" OR "bee venom acupuncture" in each database language. The search strategy was adjusted for each database.

Inclusion/exclusion criteria

We included studies of the use of acupuncture treatment in animal PD models. Trials were excluded if the study designs did not evaluate the effectiveness of acupuncture in animal PD models, or if they reported insufficient data. No search restrictions on language or publication forms were imposed. During the first stage of selection/exclusion, titles and abstracts were analyzed, and literature that had no relevance to our study was excluded. The second stage of selection/exclusion involved analyzing the full text of particular studies, because it was impossible to determine the relevance of the studies based solely on the abstracts.

Data extraction

Two reviewers (LSH and KJY) independently reviewed the data extracted from each article using a standardized data extraction form and reached consensus on all items. The extracted data included the type of animal PD models, the sex of the animal PD models, the methods used to induce PD, the types of acupuncture, the acupuncture points, and the effectiveness of the treatment.

Results

Study description

We identified 810 publications, 57 of which met the eligibility criteria (Fig. 1). The 57 articles were published from 1996 to 2014. The characteristics of the studies are summarized in Table 1 [7–12, 18, 19, 21–69].

Animals of PD models

The animals of PD models included mice (C57/BL6 and ICR) and rats (Sprague–Dawley, and Wistar) (Fig. 2). The most frequently used animal PD model was C57/BL6, which was used in 24 articles, followed by SD and Wistar, each of which were used in 15 articles, and ICR

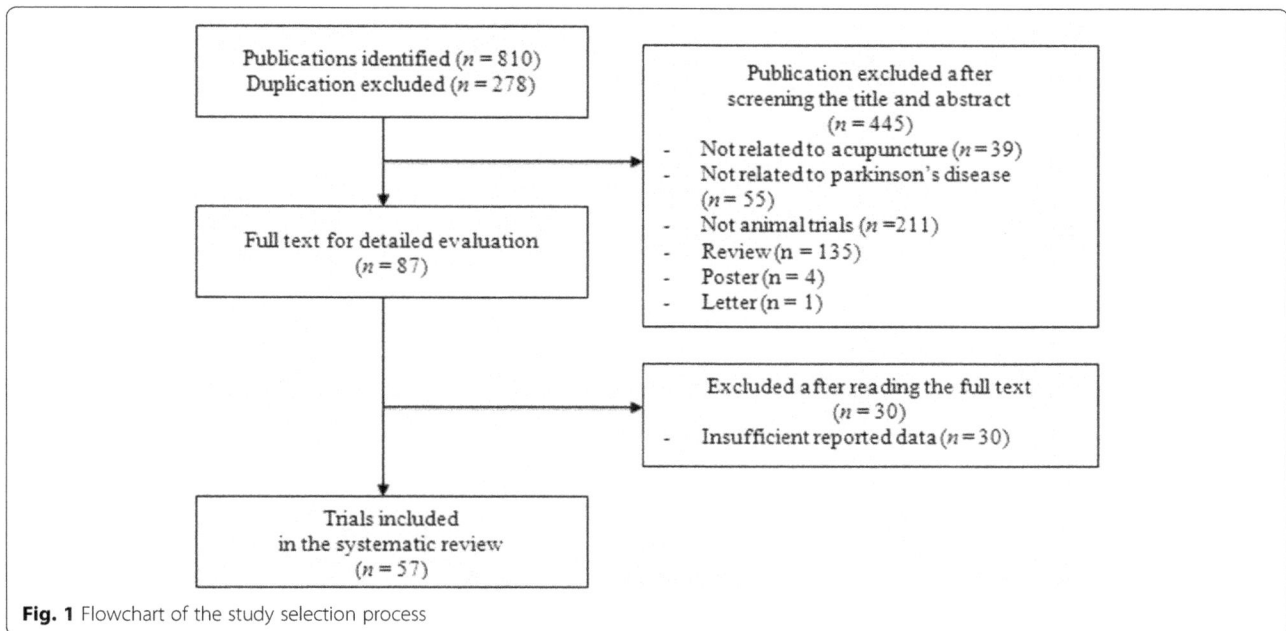

Fig. 1 Flowchart of the study selection process

and undefined animals, which were used in one article each. All of the studies using C57/BL6 animals used only males. Of the studies using SD animals, ten used males only, four used a male/female mix, and one used animals with undefined sex. Of the studies using Wistar animals, nine used a male/female mix, two used males only, three used animals with undefined sex, and one study used females only.

Methods used to induce PD

The drugs 6-hydroxydopamine (6-OHDA), 1-methyl-4-phenyl-1,2,3,6-tetrahydropyridine (MPTP), and rotenone, as well as medial forebrain bundle (MFB) transection, were used to induce PD in the animal models (Fig. 3). 6-OHDA was used in 47 % (27) of the studies, MPTP was used in 44 % (25) of the studies, and rotenone was used in 7 % (4) of the studies. MFB transection was used in 2 % (1) of the studies. Of the studies using 6-OHDA, 13 used a male/female mix, nine used only males, and five used animals with undefined sex. All of the studies using MPTP or Rotenone used only male animals. The study using MFB transection used only females. Therefore, three out of the four PD induction models studied were only used in animals of a single sex. Only the results of 6-OHDA induced animal PD models could potentially be compared between the sexes.

Types of acupuncture

Electro-acupuncture (EA) was used in 54 % (38) of the studies, manual acupuncture (MA) was used in 30 % (18) of the studies, and bee-venom (BV) acupuncture was used in 11 % (6) of the studies. Of the studies using

EA, 18 used only males, 11 used a male/female mix, three used animals of undefined sex, and one used only females. Of the studies using MA, 14 used only males, two used a male/female mix, and two used animals with undefined sex. All of the studies using BV acupuncture used only males (Fig. 4).

Acupuncture points

Regardless of the type of acupuncture, the acupuncture points used consisted mainly of LR3, GB34, GV20, GV16, and ST36 (Additional file 1). LR3 was used in 35 % (20) of the studies, and GV34 and GV20 were each used in 26 % (16) of the studies. Of the studies using LR3, 14 used only males, three used a male/female mix, and three used animals with undefined sex. Of the studies using GB34, 14 used only males, and two used a male/female mix. Of the studies using GV20, eight used only males, seven used a male/female mix, and one used animals with undefined sex. Of the studies using GV16, seven used only males, three used a male/female mix, and three used animals with undefined sex. Of the studies using ST36, four used only males, two used animals with undefined sex, and one used a male/female mix.

Behavioral test

Behavioral analyses were carried out using the rotational behavior test, the pole-climbing test, the swimming test, and locomotor counts (Additional file 2). The rotational behavior test was used in 56 % (10) of the studies, the pole-climbing test was used in 22 % (6) of the studies, and the swimming test, and locomotor counts were each used in 6 % (1) of the studies. The rotational behavior

Table 1 Summary of acupuncture for animal PD models

First author (year)	Type of animal PD models	Sex of animal PD models	Drugs used to induce PD	Types of acupuncture	Types of acupuncture points	Evaluation of the treatment effectiveness
Bai (2014a) [22]	Undefined	Undefined	6-OHDA	EA	GV20, EX-HN5	DA
Bai (2014b) [8]	Undefined	Male	6-OHDA	EA	GV20, EX-HN5	Caspase-3
Feng (2014) [10]	C57BL/6	Male	MPTP	MA	Undefined	Pole-climbing test, BDNF, TH, DA
Yeo (2013) [19]	C57BL/6	Male	MPTP	MA	GB34, LR3	TH, gene expression
Alvarez-Fischer (2013) [7]	C57BL/6	Male	MPTP	BV	Undefined	DA, DOPAC, IL-1β, IL-6, TNF-α, HVA, TH, rotational test
Ding (2013) [11]	SD	Male	6-OHDA	EA	LI4, LR3	nNOS, GFAP
Wang (2013a) [9]	SD	Male	Rotenone	EA	GV16, LR3	TH, COX-2
Wang (2013b) [23]	SD	Male	Rotenone	EA	GV16, LR3	TH, p-p38 MARK, COX-2
Wang (2013c) [12]	SD	Male	Rotenone	EA	GV16, LR3	TH, SOD, GSH, CAT, MDA
Wang (2013d) [24]	SD	Male	Rotenone	EA	GV16, LR3	UCH-L1, UBE1, Parkin, TH, α-synuclein
Ding (2012) [25]	SD	Male	6-OHDA	EA	LI4, LR3	TH, GFAP, PCNA
Huang (2012) [26]	ICR	Male	MPTP	EA	GB34	Lamp 1, α-synuclein
Lu (2012) [27]	C57BL/6	Male	MPTP	EA	GV20, GV16, GB34	Locomotor counts, swimming test, pole-climbing test
Guo (2012) [28]	SD	Male	6-OHDA	EA	GV20, GV16, GB34	GSH, SOD, MDA, GSH-Px
Yang (2011) [29]	C57BL/6	Male	MPTP	EA	PC7	Pole-climbing test, TH, DA, DOPAC, HVA
Choi (2011) [18]	C57/BL6	Male	MPTP	MA	GB34, LR3	TH, DAT, gene expression
Kim (2011) [30]	C57BL/6	Male	MPTP	BV	ST36	MAC-1, iNOS, TH
Du (2011) [31]	SD	Male	6-OHDA	EA	GV20, GV14	GABA, rotational test
Wang (2011) [32]	C57BL/6	Male	MPTP	EA	ST36, SP6	TH, DA, DOPAC, HVA, SOD, GSH, GSH-Px
Doo (2010) [33]	C57BL/6	Male	MPTP	BV	GB34	TH
Hong (2010) [34]	C57BL/6	Male	MPTP	MA	GB34	Gene expression
Jun (2010) [35]	C57BL/6	Male	MPTP	BV	BL23	TH, caspase-3, iNOS
Kim (2010) [36]	C57BL/6	Male	MPTP	EA	GB34, GB39	DA
Park (2010) [37]	C57BL/6	Male	MPTP	BV	GB39, LI11, BL23	TH, MAC-1, HSP70
Sun (2010) [38]	C57BL/6	Male	MPTP	MA	GV20, GV14	Pole-climbing test, TH, DA, DOPAC
Wang (2010a) [39]	Wistar	Undefined	6-OHDA	EA	GV16, LR3	TH, DA
Wang (2010b) [40]	Wistar	Undefined	6-OHDA	EA	GV16, LR3,CV4, ST36	GDNF
Wang (2010c) [41]	C57/BL6	Male	MPTP	MA	GV20, GV14	Pole-climbing test, TH, DA, NA, DOPAC, 5HIAA, 5HT
Yu (2010) [42]	Wistar	Male	6-OHDA	MA	GB34, LR3, ST36, SP10	Rotational test, SOD, GSH-Px, CAT, GSH, MDA
Huang (2010) [43]	Wistar	Male	6-OHDA	EA	LI4, LR3	Rotational test, BDNF, TrkB

Table 1 Summary of acupuncture for animal PD models (Continued)

Study	Strain	Sex	Model	Type	Acupoints	Outcomes
Choi (2009) [21]	C57BL6	Male	MPTP	MA	LR3, GB34	TH, DAT
Kim (2009) [44]	C57BL/6	Male	MPTP	BV	BL23	TH, MAC-1, HSP70
Wang (2009a) [45]	Wistar	Male, Female	6-OHDA	EA	GV20, EX-NH5	TH, BDNF
Wang (2009b) [46]	Wistar	Male, Female	6-OHDA	EA	GV20, EX-NH5	TH, DAT
Kim (2008) [47]	C57BL/6	Male	MPTP	MA	GB34	TH
Guan (2008) [48]	C57BL/6	Male	MPTP	EA	GV20	Fn
Wang (2008) [49]	Wistar	Male, Female	6-OHDA	EA	GV20, EX-NH5	TH
Jeon (2008) [50]	C57BL/6	Male	MPTP	EA	GB34, SI3, BL62, ST36	Pole-climbing test, TH, DA, BDNF
Xie (2007) [51]	Wistar	Undefined	6-OHDA	MA	GV20	Rotational test, MDA, NO, SOD
Kang (2007) [52]	C57BL/6	Male	MPTP	MA	GB34, LR3	TH, COX-2, iNOS, DA, DOPAC, HVA
Huang (2007) [53]	SD	Male	6-OHDA	MA	GB34, LR3	TH
Luo (2007) [54]	Wistar	Male, Female	6-OHDA	EA	GV20, EX-NH5	NOS
Wang (2007) [55]	SD	Male, Female	6-OHDA	MA	GV20, GV16, GB34	Rotational test, DA
Jin (2006a) [56]	Wistar	Male, Female	6-OHDA	EA	Undefined	GSH, GSH-Px,SOD, MDA, NOS
Jin (2006b) [57]	Wistar	Male, Female	6-OHDA	EA	Undefined	DA, HVA, DOPAC
Ma (2006) [58]	Wistar	Male, Female	6-OHDA	EA	GV16, LR3	Rotational test, DA
Tang (2006) [59]	C57BL/6	Male	MPTP	EA	LI4, LR3	BDNF
Wang (2006) [60]	SD	Male, Female	6-OHDA	EA	GV16, LR6	Glutamic acid
Kim (2006) [61]	C57BL/6	Male	MPTP	MA	LR8, LR4, LR2	TH
Kim (2005) [62]	SD	Undefined	6-OHDA	MA	ST36	Rotational test, TH
Ma (2005) [63]	Wistar	Male, Female	6-OHDA	EA	GV16, LR3	Rotational test, SOD, GSH, GSH-Px
Wang (2005) [64]	Wistar	Undefined	6-OHDA	MA	GV16, LR3, CV4, ST36	TH
Park (2003) [65]	SD	Male	6-OHDA	MA	GB34, LR3, LI4, LI11	Rotational test, TH, TrkB
Liang (2002) [66]	Wistar	Female	MFB transection	EA	GV14, GV21	TH, BDNF
Lin (2000) [67]	SD	Male, Female	6-OHDA	EA	LR3, SP6, ST36, GB34	DA, HVA, DOPAC
He (1998) [68]	SD	Male, Female	6-OHDA	EA	GV20, GV14	DA, NA, 5HT
Zhu (1996) [69]	C57BL/6	Male	MPTP	MA	GV20	DA, DOPAC

Abbreviations: BDNF Brain-derived neurotrophic factor, *BV* Bee-venom acupuncture, *CAT* Catalase, *Caspase-3:* caspase protein, *COX-2* Cyclooxygenase-2, *DA* Dopamine, *DAT* Dopamine active transporter, *DOPAC* Dihydroxyphenyl acetic acid, *EA* Electro-acupuncture, *Fn* Ferritin, *GABA* gamma-aminobutyric acid, *GDNF* Glial cell-derived neurotrophic factor, *GFAP* Glial fibrillary acidic protein, *GSH* Glutathione, *GSHpx* Glutathione peroxidase, *HSP70* 70 kilo Dalton heat shock proteins, *HVA* Homovanillic acid, *IL-1β* Interleukin-1 beta, *IL-6* Interleukin-6, *iNOS* Inducible nitric oxide synthase, *Lamp 1* Lysosomal-associated membrane protein 1, *MA* Manual acupuncture, *MAC-1* Macrophage-1 antigen, *MDA* Malondialdehyde, *NO* Nitric oxide, *nNos* Neuronal nitric oxide synthase, *MFB* Medial forebrain bundle, *MPTP* 1-methyl-4-phenyl-1,2,3,6-tetrahydropyridine, *pp38 MAPK* Phospho-p38 MAPK, *PCNA* Proliferating cell nuclear antigen, *SD* Sprague–Dawley, *SOD* Superoxide dismutase, *TH* Tyrosine hydroxylase, *TNF-α* Tumor necrosis factor alpha, *TrkB* Tropomyosin receptor kinase B, *UBE1* Ubiquitin-like Modifier Activating Enzyme 1, *UCH-L1* Ubiquitin C-terminal hydrolase, *5HIAA* 5-Hydroxyindoleacetic acid, *5HT* 5-hydroxytryptamine, *6-OHDA* 6-hydroxydopamine

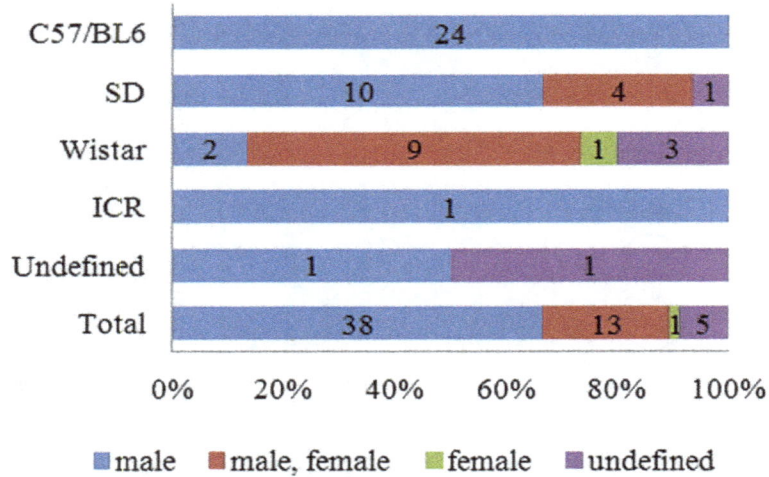

Fig. 2 Sex differences according to the types of animal used as PD model

test was mainly used in conjunction with 6-OHDA (8 studies), the pole-climbing test was used in conjunction with MPTP (6 studies), and the swimming test and locomotor counts were each used in conjunction with MPTP (Additional file 3). The rotational behavior test was used in five studies with only males, four studies with a male/female mix, and one study with animals with undefined sex. The studies using the pole-climbing test, the swimming test, and locomotor counts were each conducted with males only. Of all studies including behavioral analyses, 72 % (13) of the studies used only male animals, 22 % (4) used a male/female mix, and 6 % (1) used animals with undefined sex. In these studies, PD was induced using MPTP in 53 % (9) of the studies and 6-OHDA in 47 % (8).

Evaluation of treatment effectiveness

The effectiveness of the treatment on PD was evaluated by levels of tyrosine hydroxylase (TH), dopamine (DA),

dihydroxyphenyl acetic acid (DOPAC), homovanillic acid (HVA), superoxide dismutase (SOD), glutathione (GSH), and brain-derived neurotrophic factor (BDNF) (Additional file 4). TH was the most frequently used method to determine the effectiveness of the treatment on PD (56 % [32] of the studies). Of the studies using TH, 26 used only males, two used a male/female mix, three used animals with undefined sex, and one used only females. Of the studies using DA, ten used only males, five used a male/female mix, and two used animals with undefined sex. Of the studies using DOPAC, seven used only males, and two used a male/female mix. Of the studies using HVA and GSH, respectively, four of each used only males, and two of each used a male/female mix. Of the studies using SOD, four used only males, and two used a male/female mix. Of the studies using BDNF, four used only males, one used a male/female mix, and one used only females.

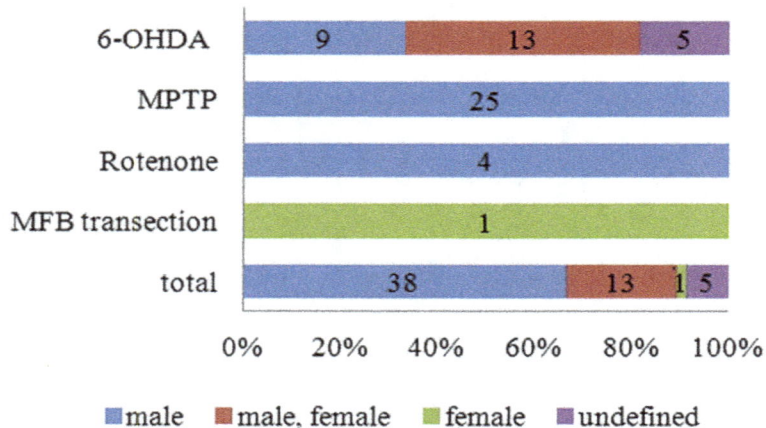

Fig. 3 Sex differences according to the method used to induce PD

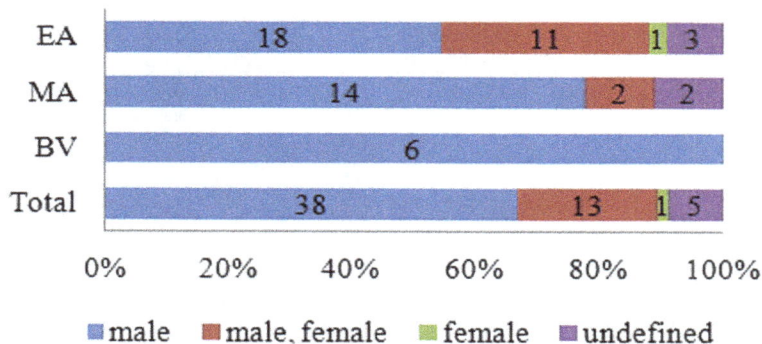

Fig. 4 Sex differences according to the type of acupuncture performed

Discussion

We analyzed sex differences among previous studies that used animal PD models of acupuncture treatment. A total of 810 potentially relevant articles were identified, 57 of which met our inclusion criteria. C57/BL6 mice were the most frequently used (42 %) animal PD models. Most of the studies evaluating the effectiveness of acupuncture treatment for PD were performed using only male animals (67 %); only one study (2 %) was performed using female animals.

Many studies have inadvertently excluded females from animal studies of acupuncture treatment for PD. Kang et al. suggested that acupuncture could be used as a neuroprotective intervention for inhibiting microglial activation and inflammatory events in the MPTP-induced male PD model [52]. Yu et al. showed that acupuncture treatment displays antioxidative and/or neuroprotective properties in the 6-OHDA lesioned male rat PD models [3]. Although a few studies were performed using a male/female mix, they could not combine and compare the results from male versus female animals. Only one report used female animals, in which was a study in which different frequencies of chronic EA stimulation were tested in a partially-lesioned female rat model of PD induced by transection of the MFB. This study suggested that long-term high frequency EA is effective in halting the degeneration of dopaminergic neurons in the substantia nigra (SN). Because the studies of male PD models generated using MFB transection are nonexistent, we could not compare the sex differences in this model. Taken together, there is currently insufficient evidence from past studies to determine whether there are sex differences in the effectiveness of acupuncture for animal PD models. In the future, studies should be performed using a male/female mix to minimize performance bias, and ideally should include a comparison of the sex differences.

Animal studies have often focused primarily on males. For the most part, examination of the differences between males and females has been disregarded in biomedical research, leaving gaps in our knowledge [42]. Recently, new drugs have been developed without considering the physiological characteristics of females or sex differences. Women have therefore been frequently exposed to dangerous side effects because the experimental studies and clinical trials had mainly used male subjects [70]. The lack of female participation in drug-development studies affects males as well as females; when side effects not seen in males during the drug safety checks appear in females, the approval of the drugs is delayed, and male patients waiting for the drugs consequently suffer. The NIH requires applicants to report their cell and animal inclusion plans as part of the preclinical experimental design. Despite this NIH policy, numerous scientific publications continue to neglect sex-based considerations and analyses in preclinical and clinical research. A stronger commitment to reporting sex-specific results will strengthen the evidence base [13]. Fortunately, sex differences are increasingly recognized as factors that influence the incidence and disease manifestations of all diseases, including neurodegenerative disorders.

Some gender differences have been documented for PD [3, 4]. Paven et al. suggested gender differences in the epidemiology, clinical features, treatment outcomes (medical and surgical/deep brain stimulation), and social impact among all available PD studies [4]. Wooten et al. performed a meta-analysis of the differences in the incidence of PD between men and women [3]. Smith et al. summarized evidence that estrogen and selective estrogen receptor modulators are neuroprotective in PD, and reviewed sex differences in basal ganglia function and dopaminergic pathways [71, 72]. Consistent with these past studies, if acupuncture research involved both males and females, additional studies of acupuncture for PD would provide a more robust conclusion about sex differences in this treatment.

Review limitations and future areas of research
A number of gaps in the reviewed literature were identified in relation to study quality and findings. Study quality could

be improved by using female animal models because they reflect the physiological characteristics of both males and females to fully evaluate the effectiveness and safety of the treatment for each sex, which is largely missing in the literature so far.

Conclusions

The results of our review suggest that acupuncture is an effective treatment for animal PD models, but there is insufficient evidence to determine whether sex differences exist in response to this treatment. Future studies should examine the effects of acupuncture in animal PD models of both sexes, to reflect the physiological characteristics of females as well as males, and to fully evaluate the effect and safety of this treatment.

Additional files

Additional file 1: Sex differences according to the acupuncture points used. (TIF 781 kb)

Additional file 2: Sex differences according to behavioral tests used. (TIF 776 kb)

Additional file 3: Behavioral tests performed categorized by the method used to induce PD. (TIF 638 kb)

Additional file 4: Sex differences according to the method of evaluation of treatment effectiveness. (TIF 842 kb)

Abbreviations

BDNF: Brain-derived neurotrophic factor; BV: Bee-venom acupuncture; DA: Dopamine; DOPAC: Dihydroxyphenyl acetic acid; EA: Electro-acupuncture; GSH: Glutathione; HVA: Homovanillic acid; MA: Manual acupuncture; MFB: Medial forebrain bundle; MPTP: 1-methyl-4-phenyl-1,2,3,6-tetrahydropyridine; SD: Sprague-Dawley; SOD: Superoxide dismutase; TH: Tyrosine hydroxylase; 6-OHDA: 6-hydroxydopamine

Acknowledgements
We would like to thank Jong-Yeop Kim for his assistance with the collection of data used for this study.

Funding
This work was supported by the Mid-Career Research Program through an NRF grant funded by the Korean government (No. 2014R1A2A1A11052795).

Authors' contributions
SHL and SL created the study background and designed the study; SHL performed data acquisition and analysis, and drafted the article; SL conducted the literature review; MvdN, PB and SL revised the article. All authors read and approved the final manuscript.

Competing interests
The authors declare that they have no competing interests.

Author details
[1]Department of Applied Korean Medicine, Graduate School, Kyung Hee University, Seoul, Republic of Korea. [2]Research Group of Pain and Neuroscience, WHO Collaborating Center for Traditional Medicine, East–west Medical Research Institute, Kyung Hee University, Seoul, Republic of Korea. [3]Donders Institute for Brain, Cognition and Behaviour, Radboud University, 6525 HR Nijmegen, The Netherlands. [4]Department of Meridian & Acupoint, College of Korean Medicine, Kyung Hee University, 26 Kyungheedae-ro, Dongdaemun-gu, Seoul 130-70102447, Republic of Korea.

References

1. Obeso JA, Rodríguez-Oroz MC, Benitez-Temino B, Blesa FJ, Guridi J, Marin C, Rodriguez M. Functional organization of the basal ganglia: therapeutic implications for Parkinson's disease. Mov Disord. 2008;23 Suppl 3:S48–59.
2. Samii A, Nutt JG, Ransom BR. Parkinson's disease. Lancet. 2004;363(9423):1783–93.
3. Wooten GF, Currie LJ, Bovbjerg VE, Lee JK, Patrie J. Are men at greater risk for Parkinson's disease than women? J Neurol Neurosurg Psychiatry. 2004; 75(4):637–9.
4. Pavon JM, Whitson HE, Okun MS. Parkinson's disease in women: a call for improved clinical studies and for comparative effectiveness research. Maturitas. 2010;65(4):352–8.
5. Wald C, Wu C. Biomedical research. Of mice and women: the bias in animal models. Science. 2010;327(5973):1571–2.
6. Haack S, Seeringer A, Thürmann PA, Becker T, Kirchheiner J. Sex-specific differences in side effects of psychotropic drugs: genes or gender? Pharmacogenomics. 2009;10(9):1511–26.
7. Alvarez-Fischer DC, Noelker F, Vulinović A, Grünewald C, et al. Bee venom and its component apamin as neuroprotective agents in a Parkinson disease mouse model. Plos One. 2013;8(4):e61700.
8. Yan B, Zhigang L, Hu B, et al. Effects of electro-acupuncture on Baihui and Taiyang points on caspase- 3 expression and apoptosis of substantia nigra dopaminergic neurons of rats with Parkinson disease. Chinese J Tradit Med Sci &Tech. 2014;21(5):534–6.
9. Wang YC, Xu YH, Ma J, et al. Effects of electric acupuncture on the oxidative stress in the rat of Parkinson's disease abductioned by rotenone. Hubei Univ of TCM. 2013;28(8):2417–9.
10. Feng J, Sun HM, Wang YY, et al. Influences of needling chorea-tremble controlled zone on expressions of dopaminergic neurons and BDNF in mice with Parkinson's disease. J Beijing Univ TCM. 2014;37(1):53–7.
11. Ding YX, Zhao J, Hou LQ. Effects of electroacupuncture on the expressions of neuroal nitric oxide synthase and astrocyte in dentate gyrus of rats with Parkinson's disease. Chin acupunct& mox. 2013;33(6):533–7.
12. Wang SJ, Fang JQ, Ma J. Effect of electroacupuncture stimulation of "Fengfu" (GV 16) and "Taichong" (LR 3) on expression of COX-2 and tyrosine hydroxylase in substantia nigra in rats with Parkinson's disease. Acupuncture Research. 2013;38(3):198–201.
13. Anita H. Gender bias in research: how does it affect evidence based medicine? J R Soc Med. 2007;100(1):2–3.
14. Clayton JA, Collins FS. NIH to balance sex in cell and animal studies. Nature. 2014;509(7500):282–3.
15. Raz L, Miller VM. Considerations of sex and gender differences in preclinical and clinical trials. Handb Exp Pharmacol. 2012;214:127–47.
16. Singh N, Pillay V, Choonara YE. Advances in the treatment of Parkinson's disease. Prog Neurobiol. 2007;81(1):29–44.
17. Walton-Hadlock J. Primary Parkinson's disease: the use of Tuina and acupuncture in accord with an evolving hypothesis of its cause from the perspective of Chinese traditional medicine–part 2. Am J Acupunct. 1999; 27(1–2):31–49.
18. Choi YG, Yeo S, Hong YM, Lim S. Neuroprotective changes of striatal degeneration-related gene expression by acupuncture in an MPTP mouse model of Parkinsonism: microarray analysis. Cell Mol Neurobiol. 2011;31(3):377–91.
19. Yeo S, Choi YG, Hong YM, Lim S. Neuroprotective changes of thalamic degeneration-related gene expression by acupuncture in an MPTP mouse model of Parkinsonism: microarray analysis. Gene. 2013;515(2):329–38.
20. Yeo S, Lim S, Choe IH, Choi YG, Chung KC, Jahng GH, Kim SH. Acupuncture stimulation on GB34 activates neural responses associated with Parkinson's disease. CNS Neurosci Ther. 2012;18(9):781–90.

21. Choi YG, Park JH, Lim S. Acupuncture inhibits ferric iron deposition and ferritin-heavy chain reduction in an MPTP-induced Parkinsonism model. Neurosci Lett. 2009;450(2):92–6.

22. Bai Y, LI ZG, Wang S, et al. Study on protective effect of different electro-acupuncture on Baihui and Taiyang points on dopaminergic neurons of rats with Parkinson Disease. Chin Med Sci Tech. 2014a;21(5):536–8.

23. Wang SJ, Fang JQ, Ma J, et al. Influence of electroacupuncture on p38-mitogen activated protein kinase in substantia nigra cells of rats with Parkinson disease model. Chin Acupunct Mox. 2013b;33(4):329–33.

24. Wang YC, He F, Ma J, et al. impacts of electroacupuncture on ubiquitin-proteasome system in rats with Parkinson's disease. Hubei Univ TCM. 2013d;33(8):725–9.

25. Ding YX, Hou LQ, Xiong KR. Effect of electroacupuncture on expression of proliferating cell nuclear antigen and glial fibrillary acidic protein in subventricular zone of Parkinson's disease rats. Acupunct Res. 2012;37(4):286–90.

26. Huang Q, Sun Y, Wang L, Zhang Y, et al. Acupuncture improve motor function in a mouse model of Parkinson's disease. Nucl Tech. 2012;35(11):877–80.

27. Lu ZY, Zhao H, Wang T. Effects of Acupuncture on Behavior and Striatal Apoptosis in Mice with Parkinson Disease. Acupunct Res. 2012;37(3):186–90.

28. Guo CX, Zhang L, Shao SJ, Hao L, et al. Oxidative stress effects of electro-acupuncture for "Baihui ", "Fengfu", "Yanglingquan " on PD model rat. Yunnan Univ TCM. 2012;35(5):26–9.

29. Yang JL, Chen JS, Yang YF, et al. Neuroprotection effects of retained acupuncture in neurotoxin-induced Parkinson's disease mice. Brain Behav Immun. 2011;25(7):1452–9.

30. Kim JI, Yang EJ, Lee MS, et al. Bee venom reduces neuroinflammation in the MPTP-induced model of Parkinson's disease. Int J Neurosci. 2011;121:209–17.

31. Du J, Sun ZL, Jia J, Wang X, et al. High-frequency electro-acupuncture stimulation modulates intracerebral γ-aminobutyric acid content in rat model of Parkinson's disease. Acta Physiol Sinica. 2011;63(4):305–10.

32. Wang H, Pan Y, Xue B, et al. The Antioxidative Effect of Electro-Acupuncture in a Mouse Model of Parkinson's Disease. PLoS ONE. 2011;6(5):e19790.

33. Doo AR, Kim ST, Kim SN, et al. Neuroprotective effects of bee venom pharmaceutical acupuncture in acute 1-methyl-4-phenyl-1,2,3,6-tetrahydropyridine-induced mouse model of Parkinson's disease. Neurolog Res. 2010;32 Suppl 1:88–91.

34. Hong MS, Park HK, Yang JS, et al. Gene expression profile of acupuncture treatment in 1-methyl-4-phenyl-1,2, 3,6- tetrahydropyridine-induced Parkinson's disease model. Neurol Res. 2010;32 Suppl 1:S74–8.

35. Jun HJ, Kim YS. Dose-dependent Effects of Bee Venom Acupuncture on MPTP-induced Mouse Model of Parkinson's Disease. J Korean Acupunct Mox Med Sci. 2010;27(5):59–68.

36. Kim ST, Moon W, Chae Y, et al. The effect of electroaucpuncture for 1-methyl-4-phenyl-1,2,3,6-tetrahydropyridine induced proteomic changes in the mouse striatum. J Physiol Sci. 2010;60:27–34.

37. Park W, Kim JK, Kim JI, et al. Neuroprotective and Anti-inflammatory Effects of Bee Venom Acupuncture on MPTP-induced Mouse. J Korean Acupunct Mox Med Sci. 2010;27(3):105–16.

38. Sun H, Wu H, Xu H, et al. Protective effect of acupuncture in acupoints of Governor Vessel on dopaminergic neurons protection and influence on ultrastructure in mice with Parkinson's disease. Beijing Univ TCM. 2010;33(4):257–62.

39. Wang YC, Cheng YH, Ma J, et al. Effect of electroacupuncture on morphological changes and apoptosis of substantia nigra cells in Parkinson's disease rats. Acupunct Res. 2010a;35(6):415–21.

40. Wang YC, Cheng YH, Ma J, et al. Effects of electroacupuncture on the expression of GDNF and Ret in Parkinson's disease model rats. Hubei Univ TCM. 2010b;30(9):739–43.

41. Wang YY, Sun HM, He X, et al. The protection effect of acupuncture of baihui and dazhui points on the dopaminergic neurons in PD mice. Prog Anatomic Sci. 2010c;16(1):16–20.

42. Yu YP, Ju WP, Li ZG, Wang DZ, Wang YC, Xie AM. Acupuncture inhibits oxidative stress and rotational behavior in 6-hydroxydopamine lesioned rat. Brain Res. 2010;1336:58–65.

43. Huang PP, Ma J, Wang Y, et al. Effect of electroacupuncture on the expression of BDNF and TrKB in mesenchpic substantia nigra of the Parkinson 's disease model rats. J Hubei Univ Chin Med. 2010;12(2):3–5.

44. Kim CY, Lee JD, Lee SH. Anti-inflammatory Effect of Bee Venom Acupuncture at Sinsu (BL23) in a MPTP Mouse Model of Parkinson Disease. J Korean Acupunct Mox Med Sci. 2009;26(4):49–58.

45. Wang S, Jiang H, Qu L. Study on the mechanism of electroacupuncture scalp point penetration therapy in action on apoptosis in the Parkinson's disease rat model. Chin Acupunct Mox. 2009a;29(4):309–13.

46. Wang S, Qi XJ, Han D. Effect of electroacupuncture scalp point-through-point therapy on the expression of tyrosine hydroxylase and dopamine transporter mRNAs in substantia nigra of Parkinson's disease model rats. Chin Acupunct Mox. 2009b;29(5):391–4.

47. Kim YJ, Kim BS, Park HJ. Acupuncture at GB34 modulates laminin expression in 1-methyl-4-phenyl-1,2,3,6-tetrahydropyridine (MPTP) induced PD mouse model. J Acupunct Acupoint. 2008;25(1):155–64.

48. Guan T, Sun H, Zhang L, et al. The effects of electroacupuncture for iron protein and stained cells in the substantia nigra in Parkinson 's disease model mice. Chin J Histochem Cytochem. 2008;17(5):427–31.

49. Wang S, Qi XJ, Han D. Impacts of penetration therapy with head electrical acupuncture on proliferation of neural stem cells in substantia nigra of rat model of Parkinson. World J Acu-Mox. 2008;18:23–30.

50. Jeon S, Kim YJ, Kim ST, et al. Proteomic analysis of the neuroprotective mechanisms of acupuncture treatment in a Parkinson's disease mouse model. Proteomics. 2008;8(22):4822–32.

51. Xie XX, Kou ST, Pu ZH, et al. Effects of scalp catgut embedding on SOD, NO, MDA in the rat with Parkinson's disease. Zhongguo Zhen Jiu. 2007;27(10):753–6.

52. Kang JM, Park HJ, Choi YG, Choe IH, Park JH, Kim YS, Lim S. Acupuncture inhibits microglial activation and inflammatory events in the MPTP-induced mouse model. Brain Res. 2007;1131(1):211–9.

53. Hwang JY, Choi IH, Park JH, et al. Acupuncture inhibits microglial activation in the rat model of Parkinson's disease. Korean J Meridian Acupoint. 2007;24(1):131–44.

54. Luo EL, Zhao FZ, Li GZ, et al. Effects of acupuncture on NOS of the medial part of the globus pallidus in rat model of Parkinson's disease. J Clinic Acupunct Mox. 2007;23(1):54–5.

55. Wang Q, Tang CZ, Chen XH, et al. Effects of acupuncture on dopaminergic neurons in rats with Parkinson Disease. Chin J Basic Med Tradit Chin Med. 2007;13(8):621–2.

56. Jin Z, Liu TT, Zhou BX. Changes of the anti-oxidation capability of rat model of Parkinson disease after acupuncture at subthalamus. Chin J Clinic Rehabil. 2006a;10(23):188–90.

57. Jin Z, Liu TT, Jiang XC, et al. Effects of electroacupuncture at subthalamus on dopamine homovanillic acid and dihydroxy-phenyl acetic acid of rats with Parkinson disease. Chin J Clinic Rehabil. 2006b;10:128–9.

58. Ma J, Wang YC, Gan SY. Effects of electroacupuncture on behaviors and dopaminergic neurons in the rat of Parkinson's disease. Chin Acupunct Mox. 2006;26(9):655–7.

59. Tang Y, Yu S, Chen J. Effect of Electroacupuncture on the Expression of BDNF and BDNF mRNA in Parkinson's Disease Mice. Acupunct Res. 2006;31(1):38–42.

60. Wang YC, Ma J, Wang H. Changes of content of glutamic acid in striatum of rats with Parkinson disease after electroacupuncture stimulation at acupoints. Chin J Clinic Rehabil. 2006;10:183–5.

61. Kim ST, Park HJ, Chae YB, et al. Acupuncture at Liver Meridian Protects the Dopaminergic Neuronal Damage in the 1-methyl-4-phenyl-1,2,3,6-tetrahydropyridine-induced Parkinson's Disease Mouse Model. Korean J Acupunct. 2006;23(4):169–76.

62. Kim YK, Lim HH, Song YK, et al. Effect of acupuncture on 6-hydroxydopamine-induced nigrostratal dopaminergic neuronal cell death in rats. Neurosci Lett. 2005;384(1-2):133–8.

63. Ma J, Zhu SX. Effect of electroacupuncture on anti-oxidase in mesencephalic substantia nigra in rats with Parkinson disease. Chin J Clin Rehabil. 2005;9:120–1.

64. Wang YD, Ma J, Wang H. Experimental study of the protective effect on dopaminergic neurons in substance nigra of the Parkinsonian rats by the acupuncture therapy of 'Shuanggu Yitong'. J Hubei College TCM. 2005;7(3):25–6.

65. Park HJ, Lim S, Joo WS, et al. Acupuncture prevents 6-hydroxydopamine-induced neuronal death in the nigrostriatal dopaminergic system in the rat Parkinson's disease model. Exp Neurol. 2003;180(1):92–7.

66. Liang XB, Liu XY, Li FQ, et al. Long-term high-frequency electro-acupuncture stimulation prevents neuronal degeneration and up-regulates BDNF mRNA in the substantia nigra and ventral tegmental area following medial forebrain bundle axotomy. Brain Res Mol Brain Res. 2002;108:51–9.

67. Lin Y, Lin X. Comparative study of D2 receptors and dopamine content in striatum before and after electro-acupuncture treatment in rats. J Chin Med. 2000;113(5):408–11.

68. He C, Wang L, Dong H, et al. Effects of Acupuncture - Moxibustion on the Contents of Monoamine Transmitters in the Striatum of Rats in Parkinson's Disease. Acupunct res. 1998;1:44–8.
69. Zhu W, Xi G, Ju J. Effect of acupuncture and Chinese medicine treatment on brain dopamine level of MPTP-lesioned C57BL mice. Acupunct Res. 1996;4:46–9.
70. Beery AK, Zucker I. Sex bias in neuroscience and biomedical research. Neurosci Biobehav Rev. 2011;35(3):565–72.
71. Martin RM, Biswas PN, Freemantle SN, Pearce GL, Mann RD. Age and sex distribution of suspected adverse drug reactions to newly marketed drugs in general practice in England: analysis of 48 cohort studies. Br J Clin Pharmacol. 1998;46(5):505–11.
72. Smith KM, Dahodwala N. Sex differences in Parkinson's disease and other movement disorders. Exp Neurol. 2014;259:44–56.

4

The quality of reporting of randomized controlled trials of electroacupuncture for stroke

Jing-jing Wei, Wen-ting Yang, Su-bing Yin, Chen Wang, Yan Wang and Guo-qing Zheng[*]

Abstract

Background: Electroacupuncture (EA), as an extension technique of acupuncture based on traditional acupuncture combined with modern electrotherapy, is commonly used for stroke in clinical treatment and researches. However, there is still a lack of enough evidence to recommend the routine use of EA for stroke. This study is aimed at evaluating the quality of reporting of randomized controlled trials (RCTs) on EA for stroke.

Methods: RCTs on EA for stroke were evaluated by using CONSORT guidelines and STRICTA guidelines. Microsoft Excel 2010 and the R software were used for descriptive statistics analyses.

Results: Seventy studies involving 5468 stroke patients were identified. The CONSORT scores ranged from 16.2 to 67.6% and STRICTA scores from 29.4 to 82.4%. The central items in CONSORT as eligibility criterion, sample size calculation, primary outcome, method of randomization sequence generation, allocation concealment, implementation of randomization, description of blinding, and detailed statistical methods were reported in 100, 6, 68, 37, 14, 10, 16, and 97% of trials, respectively. The reporting of items in STRICTA as acupuncture rationale was 1a (91%), 1b (86%) and 1c 0%; needling details 2a (33%), 2b (97%), 2c (29%), 2d (64%), 2e (100%), 2f (55%) and 2 g (66%); treatment regimen 3a (69%) and 3b (100%); other components of treatment 4a (86%) and 4b (13%); practitioner background item 5 (16%); control intervention(s) 6a (93%) and 6b (10%).

Conclusions: The quality of reporting of RCTs on EA for stroke was generally moderate. The reporting quality needs further improvement.

Keywords: Electroacupuncture, Stroke, Randomized controlled trial, Methodology

Background

Stroke is a major cause of death and disability in both developed and developing countries worldwide. Thrombolysis with intravenous recombinant tissue-type plasminogen activator therapy remains the only proven effective pharmacological treatment for selected acute ischemic stroke patients within a relatively short therapeutic time window of 3 to 4.5 h after the onset of stroke symptoms [1]. Furthermore, the major risk of intravenous thrombolysis treatment also remains the symptomatic intracranial hemorrhage, which is a devastating complication with high mortality. What's more, the enormous morbidities of ischemic stroke result from the interplay between the resulting neurological impairment, the emotional and social consequences of that impairment, and the high risk for recurrence [2]. Owing to the significant health risk of stroke and the limitations of currently available conventional therapies, unprecedented attention has been attached to complementary and alternative medicine (CAM) worldwide due to its potential efficacy on stroke.

Acupuncture is one of the most commonly used CAM therapies for stroke around the world. Up to now, at least 24 systematic reviews have been published, the available evidence suggests that acupuncture is effective for improving some aspects of poststroke neurological impairment and dysfunction, although there was insufficient evidence for stroke in preventing poststroke death [3]. Especially, electroacupuncture (EA) is an extension technique of acupuncture based on traditional acupuncture

* Correspondence: gq_zheng@sohu.com
Department of Neurology, the Second Affiliated Hospital and Yuying Children's Hospital of Wenzhou Medical University, Wenzhou, China

combined with modern electrotherapy [4]. There are many advantages of EA such as the readily quantifiable parameters for stimulation as frequency, intensity and duration, and the therapeutic benefit of EA is commonly identified to be equivalent to manual acupuncture [5]. In some situations, EA has been shown to be more effective than manual acupuncture, particularly when strong, continued stimulation was required, as when treating stroke [6]. Thus, EA is commonly used in current clinic and research. A systematic review from our team has indicated that the available evidence potentially supported the use of EA for acute ischemic stroke [4]. However, there is still a lack of enough evidence to recommend the routine use of EA for stroke.

Both systematic reviews of high-quality randomized controlled trials (RCTs) and RCT itself, especially those with double-blind placebo controls, are commonly regarded the highest level of evidence in judging the treatment efficacy and safety of interventions. The credibility of the evidence in support of a treatment approach depends on the quality of RCTs. However, a large body of evidence indicated that the quality of reporting of RCTs remains sub-optimal [7]. Researchers have accumulated and suggested that the RCTs which were of poor methodological quality tend to exaggerate the treatment effects and result in misleading in health care at all levels [8]. So far, two studies have already been conducted to evaluate the quality of reporting of RCTs on acupuncture for stroke. In 2006, one study [9] demonstrated that the quality of reporting of 74 RCTs on acupuncture for acute stroke was generally poor. In 2014, another study [10] indicated that the quality of reporting of only 15 RCTs on acupuncture for subacute and chronic stroke was improved but some central items were still insufficiently or inadequately reported in most of the studies. However, no study has yet been conducted to assess the quality of reporting RCTs on EA for stroke. Thus, this study aimed at evaluating the quality of reporting of RCTs on EA for stroke according to the consolidated standards of reporting trials (CONSORT) statement [11] and the standards for reporting interventions in clinical trials of acupuncture (STRICTA) statement [12].

Methods
Information sources and search
Eight English and Chinese databases were electronically searched from their inceptions to June 2014. They are Cochrane Controlled Trials Register, PubMed, EMBASE, AMED, China National Knowledge Infrastructure(CNKI), VIP Journals Database, Wanfang Database and Chinese Biomedical Database(CBM). The search terms were listed as follows: "electroacupuncture AND (stroke OR apoplexy OR cerebrovascular accident OR cerebrovascular attack

OR cerebral infarction OR intracerebral hemorrhage OR cerebral vascular disease)". Chinese databases were also searched using the above corresponding search terms in Chinese.

Eligibility criteria
All RCTs on EA as monotherapy or adjunct therapy for stroke compared with at least one control group as no treatment, sham/placebo EA or conventional treatment, regardless of publication status or language, were selected. The diagnostic criteria of stroke were clinically in accordance with the World Health Organization definition [13]. The diagnosis of stroke was confirmed by CT and/or MRI.

Exclusion criteria
Studies concerning EA therapy for paresthesia, post-strokedepression, bulbar paralysis and other non-functional dysfunction were excluded. Additional exclusion criteria were animal experiment, case report, review, single-arm study, retrospective study and historical control study, duplicated publications, and quasi-randomized trial. Crossover and cluster RCTs were excluded because of the employment of the CONSORT guidelines for parallel RCTs. Searches were limited to English and Chinese publications.

Data extraction
Two investigators underwent training in studying every item and multiple subitems listed in CONSORT2010 and STRICTA2010 to ensure the proper understanding of each standard. Each report was reviewed by two independent investigators. They extracted information according to CONSORT2010 and STRICTA2010 checklists. "1"or "0" was scored by the two authors independently to represent whether the RCT had reported the relevant item/subitem or not. "0" indicates no description of the corresponding item/subitem and "1" indicates that the author had mentioned the description of the item/subitem in the report. Investigators resolved discrepancies by consensus or consultations during the data-extraction process.

Data analyses
Microsoft Excel 2010 and R software (Version 3.1.1) were used for descriptive statistics analyses. The overall number of RCTs which corresponded with each item was counted. Subsequently results were represented as the percentage, and 95% confidence interval (CI) of each overall rate was calculated. We also classified the included studies into two groups according to which language they were published in Chinese or English. Proportions of reported items in two groups were compared using independent sample Student's t-test. Statistical calculations

were performed by using SPSS (version 17.0). Level of significance was set at $P < 0.05$.

Results

Study selection

A total of 2662 potentially relevant articles were identified. By reviewing titles and abstracts, 2168 papers were excluded for at least one of following reasons: (1) duplicate publication, (2) animal study, (3) not clinical trial, and (4) case report. After examining the remaining 494 literatures through reading the full text, we removed 424 papers. Of which, 61 were non-randomized controlled trials, 11 were not focusing on functional rehabilitation or with other indicators, 41 were about other diseases or using an ambiguous diagnostic criteria, 17 duplicate publications, and 294 studies with other reasons. Eventually, 70 eligible RCT studies [14–83] were selected for the final analysis (Fig. 1).

Study characteristics

Seventy studies (one article was designed with 2 comparisons) involving 5468 stroke patients were identified. For the 5468 patients, there were 2420 male and 1739 female, and with the ages ranging from 24 to 89 years old. However, the gender and age of the remaining 1309

participants could not be obtained from the primary data. Sample sizes ranged from 6 to 160 participants. In 40 studies EA was used for cerebral infarction, while in the other 30 studies EA was used for both cerebral infarction and intracerebral hemorrhage (ICH). Seventeen studies were published in English, and the other 53 studies were published in Chinese. Six studies were online Master's thesis and not formally published [17, 40, 64, 65, 81, 82]. For the control group, WCTs were used in 62 studies and sham EA plus WCTs in 8 studies. The duration of treatment varied from 10 days to 12 weeks. Six studies conducted follow-up assessment with duration from 6 weeks to 12 months. Four studies conducted sample size calculation [20, 23, 34, 63]. Twenty-one studies reported adverse effects. In 11 studies, the discripion of the professional acupuncturists who participated in the studies was very simple and without detailed background. Nine studies reported informed consent from patients [20, 23, 24, 27, 33, 34, 64, 65, 71]. Only 6 study [27, 50, 62, 64, 65, 74] reported ethical approval. Key data are summarized in Table 1.

Items reported according to CONSORT statement

The items reported from the 70 RCTs according to CONSORT statement are summarized in Table 2.

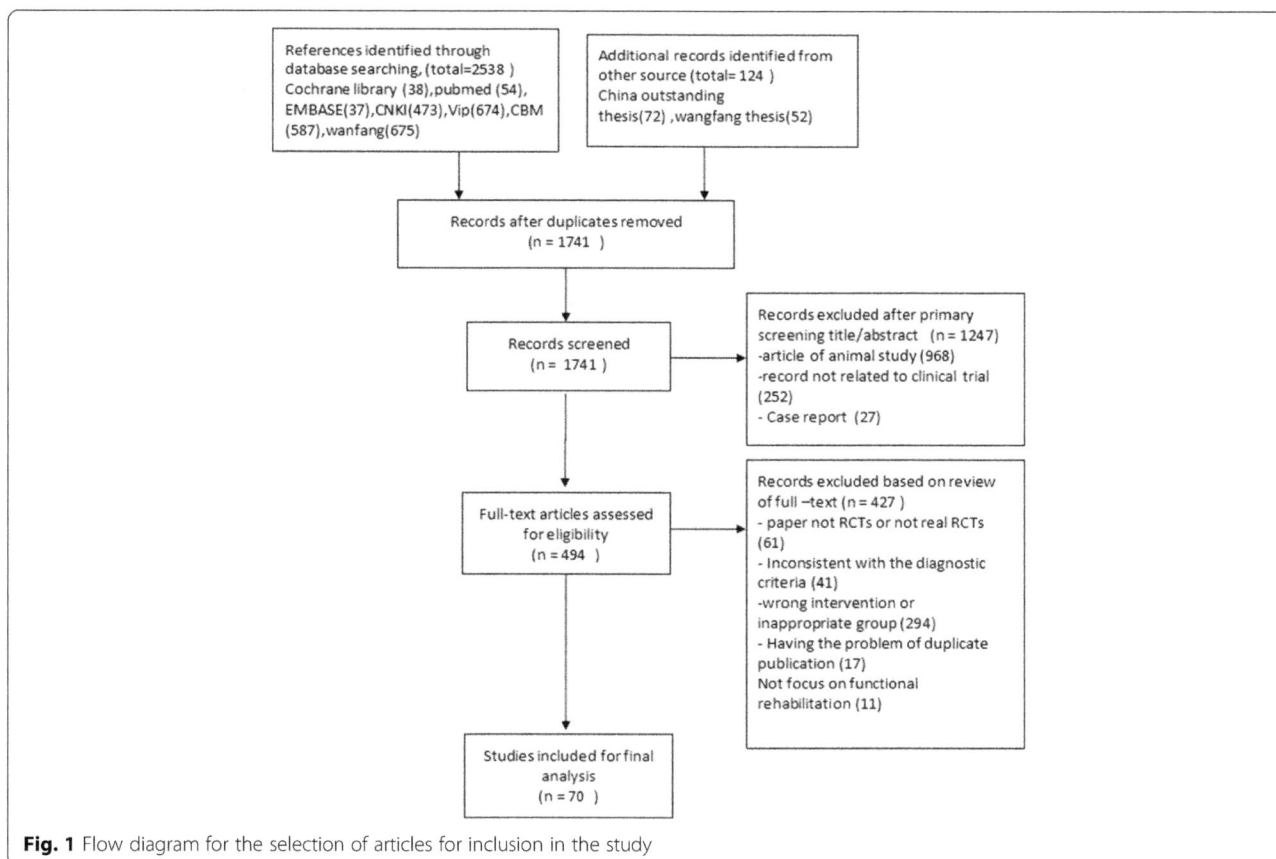

Fig. 1 Flow diagram for the selection of articles for inclusion in the study

Table 1 The characteristics of the included 70 studies

Included Trials	Publicati-on language	Type of stroke	Study designs	Sample size calculation	No. of Participants (male/female); age(y) Trial	No. of Participants (male/female); age(y) Control	Course of disease	Interventions(n)Drug/dosage Trial	Interventions(n)Drug/dosage Control	Course of treatment
Cao 2012 [14]	Chinese	infarction	RCT	No	40(22/18); 57.5 ± 9.8	40(24/16); 57.2 ± 9.5	<3d	electro-scalp-body-Ac	WCTs* (general supportive care, antiplatelet agents, neuroprotective agents, treatment of acute complications)	4w
Chen 2001 [15]	English	infarction	RCT	No	21(14/7); Mean 64.8	16(10/6); Mean 66.1	<3d	electro-scalp-body-Ac + WCTs#	WCTs*(specialized care)	4w
Chen 2010 [16]	Chinese	infarction	RCT	No	40 (27/13); Mean 54.4	38(28/10); Mean 55.4	≤7d	electro-body-Ac + WCTs#	WCTs* (general supportive care, antiplatelet agents, anticoagulants, neuroprotective agents)	4w
Chen C L (Unpublished Master's thesis, 2008) [17]	Chinese	infarction ICH	RCT	No	32(20/12); 50–75	32(18/14); 50–75	<6 m	electro-body-Ac + WCTs#	Ac + WCTs* (general supportive care, specialized care, stroke rehabilitation)	4w
Dong 2011 [18]	Chinese	infarction ICH	RCT	No	75(45/30); Mean 67	75(48/27); Mean 65	<2w	electro-body-Ac + WCTs#	WCTs* (, stroke rehabilitation)	10d
Er 2010 [19]	Chinese	infarction ICH	RCT	No	30(16/14); Mean 54.2	30(18/12); Mean 56.1	1 m–3 m	electro-body-Ac + WCTs#	WCTs* (stroke rehabilitation)	6w
Fu 2010 [20]	Chinese	infarction	RCT	No	80(41/39); Mean 62.8	80(43/37); Mean 63.3	<1 m	electro-body-Ac + WCTs#	WCTs* (general supportive care, antiplatelet agents aspirin 0.1 g po qd, treatment of acute complications, stroke rehabilitation)	4w
Gao 2012 [21]	Chinese	infarction	RCT	No	82(45/37); Mean 62.4	78(42/36); Mean 62.7	3–74d	electro-scalp-body-Ac + WCTs#	WCTs* (antiplatelet agents aspirin 0.1 g po qd.)	4w
Gong 2008 [22]	Chinese	infarction; ICH	RCT	No	32 (15/17); Mean 52	31(16/15); Mean 51.4	Mean 36–38d	electro-body-Ac + WCTs#	WCTs*(stroke rehabilitation)	6w
Gosman-Hedstrom 1998 [23]	English	infarction	RCT	No	37(20/17); Mean 76.1	33(9/24); Mean 76.9	<7d	electro-scalp-body-Ac + WCTs#	WCTs*(stroke rehabilitation)	4w
Gosman-Hedstrom 1998 [23]	English	infarction	RCT	No	37(20/17); Mean 76.1	34(17/17); Mean 79	<7d	electro-scalp-body-Ac + WCTs#	Sham Ac + WCTs* (stroke rehabilitation)	10w
Guo 2009 [24]	Chinese	infarction	RCT	No	30(17/13); Mean 56.3	30(21/9); Mean 55.6	<7d	electro-body-Ac + WCTs#	WCTs* (antiplatelet agents aspirin 0.3 g po qd, a week later recuced to 0.1 g po qd, stroke rehabilitation)	14d
Hopwood 2008 [25]	English	Infarction; ICH	RCT	No	57(19/38); Mean 70.5	48(26/22); Mean 74.4	4–10d	electro-scalp-body-Ac	Sham Ac	4w
Hsing 2012 [26]	English	infarction	RCT	No	35; Mean 50	27; Mean 52	>18 m	electro-scalp-Ac	Sham Ac	5w
Hsieh 2007 [27]	English	infarction	RCT	No	30(12/18); Mean 68.8	33(20/13); Mean 70.7	<2w	electro-body-Ac + WCTs#	WCTs* (stroke rehabilitation)	4w
Hu 1993 [28]	English	infarction	RCT	No	15(15/0); 63.6 ± 6.7	15(13/2); 62.8 ± 8.0	<36 h	electro-scalp-body-Ac + WCTs#	WCTs* (general supportive care, stroke rehabilitation)	4w
Huang 2008 [29]	Chinese	infarction	RCT	No	40(21/19); Mean 63.6	40(20/20); Mean 59.9	14–90d	electro-body-Ac + WCTs#	WCTs* + ENS	4w

Table 1 The characteristics of the included 70 studies (Continued)

Study	Language	Type	Design	Blinding	Group 1	Group 2	Time	Intervention	Control	Duration
Huang 2011 [30]	Chinese	infarction ICH	RCT	No	35(22/13); Mean 63.2	35(19/16); Mean 65.3	Mean 7.3–8.1d	electro-scalp-body-Ac	Ac	6w
Huang 2012 [31]	Chinese	infarction	RCT	No	32(12/20) 66.59 ± 10.482;	26(16/10) 68.92 ± 10.53	<6d	electro-body-Ac + WCTs#	WCTs* (general supportive care)	4w
Jahansson 1993 [32]	English	infarction	RCT	No	38; Mean 76	40; Mean 75	<10d	electro-body-Ac + WCTs#	WCTs* (stroke rehabilitation)	10w
Jahansson 2001 [33]	English	infarction	RCT	Yes	48(29/19); Mean 76	51(25/26); Mean 76	<10d	electro-scalp-body-Ac + WCTs#	sham Ac + WCTs* (antiplatelet agents, anticoagulants, stroke rehabilitation)	10w
Jin 1999 [34]	Chinese	infarction	RCT	No	60; Mean 68	60; Mean 68	<1 m	electro-scalp-body-Ac + WCTs#	WCTs* (specialized care)	6w
Jiu 2008 [35]	Chinese	infarction ICH	RCT	No	40(23/17); Mean 62.7	40(22/18); Mean 63	<2w	Electro-body-Ac + WCTs#	WCTs* (stroke rehabilitation)	2 m
Lei 2013 [36]	Chinese	infarction ICH	RCT	No	40(19/21); 48-61	40(25/15); 43–64	4–31 m	electro-body-Ac + WCTs#	WCTs* (general supportive care, stroke rehabilitation)	4w
Li 2006 [37]	Chinese	infarction	RCT	No	52(34/18); 66.8 ± 4.7	50(35/15); 67.1 ± 3.9	<1 m	electro-scalp-body-Ac + WCTs#	WCTs* (general supportive care)	3w
Li 2011 [38]	Chinese	infarction	RCT	No	30(14/16) Mean 54.4	30(13/17) Mean 55.4	<1 m	electro-body-Ac + WCTs#	WCTs* (treatment of acute complications, stroke rehabilitation)	4w
Li X Z (unpublished Master's thesis, 2005) [39]	Chinese	infarction	RCT	No	35(18/17); Mean 61.5	35(20/15); Mean 59.7	<3d	electro-scalp-Ac + WCTs#	WCTs* (general supportive care, anticoagulant,slow molecular heparin, treatment of acute complications)	10d
Liu 2007 [40]	Chinese	infarction ICH	RCT	No	38(25/13); Mean 59.4	37(14/23); Mean 56.4	<2w	Electro-body-Ac + WCTs#	WCTs* (specialized care, stroke rehabilitation)	3w
Liu 2010 [41]	Chinese	infarction ICH	RCT	No	50(32/18); Mean 61	50(35/15); Mean 63	2d–6 m	electro-scalp-Ac + WCTs#	WCTs* (stroke rehabilitation)	1 m
Long 2004 [42]	Chinese	infarction ICH	RCT	No	43(30/13); Mean 60	41(27/14); Mean 62	<7d	electro-scalp-body-Ac + WCTs#	WCTs*	7w
Luo 2012 [43]	Chinese	infarction ICH	RCT	No	10(5/5); Mean 60.5	9(5/4); Mean 62.3	2w–1 m	electro-body-Ac + WCTs#	WCTs* (stroke rehabilitation)	6w
Lv 2003 [44]	Chinese	infarction	RCT	No	29; 52–79	26; 52–79	<5d	electro-scalp-body-Ac + WCTs#	WCTs* (general supportive care, volume expansion and vasodilators, neuroprotective agents, treatment of acute complications)	1 m
Naeser 1992 [45]	English	infarction	RCT	No	10	6	1–3 m	electro-scalp-body-Ac	Sham Ac	4w
Pei2001 [46]	English	infarction	RCT	No	43(28/15); Mean 71.6	43(24/19); Mean 69.3	<7d	electro-scalp-body-Ac + WCTs#	WCTs*	4w
Peng 2007 [47]	Chinese	infarction	RCT	No	40; Mean 54	40; Mean 54	≤7d	electro-body-Ac + WCTs#	WCTs* (general supportive care, stroke rehabilitation)	12w
Peng 2009 [48]	Chinese	infarction ICH	RCT	No	30; 18–70	30; 18–70	Mean 2–3 m	electro-scalp-body-Ac	Ac	45d

Table 1 The characteristics of the included 70 studies (*Continued*)

Study	Language	Cerebral vascular disease	Design	Randomized	Treatment group (n(M/F); age)	Control group (n(M/F); age)	Time since onset	Intervention	Control	Duration
Qi 2012 [49]	Chinese	Cerebral vascular disease	RCT	No	39(20/19); 60.12 ± 6.34	39(19/20); 60.23 ± 6.45	<12 m	electro-du-meridian-Ac	manual-body-Ac	20d
Sallstrom 1996 [50]	English	infarction ICH	RCT	No	26; Median 57	23; Median 58	15–71d	electro-scalp-body-Ac + WCTs#	WCTs* (stroke rehabilitation)	6w
Sang 2011 [51]	Chinese	infarction	RCT	No	40; 38–75	40; 38–75	<7d	electro-body-Ac + WCTs#	WCTs* (neuroprotective agents cerebrolysin vial 30 ml ivgtt qd, treatment of acute complications)	14d
Schaechter 2007 [52]	English	infarction	RCT	No	4(3/1); 28–80	4	1–10.2y	electro-scalp-body-Ac	Sham Ac	10w
Schuler 2005 [53]	English	infarction	RCT	No	41; Mean 77.5	40; Mean 78.7	3–35d	scalp-body-Ac	Sham Ac	4w
Si 1998 [54]	English	infarction	RCT	No	20(15/5); 68 ± 10	22(18/4); 67 ± 8	<7d	electro-scalp-body-Ac + WCTs#	WCTs* (specialized care)	7d
Su 2002 [55]	Chinese	infarction ICH	RCT	No	43(27/16); 58 ± 4	40(23/17); 57 ± 5	<12 m	electro-body-Ac + WCTs#	WCTs* (general supportive care, stroke rehabilitation)	20–30d
Sun 2005 [56]	Chinese	infarction	RCT	No	40(27/13)	43(29/14)	<12 h	electro-scalp-Ac + WCTs#	WCTs* (specialized care)	12d
Sun 2012 [57]	Chinese	infarction	RCT	No	35(23/12); Mean 57.5	35(17/18); Mean 56	<3d	electro-scalp-body-Ac + WCTs#	WCTs* (specialized care)	14d
Wang 1998 [58]	Chinese	infarction	RCT	No	80; Mean 68	80; Mean 68	Mean 24d	electro-scalp-body-Ac + WCTs#	WCTs*	20d
Wang 2001 [59]	Chinese	infarction ICH	RCT	No	106; 35–80	54; 35–80;	<1y	Electro-body-Ac	Ac	6w
Wang 2003 [60]	Chinese	infarction ICH	RCT	No	32; 46–77	32; 46–77	<14d	electro-body-Ac + WCTs#	WCTs*	20d
Wang 2008 [61]	Chinese	ICH	RCT	No	45(30/15); Mean 62	45(29/16); Mean 63	<7d	electro-scalp-body-Ac + WCTs#	WCTs* (general supportive care, specialized care)	4w
Wang 2009 [62]	Chinese	infarction	Quasi-RCT	No	65(33/32); Mean 72.2	50(26/24); Mean 70.1	≤3d	electro-body-Ac + WCTs#	ENS + WCTs* (antiplatelet agents aspirin 0.1 g po qd, stroke rehabilitation)	4w
Wang Q (unpublished Master's thesis, 2009) [63]	Chinese	infarction	RCT	Yes	24(15/9); Mean 62.4	22(14/8); Mean 57.1	<2w	electro-body-Ac + WCTs#	WCTs* (general supportive care)	4w
Wang X W (unpublished Master's thesis, 2011) [64]	Chinese	infarction	RCT	No	31(17/14); Mean 57.4	30(19/11); Mean 60.3	<3d	electro-body-Ac + WCTs#	WCTs* (general supportive care, antiplatelet agents aspirin 0.1 g po qd, treatment of acute complications)	14d
Wayne 2005 [65]	English	infarction ICH	RCT	No	16(12/4); 38–89	17(12/5); 42–69	>6 m	electro-scalp-body-Ac	Sham Ac	10w
Wei 2008 [66]	Chinese	infarction ICH	RCT	No	46(29/17); Mean 59.4	44(23/21); Mean 56.4	2–7d	electro-body-Ac + WCTs#	WCTs* (general supportive care, specialized care, stroke rehabilitation)	5w
Wong 1999 [67]	English	infarction ICH	RCT	No	59(38/21); Mean 60.4	59(42/17); Mean 60.6	<14d	electro-body-Ac + WCTs#	WCTs*	2w
Wu 2008 [68]	Chinese	infarction ICH	RCT	No	30; 46–75	30; 46–75	>1 m	electro-body-Ac + WCTs#	WCTs* (stroke rehabilitation)	30d

Table 1 The characteristics of the included 70 studies (*Continued*)

Study	Language	Type	Design	Blinding	Treatment group n(M/F); Mean age	Control group n(M/F); Mean age	Onset time	Intervention	Control	Duration
Wu 2009 [69]	Chinese	infarction	RCT	No	29(16/13); Mean 56.7	29(17/12); Mean 58.5	<14d	electro-body-Ac + WCTs#	WCTs* (general supportive care, specialized care, antiplatelet agents aspirin 0.1 g po qd)	14d
Wu 2011 [70]	Chinese	infarction ICH	RCT	No	30(18/12)	30(19/11)	>3w	electro-body-Ac + WCTs#	WCTs* (general supportive care, specialized care, stroke rehabilitation)	6w
WuXL 2008 [71]	Chinese	infarction	RCT	No	32(20/12); Mean 67.2	29(19/10); Mean 66.6	<7d	electro-scalp-body-Ac + WCTs#	WCTs* + Ac	3 m
Xue 2007 [72]	Chinese	infarction; ICH	RCT	No	18(14/4); Mean 66.1	18(15/3); Mean 64.2	<2w	electro-body-Ac + WCTs#	WCTs* (stroke rehabilitation)	4w
Yu 2005 [73]	Chinese	infarction	RCT	No	16(10/6); 40–76	14(8/6); 40–75	<3d	electro-scalp-body-Ac + WCTs#	WCTs* (vasodilators, neuroprotective agents)	2w
Yue 2012 [74]	Chinese	infarction ICH	RCT	No	33(21/12); Mean 70.4	31(18/13); Mean 69.8	80–163d	electro-body-Ac	Ac	1 m
Zhang 1995 [75]	Chinese	infarction	RCT	No	40(23/17); Mean 65.8	40(22/18); Mean 68.7	<7d	electro-scalp-Ac + WCTs#	WCTs* (specialized care)	20d
Zhang 2006 [76]	Chinese	infarction ICH	RCT	No	32(17/15); Mean 62.7	25(15/10); Mean 64.5	<6 m	electro-body-Ac + WCTs#	WCTs* + Ac	30d
Zhang 2008 [77]	Chinese	infarction ICH	RCT	No	49(26/23); Mean 51.5	49(24/25); Mean 54.7	<2w	Electro-body-Ac + WCTs#	WCTs* (general supportive care, specialized care, stroke rehabilitation)	2 m
Zhang 2009 [78]	Chinese	infarction ICH	RCT	No	30(12/18); Mean 55.7	30(15/15); Mean 58.4	<3y	Electro-body-Ac + WCTs#	WCTs*(stroke rehabilitation)	1 m
Zhang 2013 [79]	Chinese	infarction	Quasi-RCT	No	45(27/18); Mean 65.5	45(30/15); Mean 63.2	<3d	electro-scalp-body-Ac + WCTs#	WCTs* (general supportive care, specialized care, neuroprotective agents)	4w
Zhang SS (unpublished Master's thesis, 2009) [80]	Chinese	infarction	RCT	No	29(17/12); Mean 62.9	29(16/13); Mean 63.6	<10d	electro-body-Ac + WCTs#	WCTs* (general supportive care, treatment of acute complications, stroke rehabilitation)	3w
Zhang X, (unpublished Master's thesis, 2008) [81]	Chinese	infarction	RCT	No	60(33/27); 40–80	30(17/13); 40–80	<2w	electro-body-Ac + WCTs#	WCTs* (general supportive care, antiplatelet agents aspirin 0.1 g po qd, treatment of acute complications, stroke rehabilitation)	2w
Zhao 2005 [82]	Chinese	infarction ICH	RCT	No	60(36/24); Mean 63.0	60(31/29); Mean 67.4	<2w	electro-scalp-body-Ac + WCTs#	WCTs* (general supportive care, specialized care, (treatment of acute complications, stroke rehabilitation)	1 m
Zhu 2012 [83]	Chinese	infarction ICH	RCT	No	40; 32–69	40; 32–69	<2w	Electro-body-Ac + WCTs#	WCTs* (general supportive care, specialized care)	1 m

Ac acupuncture, *d* day, *ICH* Intracerebral Hemorrhage, *m* month, *RCT* randomizedcontrolledtrial, *SA* scalp acupuncture, *w* week, *WCTs* western conventional treatments, *y* year. #: the same as the control group; *WCT** refer to the combination of needed therapies of the following aspects: (1) General supportive care mainly include: A. airway, ventilatory support and supplemental oxygen, B. cardiac monitoring and treatment, C. temperature, D. blood pressure, E. blood sugar and F. nutrition; (2) Specialized care mainly include a variety of measures to improve cerebral blood circulation (such as antiplatelet agents, anticoagulants, fibrinogen-depleting agents, volume expansion and vasodilators, except thrombolytic agents) and neuroprotective agents; (3) Treatment of acute complications mainly include: A. brain edema and elevated intracranial pressure, B. seizures, C. dysphagia, D. pneumonia, E voiding dysfunction and urinary tract infections and F. deep vein thrombosis,(4) Stroke rehabilitation

Table 2 The reporting number and percentage for each item of the CONSORT checklist of the included 70 studies

Section/Topic	Item No	Checklist item	n	% (n /70)	95%CI
Title and abstract	1a	Identification as a randomized trial in the title	12	17	[9 to 28]
	1b	Structured summary of trial design, methods, results, and conclusions (for specific guidance see CONSORT for abstracts)	54	77	[66 to 86]
Introduction					
Background and objectives	2a	Scientific background and explanation of rationale	63	90	[80 to 96]
	2b	Specific objectives or hypotheses	65	93	[84 to 98]
Methods					
Trial design	3a	Description of trial design (such as parallel, factorial) including allocation ratio	58	83	[72 to 91]
	3b	Important changes to methods after trial commencement (such as eligibility criteria), with reasons	0	0	[0 to 5]
Participants	4a	Eligibility criteria for participants	70	100	[95 to 100]
	4b	Settings and locations where the data were collected	58	83	[72 to 91]
Interventions	5	The interventions for each group with sufficient details to allow replication, including how and when they were actually administered	70	100	[95 to 100]
Outcomes	6a	Completely defined pre-specified primary and secondary outcome measures, including how and when they were assessed	68	97	[90 to 100]
	6b	Any changes to trial outcomes after the trial commenced, with reasons	1	1	[0 to 8]
Sample size	7a	How sample size was determined	4	6	[2 to 14]
	7b	When applicable, explanation of any interim analyses and stopping guidelines	7	10	[4 to 20]
Randomisation					
Sequence generation	8a	Method used to generate the random allocation sequence	26	37	[26 to 50]
	8b	Type of randomization; details of any restriction (such as blocking and block size)	20	29	[18 to 41]
Allocation concealment mechanism	9	Mechanism used to implement the random allocation sequence (such as sequentially numbered containers), describing any steps taken to conceal the sequence until interventions were assigned	10	14	[7 to 25]
Implementation	10	Who generated the random allocation sequence, who enrolled participants, and who assigned participants to interventions	7	10	[4 to 20]
Blinding	11a	If done, who was blinded after assignment to interventions (for example, participants, care providers, those assessing outcomes) and how	11	16	[8 to 27]
	11b	If relevant, description of the similarity of interventions	6	9	[3 to 18]
Statistical methods	12a	Statistical methods used to compare groups for primary and secondary outcomes	68	97	[90 to 100]
	12b	Methods for additional analyses, such as subgroup analyses and adjusted analyses	0	0	[0 to 5]
Results					
Participant flow (a diagram is strongly recommended)	13a	For each group, the numbers of participants who were randomly assigned, received intended treatment, and were analysed for the primary outcome	5	7	[2 to 16]
	13b	For each group, losses and exclusions after randomization, together with reasons	15	21	[13 to 33]
Recruitment	14a	Dates defining the periods of recruitment and follow-up	44	63	[50 to 74]
	14b	Why the trial ended or was stopped	2	3	[0 to 10]
Baseline data	15	A table showing baseline demographic and clinical characteristics for each group	23	33	[22 to 45]
Baseline data	16	For each group, number of participants (denominator) included in each analysis and whether the analysis was by original assigned groups	57	81	[70 to 90]

Table 2 The reporting number and percentage for each item of the CONSORT checklist of the included 70 studies *(Continued)*

Outcomes and estimation	17a	For each primary and secondary outcome, results for each group, and the estimated effect size and its precision (such as 95% confidence interval)	2	3	[0 to 10]
	17b	For binary outcomes, presentation of both absolute and relative effect sizes is recommended	0	0	[0 to 5]
Ancillary analyses	18	Results of any other analyses performed, including subgroup analyses and adjusted analyses, distinguishing pre-specified from exploratory	1	1	[0 to 8]
Harms	19	All important harms or unintended effects in each group (for specific guidance see CONSORT for harms)	21	30	[20 to 42]
Discussion					
Limitations	20	Trial limitations, addressing sources of potential bias, imprecision, and, if relevant, multiplicity of analyses	10	14	[7 to 25]
	21	Generalisability (external validity, applicability) of the trial findings	13	19	[10 to 30]
Interpretation	22	Interpretation consistent with results, balancing benefits and harms, and considering other relevant evidence	22	31	[21 to 44]
Other information					
Registration	23	Registration number and name of trial registry	0	0	[0 to 5]
Protocol	24	Where the full trial protocol can be accessed, if available	1	1	[0 to 8]
Funding	25	Sources of funding and other support (such as supply of drugs), role of funders	14	20	[11 to 31]
Total mean score[a]				13.0 ± 4.0	

[a]Mean ± SD

Title and abstract

Twelve (18%) trials can be identified as random trials after reviewing the title (1a), among which 8 were in English. Fifty-four (77%) articles had abstracts that were comprised of objective, methods, results and conclusions (1b).

Introduction

Of the included studies, 90% provided the detailed description of backgrounds (2a). The proportion of studies with objectives (2b) was 93%.

Methods

Only 2 CONSORT items were described in all the included articles. One was the eligibility criterion for participants (4a) and the other was the interventions for each group with sufficient details to allow replication, including how and when they were actually administered (5). However, the proportion on the description of the patient's allocation ratio was 58% (3a). None of the articles (0%) described the important changes after the beginning of the trial because of the recruitment (3b). Fifty-eight reports (83%) described the settings and locations where the data were collected (4b). The proportion on the description of definition of primary/secondary outcomes was 68% (6a). Four (6%) reports mentioned the method of how to determine the sample size (7a). Items on incomplete reporting were 1% (subitem 6b) and 10% (subitem 7b).

Randomization

Twenty studies (29%) mentioned the type of randomization as the simple random method (8b). However, the proportion of the description on sequence generation was 37% (8a), which used computer or random number table. Ten articles (14%) described the hidden mechanism by the use of opaque envelopes aiming to implement the allocation concealment (9). The detailed implementation was given in 7 articles (10%) (10). A total of 11 articles (16%) provided the description of blinding (11a), among which one was double blind (participants and evaluators) and the others were single-blind assessment. Sixty-eight studies (97%) provided the description of detailed statistical methods (12a), but no one provided methods for additional analyses (12b).

Result and discussion

Nine studies (13%) described the treatment progress of participants by a diagram (13a). Fifteen (21%) of these articles mentioned the number of the losses and exclusions after randomization with explanations (13b). Forty-four studies (63%) mentioned the periods of recruitment, but only 6 studies described the follow-up duration (14a). Two articles had reported a temporal interruption of the therapy because of the drop out of participants with personal reasons. Thirty-four reports (49%) offered the description of baseline data that included underlying disease or basic demographic or clinical characteristics, among which 23 studies (33%) represented the data in the form of a table (15). Fifty-seven studies (81%) described the statistics methods, including the use of intention-to-treat analysis (16). Almost all outcomes of the included reports were presented as the ratio of efficiency or means ± SD. Two papers (3%) applied 95% CI to describe the estimated value of the effect and its precision (17a). No study reported binary outcomes (17b). One study provided a kind of secondary analyses as "error type I" in statistics (18). In discussion section, 21 papers (30%) reported the occurrence of adverse events, such as acupuncture syncope, infection of puncture site and death (19). The proportions of papers reporting limitation (20), generalisability (21) and interpretation (22) were 14, 19, and 31%, respectively.

Other information: None of the papers reported the registration (23). Only 1 report (1%) gave the relevant electronic links for the obtainment of protocol (24). The proportion of paper with reporting of funding (25) was 420%.

Items reported according to STRICTA statement

The items reported from the 70 RCTs according to STRICTA statement are summarized in Table 3.

Acupuncture rationale

Apart from several English articles, majority of the other included articles (91%) used the style of acupuncture from Traditional Chinese Medicine (1a). Eighty-six percent of the reports provided reasons for treatment based on historical context, literature sources, citing references where appropriate, and so on (1b). None of the studies had mentioned any alteration of the treatment after the beginning of the experiments (1c).

Needling details

Various intervention methods were used in EA treatment group, and were mainly as follows: EA plus conventional theory, EA plus acupoint injection, scalp EA plus acupoint injection, and EA plus internal carotid injection. All the 70 included reports provided the type of needle stimulation, including electrical acupuncture or electrical acupuncture combined with manual acupuncture (2e). Ninety seven percent of articles listed the names (or location if no standard name) of acupoints used at the uni/bilateral sides (2b); however, only 33% articles mentioned the number of needles, 33% (2a). Twenty nine percent of studies mentioned the depth of needle insertion (2c). The other STRICTA items on needling details were response elicited (*de qi* or muscle twitch response), 64% (2d), needle retention time, 55% (2f) and needle type, 66% (2 g).

Treatment regimen

All the reports mentioned the frequency and duration of treatment sessions (3b), whereas 69% articles provided the number of treatment sessions (3a).

Cointerventions

One item, details of other interventions, was mentioned in more than half of the reports, 86% (4a). Nine reports (13%) described some relevant information and explanations to patients, including informed consent (4b).

Practitioner background

Eleven articles (16%) provided vague and unspecific description on the background of acupuncturist which included expertise, duration of training and length of clinical experience (5). In the 11 articles, four mentioned that the acupuncturists were professionals, and the others mentioned the contents as expertise or duration of specific training.

Control intervention(s)

A total of 93% trials reported a precise description of the control or comparator (6b). Furthermore, 8 studies used sham EA as control with providing further details of items 1 to 3 in STRICTA. Ten percent of studies provided the quoted data to elucidate the rationality of contrasting and comparing other similar experiments (6a).

Comparison of reporting quality between Chinese and English studies

The total mean score in CONSORT items failed to achieve significant differences between English studies and Chinese studies (English vs. Chinese: 15.2 ± 4.3 vs. 12.3 ± 3.6, $p = 0.05$), Table 4. However, there is statistically significant improvement in three items published in English vs. in Chinese as follows: (1a) title (56% vs.6%, $p = 0.01$), (11a) blinding (44% vs. 7%, $p = 0.014$), (13b) losses and exclusions (56% vs. 11%, $p = 0.004$). As for the other items, they all showed no statistical significant differences, Table 4.

There are no differences in proportions of items in STRICTA comparing studies in Chinese with that in English (Chinese vs. English: 10.3 ± 1.8 vs. 9.6 ± 2.1, $p = 0.235$), Table 3. Studies in Chinese have statistically siginifical improvement in the item (1b) reasoning for treatment provided (93% vs. 63%, $p = 0.033$) and (2d) response sought (72% vs. 44%, $p = 0.035$) compared with studies in English, whereas studies in English in the item (5) practitioner background (6% vs. 50%, 0.004) showed significant improvement compared with studies in Chinese, Table 3.

Discussion

A wealth of evidence indicated the very inadequate reporting of clinical researches. For example, information on the method of random sequence generation, primary outcome, sample size calculation, randomization stated in title, allocation concealment, and adequate blinding was reported in 34, 53, 45, 33, 25, and 18% of

Table 3 The reporting number and percentage for each item of the STRICTA checklist of the included 70 studies

Item	Detail	Total N = 70			Chinese N = 54			English N = 16			Chinese vs. English (P-value for difference)
		n	%(n /70)	95% CI	n	%(n /54)	95% CI	n	%(n /16)	95% CI	
1. Acupuncture rationale (Explanations and examples)	1a) Style of acupuncture (e.g. Traditional Chinese Medicine, Japanese, Korean, Western medical, Five Element, ear acupuncture, etc.)	64	91	[82 to 97]	50	93	[82 to 98]	14	88	[62 to 98]	0.530
	1b) Reasoning for treatment provided, based on historical context, literature sources, and/or consensus methods, with references where appropriate	60	86	[75 to 93]	50	93	[82 to 98]	10	63	[35 to 85]	0.033
	1c) Extent to which treatment was varied	0	0	[0 to 5]	0	0	[0 to 7]	0	0	[0 to 21]	–
2. Details of needling (Explanations and examples)	2a) Number of needle insertions per subject per session (mean and range where relevant)	25	36	[25 to 48]	18	33	[21 to 47]	7	44	[20 to 70]	0.452
	2b) Names (or location if no standard name) of points used (uni/bilateral)	68	97	[9 to 10]	52	96	[87 to 100]	16	100	[79 to 100]	0.442
	2c) Depth of insertion, based on a specified unit of measurement, or on a particular tissue level	20	29	[18 to 41]	18	33	[21 to 47]	2	12	[2 to 38]	0.060
	2d) Response sought (e.g. de qi or muscle twitch response)	46	66	[53 to 77]	39	72	[58 to 84]	7	44	[20 to 70]	0.035
	2e) Needle stimulation (e.g. manual, electrical)	70	100	[95 to 100]	54	100	[93 to 100]	16	100	[79 to 100]	–
	2f) Needle retention time	40	57	[45 to 69]	32	59	[45 to 72]	8	50	[25 to 75]	0.518
	2g) Needle type (diameter, length, and manufacturer or material)	46	66	[53 to 77]	38	70	[56 to 82]	8	50	[25 to 75]	0.222
3. Treatment regimen (Explanations and examples)	3a) Number of treatment sessions	48	69	[56 to 79]	38	70	[56 to 82]	10	63	[35 to 85]	0.558
	3b) Frequency and duration of treatment sessions	70	100	[95 to 100]	54	100	[93 to 100]	16	100	[79 to 100]	–
4. Other components of treatment (Explanations and examples)	4a) Details of other interventions administered to the acupuncture group (e.g. moxibustion, cupping, herbs, exercises, lifestyle advice)	60	86	[75 to 93]	49	91	[80 to 97]	11	69	[41 to 89]	0.098
	4b) Setting and context of treatment, including instructions to practitioners, and information and explanations to patients	9	13	[6 to 23]	4	7	[2 to 18]	5	31	[11 to 59]	0.073
5. Practitioner background (Explanations and examples)	5) Description of participating acupuncturists (qualification or professional affiliation, years in acupuncture practice, other relevant experience)	11	16	[8 to 26]	3	6	[1 to 15]	8	50	[25 to 75]	0.004
6. Control or comparator interventions (Explanations and examples)	6a) Rationale for the control or comparator in the context of the research question, with sources that justify this choice	7	10	[4 to 20]	4	7	[2 to 18]	3	19	[4 to 46]	0.302
	6b) Precise description of the control or comparator. If sham acupuncture or any other type of acupuncture-like control is used, provide details as for Items 1 to 3 above.	65	93	[84 to 98]	52	96	[87 to 100]	13	81	[54 to 96]	0.166
Total mean score[a]		10.1 ± 1.9			10.3 ± 1.8			9.6 ± 2.1			0.235

[a]Mean ± SD

Table 4 Comparison of reporting quality between Chinese and English studies (CONSORT)

CONSORT item	Chinese N = 54			English N = 16			Chinese vs. English (P-value for difference)
	n	%(n/54)	95%CI	n	%(n/16)	95%CI	
Title	3	6c	[1 to 15]	9	56	[30 to 80]	0.01
Methods							
Trail design	48	89	[77 to 96]	10	63	[35 to 85]	0.061
Eligibility criteria	54	100	[93 to 100]	16	100	[79 to 100]	–
Interventions	54	100	[93 to 100]	16	100	[79 to 100]	–
Primary and secondary outcome	52	96	[87 to 100]	16	100	[79 to 100]	0.442
Sample size	3	6	[1 to 15]	1	6	[0 to 30]	0.918
Generation of random sequence	22	41	[28 to 55]	4	25	[7 to 52]	0.239
Allocation concealment	6	11	[4 to 23]	4	25	[7 to 52]	0.26
Blinding	4	7	[2 to 18]	7	44	[20 to 70]	0.014
Statistical methods	53	98	[90 to 100]	15	94	[70 to 100]	0.361
Results							
Losses and exclusions	6	11	[4 to 23]	9	56	[30 to 80]	0.004
Recruitment	38	70	[56 to 82]	6	38	[15 to 65]	0.017
Numbers analysed	47	87	[75 to 95]	10	63	[35 to 85]	0.081
Harms	14	26	[15 to 40]	7	44	[20 to 70]	0.177
Limitations	4	7	[2 to 18]	6	38	[15 to 65]	0.33
Total mean score[a]		15.2 ± 4.3			12.3 ± 3.6		0.05

[a]Mean ± SD

616 reports indexed in PubMed in 2006, respectively [84]. Especially, in RCTs of traditional Chinese medicine that include herbal medicine, acupuncture and other no medication therapies, reporting of the key methods used for adequate randomization methods, adequate allocation concealment, adequate blinding, both adequate randomization methods and allocation concealment used, and all three used was only 12, 7, 19, 4, and 3% of 2580 reports, respectively [8]. Thus, several guidelines have been recommended to help incomplete and inaccurate reporting. The CONSORT statement [11] is an evidence-based, minimum set of recommendations for reporting randomized trials to alleviate the problems arising from inadequate reporting of RCTs. It offers a standard way for authors to prepare reports of trial findings, facilitating their complete and transparent reporting, and aiding their critical appraisal and interpretation. The 2010 version of STRICTA statement [12], an official extension to the CONSORT statement, is the standards for reporting interventions in clinical trials of acupuncture to facilitate transparency in published reports, enabling a better understanding and interpretation of results, aiding their critical appraisal, and providing detail that is necessary for replication.

In the present study, the quality of reporting of 70 RCTs on EA for stroke was generally moderate. The CONSORT scores achieved by the included studies ranged from 4.7 to 91.5% according to seven subdomains, and the STRICTA scores across six subdomains ranged from 16 to 84.5%. The central items in CONSORT of eligibility criterion, sample size calculation, primary outcome, method of randomization sequence generation, allocation concealment, implementation of randomization, description of blinding, and detailed statistical methods are reported in 100, 3, 68, 37, 14, 10, 16, and 97% of 70 reports, respectively. The reporting of detail items in STRICTA of acupuncture rationale is 1a (91%), 1b (86%) and 1c 0%; of needling details is 2a (33%), 2b (97%), 2c (29%), 2d (64%), 2e (100%), 2f (55%) and 2 g (66%); of treatment regimen is 3a (69%) and 3b (100%); of other components of treatment is 4a (86%) and 4b (13%); of practitioner background is item 5 (16%); of control intervention(s) is 6a (93%) and 6b (10%). Based on the results of present study, several key items need further improvement. First, a priori sample size calculation can reduce the risk of an underpowered (false-negative) result. However, in the present study sample size calculation was reported in only 3% of all the included trials. In fact, a survey of 215 studies published in 2005 and 2006 in six general medical journals with high impact factors revealed that only 34% of 73 studies adequately described sample size calculations [85]. If the trials were not conducted with pre-trial estimation of sample size, there will be a lack of statistical power to ensure appropriate estimation of the treatment effect [86]. Thus, we suggest that an effort should be made to increase transparency in sample size calculation. Second, successful randomisation reduces selection bias at trial entry, which depends on two hinge steps-adequate sequence generation and allocation concealment, and is the crucial component of high quality RCTs [87]. In the present study method of randomization sequence generation, allocation concealment, and implementation of randomization is reported in only 37, 14, and 10% of 70 RCTs, respectively. Inadequate or unclear allocation concealment can exaggerate clinical effects in 41 and 30%, respectively [88]. Thus, proper randomization should involve both random sequence generation and complete implementation of allocation concealment to minimize bias. Third, blinding is an essential method for preventing research outcomes from being influenced by either the placebo effect or the observer bias. Trials that were not double blinded yielded larger estimates of treatment effect than trials in which authors reported double blinding (odds ratios exaggerated, on average by 17%) [88]. In the present study, only 16% of 70 trials described blinding procedure. Thus, more attentions should be paid to this situation, especially in EA trials. Fourth, item 5 in STRICTA is practitioner background that required description of participating acupuncturists in qualification or professional affiliation, years in acupuncture practice, other relevant experience. However, practitioner background was reported only in 16% trials. Thus, practitioner qualifications should be completely reported, which could increase the certainty with regard to treatment quality and safe implementation of interventions.

Currently, the evidence from the study of manual and electrical needle stimulation in acupuncture researched by an executive board of the society for acupuncture research [5] demonstrated that fundamental gaps existed in the understanding of the mechanisms and relative effectiveness between manual and electrical acupuncture, and these two techniques are not interchangeable. In 2006, Zhang et al. [9] evaluated the reporting quality of 74 RCTs on acupuncture for acute ischemic stroke, indicating that the items in CONSORT of baseline demographic and clinical characteristics, method of random sequence generation, allocation concealment, blinding procedure, sample size calculation and intention-to-treat (ITT) analysis was 73, 35, 8, 11, 5, and 7% of 74 RCTs respectively; the items in STRICTA of the numbers of needles inserted, the needle type, the depths of insertion, the length of clinical experience, and the background of

the acupuncture practitioners was 5, 47, 35, 1, and 8% of 74 reports, respectively. Compared with zhang's study [9], the quality of reporting RCTs of EA for stroke in present study is better. In 2014, Zhuang et al. [10] analyzed the quality of reporting of only 15 RCTs on acupuncture for subacute and chronic stroke, indicating that poor reporting existed in terms of outcomes, sample size, outcomes and estimation, ancillary analyses, with positive rate less than 30% according to CONSORT statement. Meanwhile, based on STRICTA statement, item 4a: Details of other interventions and 4b: Setting and context of treatment, the positive rate was 20 and 33% respectively. The quality of reporting of RCTs on EA for stroke in present study is similar to the results of Zhuang's study [10]. This result indicates some improvements in the quality of reporting of RCTs on both acupuncture and EA for stroke. One probable reason is that reporting of several important aspects of trial methods improved because the endorsement of the CONSORT Statement and STRICTA statement. Another possible reason is that Zhuang [10] studied only a small number of selected RCTs, thus the conclusions may not be scientifically sound and may be misleading. For present EA study, the third possible reason is that EA is more readily controlled, standardized and objectively measurable. Additionally, EA is mainly considered as a method to provide stronger treatment for nervous and mental diseases like stroke. Thus, the use of EA for stroke research can at least in part improve the standards of published RCTs and is favored in stroke trials.

From the comparison of the included studies published in Chinese and in English, we found the compliance with CONSORT statement is unsatisfactory. Thus, reporting of RCTs both in English and in Chinese should endorse the CONSORT items as complete as possible. In particular, studies published in Chinese need to improve the reporting of (1a) title, (11a) blinding, and (13b) losses and exclusions. For the STRICTA statement, the proportions of fulfilling the items (1b) reasoning for treatment and (2d) response sought in Chinese have statistically significant increase compared with those in English. The main reasons are as follows: (1) acupuncture has been practiced in China for over 2000 years [89] and Chinese journals lay emphasis on reasoning for treatment; (2) as one of the fundamental characteristics of acupuncture, *deqi* has been used as a prerequisite for clinical effects for a long time in China [90]. However, the proportion of reporting item (5) practitioner background achieved statistically significant improvement in English compared that in Chinese. The possible reason is that English journals pay more attention to endorsing the STRICTA statement [91]. Thus, both English and Chinese journals need to endorse reporting acupuncture RCTs based on the STRICTA checklist, especially item (5) practitioner background in Chinese and items (1b) reasoning for treatment and (2d) response sought in English, thereby actualizing an improvement in reporting quality of RCTs for acupuncture.

There are some limitations in this study. First, the searching languages are limited to only Chinese and English during sample selection. The reports which are published in other languages may be left out, and may harm the reliability of our results. Second, we only discussed the reporting quality of RCTs on EA in the present study, and compared with that of RCTs on acupuncture in the previous studies. The results may be potentially misleading, and the direct comparison between the reporting qualities of RCTs on manual acupuncture for stroke with that of RCTs on EA is needed in the future. Third, we carried out data extraction based on the published paper itself. This approach meant that we were unable to capture some primary trials with truly good quality in trial methodology but poor reporting in the final publication. Thus, when assessing trial quality of such studies, reviewing research protocols and contacting trialists for more information are needed.

Conclusions

Our study indicated that the overall quality of reporting of RCTs on EA for stroke according to CONSORT and STRICTA statement was moderate and the reporting quality needs further improvement. In particular, it must be emphasized that the poor quality reporting of crucial items which includes sample size calculation, sequence generation, allocation concealment, randomization implementation, blinding, and practitioner background should be adequately involved in RCTs on EA for stroke. More attention should be given to the reporting of RCTs on EA for stroke to ensure that all items in checklist of CONSORT and STRICTA are clearly delineated, especially the central items in the methodology. In addition, the use of EA for stroke research can possibly improve the standards of published RCTs when compared with manual acupuncture trials. However, this need further direct comparative studies.

Acknowledgements

The funders had no role in study design, data collection and analysis, decision to publish, or preparation of the manuscript.

Funding

This project was supported by the grant of National Natural Science Foundation of China (81573750/81473491/81173395/H2902); the Young and Middle-Aged University Discipline Leaders of Zhejiang Province, China (2013277); Zhejiang Provincial Program for the Cultivation of High-level Health talents (2015).

Authors' contributions

Conceived and designed the experiments: GQZ and YW. Performed the experiments: JJW, SBY, CW and LS. Analyzed the data: JJW, SBY, CW and LS. Wrote the paper: GQZ, YW, JJW, SBY, CW and LS. All authors have read and approved the final version of the manuscript.

Competing interests

The authors declare that they have no competing interests.

References

1. Jauch EC, Saver JL, Adams Jr HP, Bruno A, Connors JJ, Demaerschalk BM, et al. Guidelines for the early management of patients with acute ischemic stroke: a guideline for healthcare professionals from the American Heart Association/American Stroke Association. Stroke. 2013;44(3):870–947.
2. Kernan WN, Ovbiagele B, Black HR, Bravata DM, Chimowitz MI, Ezekowitz MD, et al. Guidelines for the prevention of stroke in patients with stroke and transient ischemic attack: a guideline for healthcare professionals from the American Heart Association/American Stroke Association. Stroke. 2014;45(7):2160–23.
3. Zhang JH, Wang D, Liu M. Overview of systematic reviews and meta-analyses of acupuncture for stroke. Neuroepidemiology. 2014;42(1):50–8.
4. Liu AJ, Li JH, Li HQ, Fu DL, Lu L, Bian ZX, Zheng GQ. Electroacupuncture for acute ischemic stroke: A meta-analysis of randomized controlled trials. Am J Chin Med. 2015;46(8):1–26.
5. Langevin HM, Schnyer R, MacPherson H, Davis R, Harris RE, Napadow V, et al. Manual and electrical needle stimulation in acupuncture research: pitfalls and challenges of heterogeneity. J Altern Complem Med (New York, NY). 2015;21(3):113–28.
6. Mayor D. Electroacupuncture: An introduction and its use for peripheral facial paralysis. J Chin Med. 2007;84:1–17.
7. Turner L, Shamseer L, Altman DG, Weeks L, Peters J, Kober T, et al. Consolidated standards of reporting trials (CONSORT) and the completeness of reporting of randomised controlled trials (RCTs) published in medical journals. Cochrane DB Syst Rev. 2012;11:Mr000030.
8. He J, Du L, Liu G, Fu J, He X, Yu J, et al. Quality assessment of reporting of randomization, allocation concealment, and blinding in traditional Chinese medicine RCTs: a review of 3159 RCTs identified from 260 systematic reviews. Trials. 2011;12:122.
9. Zhang XL, Li J, Zhang MM, Yuan WM. Assessing the reporting quality of randomized controlled trials on acupuncture for acute ischemic stroke using the CONSORT statement and STRICTA. Chin J Evid Med. 2006;15(8):586–90.
10. Zhuang L, He J, Zhuang X, Lu L. Quality of reporting on randomized controlled trials of acupuncture for stroke rehabilitation. BMC Complem Altern M. 2014;14:151.
11. Moher D, Hopewell S, Schulz KF, Montori V, Gotzsche PC, Devereaux PJ, et al. CONSORT 2010 explanation and elaboration: updated guidelines for reporting parallel group randomised trials. BMJ. 2010;340:c869.
12. MacPherson H, Altman DG, Hammerschlag R, Youping L, Taixiang W, White A, et al. Revised Standards for Reporting Interventions in Clinical Trials of Acupuncture (STRICTA): Extending the CONSORT statement. J EvidMed. 2010;3(3):140–55.
13. Hatano S. Experience from a multicentre stroke register: a preliminary report. B World Health Organ. 1976;54(5):541–53.
14. Cao GJ. Clinical Efficacy and Inflammatory Cytokines Change of Combined Treatment of Stroke with Scalp Electroacupuncture and Xingnaokaiqiao Acupuncture. J Extern Ther Tradit Chin Med. 2012;21(6):32–3.
15. Chen JF, Li CP, Ding P, Ma YL. Effect of acupuncture on plasmic levels of insulin, glucagon and hypercoagulability in NIDDM complicated by acute cerebral infarction. J Tradit Chin Med. 2001;21(4):267–9.

16. Chen BW, Guo X. Clinical Observation of Early Electroacupuncture Therapy for Hemiplegia Patients with Acute Cerebral Infarction. Chin J integr med. 2010;8(2):179–81.

17. Chen CL. Clinical research on the treatment of spastic paralysis after cerebral infarction with antagonistic electric acupuncture[D]. Heilongjiang: Heilongjiang University Of Chinese Medicine; 2008.

18. Dong Y. Combined therapy and precaution for stroke hemiplegia. Chin Rural Health Serv Adm. 2011;31(10):1091–2.

19. Er ZJ, Zhao K, Su HJ, Zhang HX, Li ZY. Clinical Study of Combined Treatment of Hypermyotonia in Acute Stroke Patients with Acupuncture and Tolperisone. Sichuan J Tradit Chin Med. 2010;2(28):120–2.

20. Fu WB, Guo YQ, Chen XK, Jiang GH, He Q, Zhu XP, et al. Comprehensive therapeutic protocol of Electroacupuncture combined with Chinese herbs and rehabilitition training for treament of cerebral infarction: a multi-center randomzied controlled trail. Chin Acupunct Moxib. 2010;30(1):6–9.

21. Gao YH. Clinical observation of electroacupuncture treatment for 82 cases with cerebral infarction sequela. Chin Med Pharm. 2012;2(18):90–3.

22. Gong WJ, Zhang T, Cui LH, Yang YQ, Sun XT. Effects of electroacupuncture at zusanli (ST36) on lower limbs motor function in patients with stroke during spasm Period: a clinical research. Chin J Rehabil Theory and Pract. 2008;14(11):1057–8.

23. Gosman-Hedstrom G, Claesson L, Klingenstierna U, Carlsson J, Olausson B, Frizell M, et al. Effects of acupuncture treatment on daily life activities and quality of life: a controlled, prospective, and randomized study of acute stroke patients. Stroke. 1998;29(10):2100–8.

24. Guo JB, Yang LT, Zhu HF, Cui B, Lu HZ. Clinical observations of combining acupuncture with medicine on treatment of lower limp dysfunction in hemiplegic patients. Shanxi J Tradit Chin Med. 2009;25(4):36–7.

25. Hopwood V, Lewith G, Prescott P, Campbell MJ. Evaluating the efficacy of acupuncture in defined aspects of stroke recovery: a randomised, placebo controlled single blind study. J Neurol. 2008;255(6):858–66.

26. Hsieh RL, Wang LY, Lee WC. Additional therapeutic effects of electroacupuncture in conjunction with conventional rehabilitation for patients with first-ever ischaemic stroke. J Rehabil Med. 2007;39(3):205–11.

27. Hsing WT, Imamura M, Weaver K, Fregni F, Azevedo Neto RS. Clinical effects of scalp electrical acupuncture in stroke: a sham-controlled randomized clinical trial. J Altern Complem Med (New York, NY). 2012;18(4):341–6.

28. Hu HH, Chung C, Liu TJ, Chen RC, Chen CH, Chou P, et al. A randomized controlled trial on the treatment for acute partial ischemic stroke with acupuncture. Neuroepidemiology. 1993;12:106–13.

29. Huang F, Liu Y, Yao GX, Zhou FX, Wang XY, Yang D. Clinical observations on treatment of ischemic stroke with acupuncture at back-shu points. Shanghai J Acupunct Moxib. 2008;27(10):4–7.

30. Huang J, Peng ZL, Ding P. Effect of electroacupuncture and Xingnao Kaiqiao needling method on patients poststroke hemiplegia. Lishizhen Med Mater Med Res. 2011;22(6):1506–7.

31. Huang T, Li CX. Effect of electroacupuncture at pionts of yangming meridians on CD62p expression, D-Dimer expression, ADL and NIHSS in patients with acute cerebral infarction. Lishizhen med Mater Med Res. 2012;23(10):2665–7.

32. Johansson K, Lindgren I, Widner H, Wiklund I, Johansson BB. Can sensory stimulation improve the functional outcome in stroke patients? Neurology. 1993;43(11):2189–292.

33. Johansson BB, Haker E, von Arbin M, Britton M, Langstrom G, Terent A, et al. Acupuncture and transcutaneous nerve stimulation in stroke rehabilitation: a randomized, controlled trial. Stroke. 2001;32(3):707–13.

34. Jin ZQ, Gu FL, Chen RX, Cheng JS. Clinical investigation of acupuncture effect on acute cerebral infarction. Acupunct Res. 1999;24:5–7.

35. Jiu YQ, Yang WX. Clinical Observation of Combined Treatment of Hemiplegic Stroke Patients with Electroacupuncture and Rehabilitative treatment. Jiangsu J Tradit Chin Med. 2008;40(12):79–80.

36. Lei SF. Clinical study of neurodevelopmental therapy combined with electroacupuncture treatment of cerebrovascular disease recovery period. Chin foreign med res. 2013;25(11):1674–6805.

37. Li YT, Li B, Li Y, Dong YX. The Analysis of Curative Effect of Combined Treatment of Electroacupuncture and Medicine in Geratic Hemiplegic Stroke Patients. Chin J Gerontol. 2006;26:128–9.

38. Li WL. Clinical study on the effect of combination of electroacupuncture and rehabilitation therapy on treating hemiplegia after ischemic stroke. Jiangsu J Tradit Chin Med. 2011;43(9):68–9.

39. Li XZ. Clinical and experimental research of electroacupuncture at Baihui (GV20) and fengchi (GB20) in treating acute cerebral ischemia[D]. Shangdong: Shangdong University of Traditional Chinese Medicine; 2005.

40. Liu Y, Zou SJ. Effect of Electroacupuncture on Motor Function of Acute Stroke Patients Received Early Rehabilitation. Chin J Rehabil Theory Pract. 2007;13(10):969–70.

41. Liu WA, Wu QM, Li XR, Li DD, Lei F, Yi XC, et al. Observations on the Efficacy of Combined Treatment of Stroke Hemiplegia with Scalp Electroacupuncture and Stroke Unit. Shanghai J Acupunct Moxib. 2010; 29(3):149–51.

42. Long WQ. The observation of curative effect of early acupuncture on 84 hemiplegic patients with stroke. Chin J Integr Tradit Chin West Med Intensive Crit Care. 2004;11(4):252.

43. Luo X, Li SJ, Cui XP, Liu LA, Song C, Zhou WN. Effects of combining electroacupuncture with constraint-induced movement therapy on upper limbs functions of hemiparalysis. Guangming J Tradit Chin Med. 2012;27(6): 1183–6.

44. Lv LJ, Shen LY, Fan GQ, Zhu LP, Wu X. Clinical study on the treatment of acupuncture on cerebral infarction with upper extremity motor disfunction. Zhejiang J Integr Tradit Chin West Med. 2003;13(1):14–6.

45. Naeser MA, Alexander MP, Stiassny-Eder D, Galler V, Hobbs J, Bachman D. Real versus sham acupuncture in the treatment of paralysis in acute stroke patients: a CT scan lesion site study. Neurorehab Neural Re. 1992;6(4):163–74.

46. Pei J, Sun LJ, Chen RX, Zhu TM, Qian YZ, Yuan DJ. The effect of electro-acupuncture on motor function recovery in patients with acute cerebral infarction:a randomly controlled trial. J Tradi Chin Med. 2001;21(4):270–2.

47. Peng L, Lv J, Yan WQ, Yang DR, Zhou LZ, Ao JB, et al. Acupuncture in combination with rehabilitation treatment of acute apoplexy. J Emerg in Tradit Chin Med. 2007;16(10):1173–5.

48. Peng ZL, Lei H, Ding P, Li M, Li MX. Observations on the Efficacy of Combined Treatment of with Xingnaokaiqiao Acupuncture and Electroacupuncture in Limbs Dysfunction after stroke. J Pract Tradit Chin Med. 2009;25(10):684-684.

49. Qi J, Liu HJ, Feng SF. Clinical observation on acupuncture of Du meridian therapy for ischemic cerebral vascular disease. Guide Chin Med. 2012;10(10): 1671–8194.

50. Sällström S, Kjendahl A, Østen PE, Kvalvik, Stanghelle J, Borchgrevink CF. Acupuncture in the treatment of stroke patients in the subacute stage: a randomized, controlled study. Complement Ther Med. 1996;4(3):193–7.

51. Sang P, Wang S, Zhao JH. Clinical observation of scalp penetration acupuncture on 40 Patients with acute infarction. Chin J Tradit Med Sci Technol. 2011;18(4):330–1.

52. Schaechter JD, Connell BD, Stason WB, Kaptchuk TJ, Krebs DE, Macklin EA, et al. Correlated change in upper limb function and motor cortex activation after verum and sham acupuncture in patients with chronic stroke. J Altern Com plem Med (New York, NY). 2007;13(5):527–32.

53. Schuler MS, Durdak C, Höl NM, Klink A, Hauer KA, Oster P, Du X. Acupuncture treatment of geriatric patients with ischemic stroke: a randomized, double-controlled, single-blind study. J Am Geriatr Soc. 2005;53(3):549–50.

54. Si QM, Wu GC, Cao XD. Effects of electroacupuncture on acute cerebral infarction. Acupunct Electrother Res. 1998;23(2):117–24.

55. Su YJ. The observation of effect of electroacupuncture stimulation on the recovery of limb function of cerebral infarction. Chin J Clin Rehabil. 2002; 6(19):2936–2936.

56. Sun SJ, Zhang XH, Xu BJ. Clinical curative effect observation and effect of scalp acupuncture on S100B in patients with acute cerebral infarction. J Clin Acupunct Moxib. 2005;21(1):20–1.

57. Sun HJ. Clinical Observation of Combined Treatment of Electroacupuncture and Fasudil in Acute Ischemic Cerebrovascular Disease. Chin Med Innov. 2012;9(36):137–8.

58. Wang DJ, Zhang DJ, Tong LM, Hu YJ, Li JM. Clinical observation of the curative effect of electroacupuncture carotid drug injection on cerebrol infarction. Shanghai J Acupunct Moxib. 1998;17(5):5–6.

59. Wang XY, Xu DM, Niu J. Curative Observation of Combined Treatment of Electroacupuncture and body acupuncture in 106 cases of Hemiplegic Stroke Patients. Hebei J Tradit Chin Med. 2001;23(2):124–5.

60. Wang DS, Wang XW, Xie RM. A prospective clinical case-controlled study of electroacupuncture treatment in patients with acute stroke. Clin Med J China. 2003;10(5):639–41.

61. Wang ZH. Effect of early electroacupuncture on motor function rehabilitation in patients with acute cerebral hemorrhage. Chin J Rehabil Med. 2008;23(6):554–5.

62. Wang JL, Tan F, Ding DQ, Huang T, Wu HK, Zhang MX. Effect of electro-acupuncture combined with early rehabilitation on motor function and expressions of CD11b/CD18 and tumor necrosis factor-αin patients with acute cerebral infarction. Chin J Neuromed. 2009;8(6):569–73.

63. Wang Q. Clinical study on complex facilitation technique of electro-acupuncturing antagonistic muscle acupoint in treating extremital spasm caused by cerebral infarction hemiplegia[D]. Chengdu: Chengdu University of Traditional Chinese Medicine; 2009.

64. Wang XW. Effects of electroacupuncture on motor function in patients with acute cerebral infarction patients by Triple Stimulation Technique[D]. Guangzhou: Guangzhou University of Chinese Medicine; 2013.

65. Wayne PM, Krebs DE, Macklin EA, Schnyer R, Kaptchuk TJ, Parker SW, et al. Acupuncture for upper-extremity rehabilitation in chronic stroke: a randomized sham-controlled study. Arch Phys Med Rehabil. 2005;86(12):2248–55.

66. Wei ZJ. The application of electroacupuncture on eraly rehabilitation in stroke patients. Chin J Phys Med Rehabil. 2008;30(8):513–4.

67. Wong AM, Su TY, Tang FT, Cheng PT, Liaw MY. Clinical trial of electrical acupuncture on hemiplegic stroke patients. Assoc Acad Physiatrists. 1999;78(2):117–22.

68. Wu BF, Gao WB, Yang XY, Li XY. Acupuncture in combination with rehabilitation in treatment of 30 cases of poststroke spastic hemiplegia. J Clin Acupunct Med. 2008;24(5):24–5.

69. Wu HK, Tan F, Huang T, Zhang X, Wan SY, Ding DQ, et al. Effect of early electroacupuncture with acupoints of yangming meridians on functional recovery of the lower extremity and the expression of PAC-1 and CD62p in ACI patients. Inter Natl Med Hygiene Guidance News. 2009;15(16):90–90.

70. Wu H, Gu XD, Yao YH, Fu JM, Wang WG, Li Y. Effects of electroacupuncture combined with neuro-facilitation technique on lower limb motro function and walking ability in hemiplegic stroke patients. Chin Arch Tradit Chin Med. 2011;29(10):2372–4.

71. Wu XL, Lu BJ, Hu GR, Li YH. Effect of different acupuncture manipulation on neurological function rehabilitation in hemiplegic patients with acute cerebral infarction. Hebei J Tradit Chin Med. 2008;30(5):511–2.

72. Xue Q, Xiong GX, Huo GM, Li SP. Effect of electroacupuncture at pionts of yangming meridians on motor function in hemiplegic patients. Chin J Rehabil Theory Pract. 2007;13(11):1056–7.

73. Yu L, Huang XL, Wang W, Yu ZY. Effect of electroacupuncture on content of serum NSE and neurological dysfunction in patients with acute cerebral infarction. Chin J Phys Med Rehabil. 2005;27(2):103–5.

74. Yue ZH, Li L, Chang XR, Jiang JM, Chen LL, Zhu XS. Comparative study on effects between electroacupuncture and acupuncture for spastic paralysis after stroke. Chin Acupunct Moxib. 2012;32(7):582–6.

75. Zhang XJ. Clinical observation of the curative effect of Scalp Acupuncture on cerebral infarction. Chin J Rehabil Med. 1995;10(2):85–6.

76. Zhang SJ, Gao WB. Clinical study on electroacupuncture for poststroke spastic hemiplegia. J Clin Acupunct Med. 2006;22(11):36–7.

77. Zhang H, Li L. Effect of Early Electro-acupuncture on Locomotion of Hemiplegia Patients after Stroke. Chin J Rehabil Theory Pract. 2008;14(9):824–5.

78. Zhang MX, Tan F. Clinical Observation of Combined Treatment of Electroacupuncture and neurodevelopment therapy in Convalescence in Acute Ischemic Cerebrovascular Disease. Chin Community Doctors. 2009;11(225):153.

79. Zhang C, Liu J, Lin QH, Zeng TJ, Gu MG. Clinical Observation of EA in the Treatment of Acute Cerebral Infarction. Mod Diagn Treat. 2013;24(13):2913–4.

80. Zhang SS. The influences of two different intervening periods of acupuncture therapy on the limbs motor function in patients[D]. Guangzhou: Guangzhou University of Chinese Medicine; 2009.

81. Zhang X. Effects of electric acupuncture with acupoints of yangming meridians on the expression of PAC-1 and CD62p in acute cerebral infarct patients[D]. Guangzhou: Guangzhou University of Chinese Medicine; 2008.

82. Zhao DG, Mu JP. Clinical study on scalp acupuncture combined with sports therapy for rehabilitation of poststroke hemiplegia. Chin Acupunct Moxib. 2005;25(1):19–20.

83. Zhu BH. The study of curative effect on rehabilitation of hemiplegic stroke patients. ASIA-Pacific Tradit Med. 2012;8(10):68–9.

84. Hopewell S, Dutton S, Yu LM, Chan AW, Altman DG. The quality of reports of randomised trials in 2000 and 2006: comparative study of articles indexed in PubMed. BMJ. 2010;340:c723.

85. Charles P, Giraudeau B, Dechartres A, Baron G, Ravaud P. Reporting of sample size calculation in randomised controlled trials: review. BMJ. 2009;338:b1732.

86. Schulz KF, Grimes DA. Sample size calculations in randomised trials: mandatory and mystical. Lancet. 2005;365(9467):1348–53.

87. Altman DG. Randomisation. BMJ. 1991;302(6791):1481–2.

88. Schulz KF, Chalmers I, Hayes RJ, Altman DG. Empirical evidence of bias. Dimensions of methodological quality associated with estimates of treatment effects in controlled trials. JAMA. 1995;273(5):408–12.

89. Consensus Conference NIH. Acupuncture. JAMA. 1998;280(17):1518–24.

90. Yang XY, Shi GX, Li QQ, Zhang ZH, Xu Q, Liu CZ. Characterization of deqi sensation and acupuncture effect. Evid Based Complement Alternat Med. 2013;2013:319734.

91. MacPherson H, White A, Cummings M, Jobst K, Rose K, Niemtzow R. Standards for reporting interventions in controlled trials of acupuncture: the STRICTA recommendations. Complement Ther Med. 2001;9(4):246–9.

5

Coarse needle surface potentiates analgesic effect elicited by acupuncture with twirling manipulation in rats with nociceptive pain

Sunoh Kwon[1,3,4], Yangseok Lee[1,2], Hi-Joon Park[1,2] and Dae-Hyun Hahm[1,2*]

Abstract

Background: Biomechanical phenomenon called "needle grasp" through the winding of connective tissue has been proposed as an action mechanism of acupuncture manipulation. The aim of the present study is to verify whether the needle grasp force affects the pain-relieving activity of acupuncture in the tail-flick latency (TFL) and the rat paw formalin tests.

Methods: In order to make different roughness on the acupuncture needle surface, the needles with 0.2 mm-diameter were scratched using silicon carbide sandpapers with the grit numbers of 600 (mild coarse) and 200 (extra coarse). The surface roughness and rotation-induced torque of the scratched needles were then measured by atomic force microscope and Acusensor®, respectively. Rat abdominal wall tissues including insertion site of acupuncture needle were excised after 5 unidirectional rotations of the needles having various degrees of roughness, and the morphological changes of connective tissues were analyzed using hematoxylin and eosin (H-E) staining. Finally, the effects of coarse needle surface on anti-nociception induced by twirling manipulation were tested in rat TFL and formalin test.

Results: It was observed that the rougher the needle surface, the stronger the needle grasp force and thickness of subcutaneous connective tissue while rotating. TFL increased in proportion to surface roughness of the ground needles 10 min after acupuncture into the Zusanli acupoint (ST36) on rat's legs. In the rat formalin test, the rougher needle also significantly exerted the larger analgesic effect during both early and late phases compared to non-ground normal needle.

Conclusion: Surface roughness of the acupuncture needle enhanced an anti-nociceptive activity of acupuncture therapy in rats, which partially supports the mechanical signaling theory through connective tissues in acupuncture manipulation.

Keywords: Acupuncture, Manipulation, Needle surface roughness, Connective tissue, Analgesia

Background

Acupuncture has become increasingly popular in the Western world as a therapy for a wide range of pain difficult to manage with conventional treatments [1], however the mechanisms related to the therapeutic effect of acupuncture remains largely unknown [2].

To achieve therapeutic effect, acupuncture needles are manually manipulated after their insertion into the body. Acupuncture manipulation typically consists of rapid rotation (back-and-forth or uni-direction) and/or pistoning (up-and-down motion) of the needle [3]. A characteristic symptoms and reactive phenomenon linked to acupuncture manipulation is known as *de qi*, widely considered essential to acupuncture's therapeutic effect [4–6]. *De qi* emphasizes a sensory component experienced by the patient as an aching sensation in the area of the inserted needle as well as a teasing sensation through the inserted needle that the acupuncturist feels as if the

---

* Correspondence: dhhahm@khu.ac.kr
[1]Acupuncture and Meridian Science Research Center, College of Korean Medicine, Kyung Hee University, 26, Kyungheedae-ro, Dongdaemun-gu, Seoul 02447, Republic of Korea
[2]Department of Basic Science of Korean Medicine, Graduate School, Kyung Hee University, 26, Kyungheedae-ro, Dongdaemun-gu, Seoul 02447, Republic of Korea
Full list of author information is available at the end of the article

tissue is contracting around the needle, such that there is increased resistance to further motion of the needle [1, 4, 5, 7].

The theory quoted for needle manipulation is that it is due to a contraction of skeletal muscle [6, 8, 9], however this theory has not been supported by quantitative data regarding muscle contraction. As an alternative, Langevin et al. have previously hypothesized that a different and novel mechanism for needle grasp might involve the contraction of connective tissue, and proposed that the winding connective tissue during needle rotation creates a tight mechanical coupling between needle and tissue, which might allow needle manipulation to deliver a powerful mechanical signal into the tissue [10]. This hypothesis was supported by histological observations in rat tissue explants that showed marked thickening of subcutaneous tissue and a whorl of dense connective tissue around the rotated needle [10]. Whereas the importance of grasp force by winding connective tissues was elucidated by showing the morphological changes of tissues or neighboring cells around the pricking point of acupuncture manipulation in an ex vivo system, there have been no reports precisely explaining how the friction-induced grasp force between the needle surface and the contacting tissues correlates with alleviating the symptoms of diseases.

Manual manipulation of the needle (e.g., rotation, or pistoning) is used to clinically enhance needle grasp [4], and the needle grasp can be quantified by measuring the amount of force necessary to pull the acupuncture needle out of the skin (pullout force) [11]. We have previously reported that both twirling and lifting–thrusting manipulation potentiated acupuncture at acupoint ST36-induced analgesic effect in formalin-induced rats and that twirling had the more potentiation rather than lifting–thrusting [12]. Taken together, we hypothesized that twirling-induced frictional force between needle surface and adjacent tissues might be increased as the surface roughness of the acupuncture needle becomes coarser and that this frictional force affects acupuncture-elicited analgesic effect in rats with nociception. Thus, we used silicon carbide sandpapers with different grit numbers to manipulate the needle grasp force by changing surface roughness. We confirmed the different surface roughness and rotation-induced torques of the scratched acupuncture needles using atomic force microscope and Acusensor®, respectively. Under the various conditions of grasp force, it was also investigated whether the rotation manipulation of acupuncture with coarser surface at acupoint ST36 has more analgesic effects on tail-flick latency (TFL) test and formalin-induced pain behavior.

Methods

Animals

Male Sprague–Dawley rats, weighing 200–250 g, were purchased from Samtaco Animal Co. (Osan, Kyungki-do, Korea). All rats were housed in a limited access rodent facility with up to five rats per polycarbonate cage. The room controls were set to maintain the temperature at 22 ± 2 °C and the relative humidity at $55 \pm 15\%$, the cages were lit by artificial light for 12 h each day, and sterilized drinking water and a standard chow diet were supplied ad libitum throughout the study. All animal experiments began a minimum of 7 days after the animals arrived, were conducted in accordance with the *Guide for the Care and Use of Laboratory Animals Eighth Edition* (by the National Research Council of the National Academies, revised in 2011), and were approved by the Kyung Hee University Institutional Animal Care and Use Committee. All efforts were made to minimize the number and suffering of animals.

Generation of different surface roughness of acupuncture needle

A disposable stainless steel needle (silicone coated, ø0.20 × 60 mm) was purchased from Dongbang Acupuncture Ltd. (Kyunggi-do, Korea). The total length of the needle was 60 mm from which the handle part was 20 mm and the body part was 40 mm. In order to produce different surface roughness, premium silicon carbide discs having the grit numbers of 200 (80 µm) and 600 (15 µm) (3 M Korea Co., Seoul, Korea) was used to grind the surface of the body part. The scrapes on the needle surface were generated by pulling once as holding the handle part while the body part was strongly embedded by sandpaper, parallel to the needle axis. The scratch was confirmed by observing distal end of the needle tip using a microscope (BX51; Olympus Ltd., Tokyo, Japan), and subsequently photographed to compare their uniformity (200×).

Atomic force microscope (AFM) observation of acupuncture needle surface

The AFM images were obtained using Nanostation II™ (Surface Imaging Systems, Herzogenrath, Germany) in non-contact mode. The Nanostation II™ was equipped with 92.5 µm XY/6 µm Z scanner and an optical microscope, Zeiss Epiplan 50× (Carl Zeiss, Oberkochen, Germany). The AFM was placed on top of the active vibration isolation table (TS-150, S.I.S., Herzogenrath, Germany), which was located inside of the passive vibration isolation table (Pucotech., Seoul, Korea) to eliminate external noise such as vibration. Data acquisition and processing were performed by the SPIP™ (Scanning Probe Image Processor, version 4.1, Image Metrology,

Denmark). The reflex coated silicon cantilevers for non-contact mode (PR-NC, S.I.S., Germany) had the following characteristics: (manufacturer's specifications: F = 146 ~ 236 kHz, C = 21-98 N/m, L = 225 μm and R = 0.01 ~ 0.02 Ohm·cm). Samples were scanned at the resolution of 256 × 256 pixel with scan speed of 1 line/s.

Rotation-elicited torque measurement of acupuncture needle using Acusensor®

The measurement of acupuncture needle torque was performed using Acusensor® (Stromatec, Burlington, VT, USA) according to the protocol by RT Davis, DL Churchill, GJ Badger, J Dunn and HM Langevin [3]. Acusensor measurement system consists of two units: a needle motion sensor and a needle force (torque) sensor. Both sensors were cooperatively operated to quantitatively analyze rotational (back-and forth or one direction) and/or pistoning (up-and-down motion) manipulations. After the acupuncture needle was inserted at a depth of 5 mm perpendicularly to the skin using insertion tube of the needle motion sensor, the needle was manually rotated 3 times in one direction and the torque was measured in every 360° clockwise rotation.

Experimental groups and acupuncture treatment

Animals were randomly divided into four treatment groups: the normal group without any treatments (NOR, $n = 7$), the plain acupuncture group without scraping of needle surface (ACU, $n = 7$), the acupuncture group with needle surface of low roughness (ACU600, $n = 7$), the acupuncture group with needle surface of high roughness (ACU200, $n = 7$), and morphine (10 mg/kg, $i.p.$)-treated group (MOR10, $n = 7$).

TFL test and formalin test were performed immediately after the acupuncture treatment or morphine administration. Morphine was used as the positive control and its dose was adopted according to the previous study [13]. The needle was inserted into the acupoint ST36 on the dextral side at a depth of 5 mm and then manually twirled 360° clockwise and counterclockwise as one cycle, three cycles per second for the total duration of three seconds. The acupoint ST36 is located at the proximal one fifth point on the line from the depression lateral to the patella ligament to the anterior side of ankle [14].

Histochemical staining of abdominal skin tissue

In order to verify the histological changes of the abdominal skin layers including epidermis, dermis, subcutaneous tissue and abdominal wall muscle, caused by acupuncture needle twisting, an acrylic equipment was designed tightly to hold the skin explant. While anesthetizing with a sodium pentobarbital (80 mg/kg, i.p.), rat

abdominal skin including the skin abdominal wall, with a liberal margin of surrounding skin, was excised to a depth to include the underlying connective tissue above the external fascia of the dorsal muscles wall with an appropriate size (30 mm × 30 mm) using a surgical knife, washed in phosphate buffered saline (PBS) for 5 min, and tied up to the acrylic plastic frame using clamps. Subsequently the needles with various surface roughness were inserted at a depth of 5 mm into the ex vivo abdominal skin and uni-directionally rotated 5 consecutive cycles. The schematic of the needle rotation for histology with the acupuncture needle inserted to the abdominal skin is depicted in Fig. 1. We picked up the abdominal skin tissues instead of the anterior tibialis skin tissues (ST36 region) to observe the morphological intorsion of connective tissue induced by twirling manipulation. The abdominal tissues are wider and softer, which helps to execute tissue biopsy easily and to maximize the visualization, whereas the anterior tibialis tissue is too narrow to cut off so it was impossible to show the intorsion due to technical limitation. Nevertheless, we can suppose the morphological change by twirling manipulation might be occurred in the anterior tibialis tissue as the same aspect in the abdominal tissue, although we cannot observe visually.

These biopsy specimens were fixed in 4% paraformaldehyde overnight, dehydrated through a graded ethanol series, embedded in paraffin, sectioned parallel to the needle axis at 10 μm thickness using a rotatory microtome, Shandon Finesse 325 (Thermo Fisher Scientific Inc., MA USA), and mounted on slides. Before staining, slides were deparaffinized. For demonstrating morphologic changes and eosinophil

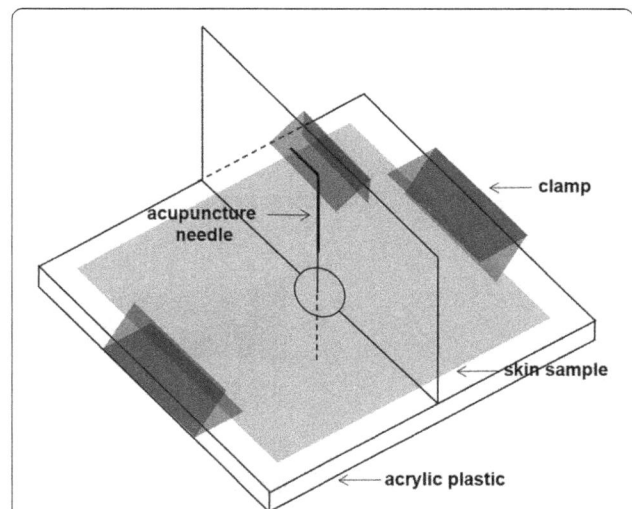

Fig. 1 Schematic diagram of the equipment to tightly hold and spread the skin tissue and to fix an acupuncture needle inserted into the skin perpendicularly and rotated uni-directionally

infiltration, the slides were stained with hematoxylin (Merck Co., Darmstadt, Germany) and 1% eosin (Sigma-Aldrich Co., St. Louise, MO, USA). The slides were bathed in hematioxylin for 7 min, distilled water for 5 min, 1% HCL tapping for 3 times, 80% ethanol (EtOH) for 3 min, 100% EtOH for 3 min, 1% eosin for 1 min, 80% EtOH for 1 min, 90% EtOH for 5 min and 100% EtOH for 5 min, continuingly. The slides were finally put into 100% xylene for 3 min and this procedure was repeated three times. Then, 2–3 drops of permount were dropped directly to the tissues on the slide, and a cover slip was gently placed over the tissues after pressing out the bubbles with tweezers. These slides were air-dried and cover-slipped for microscopic observation. All slides (40× magnification) were observed, photographed using a microscope (BX51; Olympus Ltd., Tokyo, Japan).

Tail flick latency and formalin tests

Anti-nociception was assessed using TFL and the rat formalin tests. TFL test was conducted using a model 33 tail flick analgesia meter (IITC Life Science Inc., Woodland Hills, CA) with the beam intensity set at 4.0 (Fig. 5.). All rats were habituated for 30 minutes in the procedure room prior to testing. During the TFL, rats were wrapped with a soft paper towel with the whole tail length exposed, and handheld with appropriate strength.

To perform the formalin test, 50 µL of 5% formalin was injected subcutaneously into the plantar surface of the right hind paw with a 30-gauge needle, then pain behaviors of the rats were examined for 60 min after formalin injection. Nociceptive behaviors were quantified by counting the number of times the animal licked, bit, or shaked the formalin-injected paw at 5-min intervals. Two phases of spontaneous nociceptive behavior were observed: an initial acute phase (early phase, duration of the first 10 min after formalin injection) was followed by a relative short quiescent period and then by a prolonged tonic response (late phase, duration of 50 min after the early phase). The analgesic effect of acupuncture with rough needle surface was compared with that of morphine (10 mg/kg, *i.p.*), an opioid analgesic drug, in both tests.

Statistical analysis

The experimental results were expressed as the mean ± standard error (SEM). The behavioral data were calculated and analyzed by repeated measures analysis of variance (ANOVA) and one-way ANOVA followed by Tukey's *post hoc* test using SPSS (Version 13.0; SPSS Inc., Chicago, USA). In all analyses, $p < 0.05$ was considered significant.

Results

Generation of different surface roughness of acupuncture needle surface

In order to increase the grasp force of needle differently, silicon carbide sandpapers with different grit numbers were used to make different longitudinal scratches on the needle surfaces. As shown in Fig. 2, long scratches were evidently observed on the ground needle surface along the needle axis and even some splinters in case of extra coarse sandpaper (grit number 200 in ACU200) while the surface of normal needle tip was observed slick and smooth.

Atomic force microscope (AFM) observation of scratched acupuncture needle surface

AFM is one of the foremost imaging tools by which we can measure and manipulate matters at the nanoscale by using a high-resolution scanning probe (tip), and it is generally used to scan the specimen surfaces. In order to verify the scratches on the needle surface

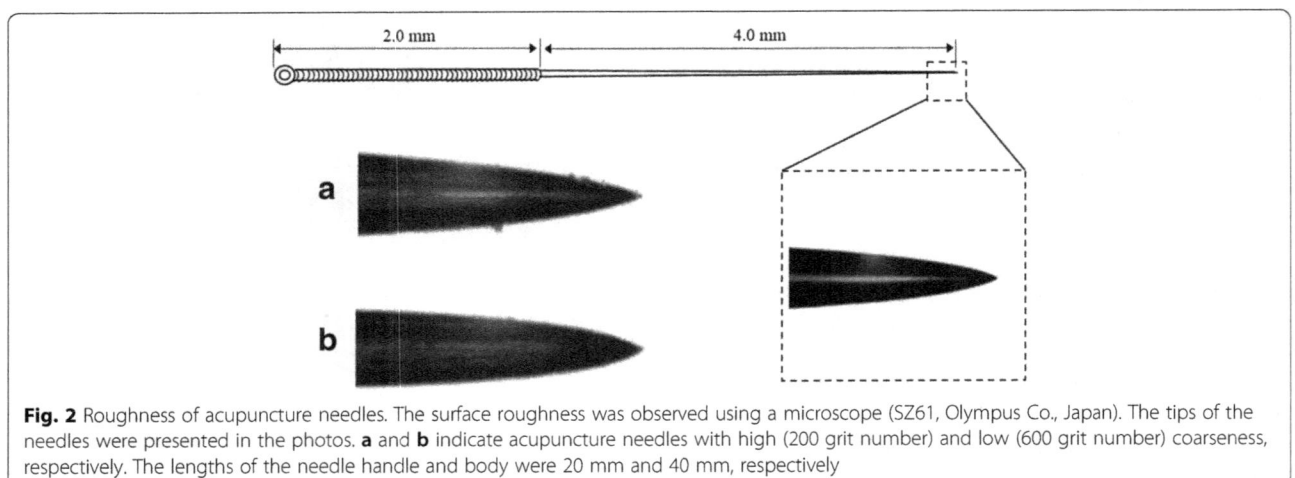

Fig. 2 Roughness of acupuncture needles. The surface roughness was observed using a microscope (SZ61, Olympus Co., Japan). The tips of the needles were presented in the photos. **a** and **b** indicate acupuncture needles with high (200 grit number) and low (600 grit number) coarseness, respectively. The lengths of the needle handle and body were 20 mm and 40 mm, respectively

analytically, the shape and depth of the scratch were analyzed using an AFM. Stereomicroscopic images of normal, lightly scraped and deeply scraped needle surfaces were shown in Fig. 3. The surface of normal needle was flat and smooth even though there were several small bumps with various sizes but less than 0.5 μm height. Lightly scraped needle obviously showed the stripe-shaped artificial scratches with about 2 μm interval whereas deeply scraped needle had the deeper scratches with about 10 μm interval. Most of surfaces of scraped needles had significant abrasion compared with the smooth surface of normal needle as shown in Fig. 4. The maximum depth of the scratches on the surfaces of lightly scraped and deeply scraped needles were about 0.625 and 1.625 μm, respectively even though the patterns of scratches of both needles were irregular.

Measurement of twirling-elicited torque in scratched acupuncture needle using Acusensor®

In order to quantify acupuncture needle manipulation according to the rotation number in uni-direction, Acusensor® was used for measuring the torque, a

mechanical load developed by skin tissue that has tendency of resisting against the twirling needle. Uni-directional rotation of deeply scraped needles significantly increased torque as the rotation number was increased from 1 to 3. In the second and third rotation, the torque developed by rotating scraped needles was consistently greater than that by normal one, and the torque by deeply scraped needle was also greater that that by lightly scraped one (Fig. 5).

Histochemical changes of abdominal skin tissues after twirling manipulation of scratched acupuncture needle

Histological examination of tissue sections revealed that acupuncture needle penetrated epidermis, dermis, subcutaneous and muscle layers of skin, and that marked rise and thickening of skin tissue layers were observed along the axis of the deeply scraped needle (Fig. 6d) whereas slight thickening and deformity of subcutaneous and muscle layers were observed in the vicinity of the lightly scraped needle (Fig. 6c). Deformity of dermal and subcutaneous layers harboring skin fibroblast cells was remarkable among the skin layers observed. In case of deeply scraped needle, arrangements of various cells and

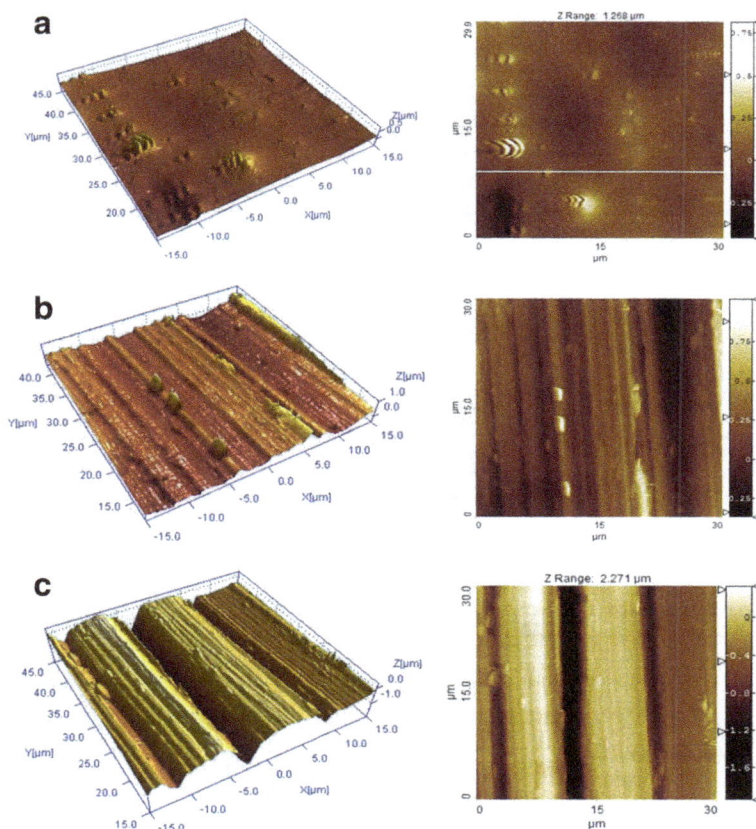

Fig. 3 The different shapes of the scratches on the differently scraped needle surfaces in the stereomicroscope images were obtained by using atomic force microscope (AFM). The normal (ACU, **a**), lightly scraped (ACU600, **b**), and deeply scraped (ACU200, **c**) acupuncture needles

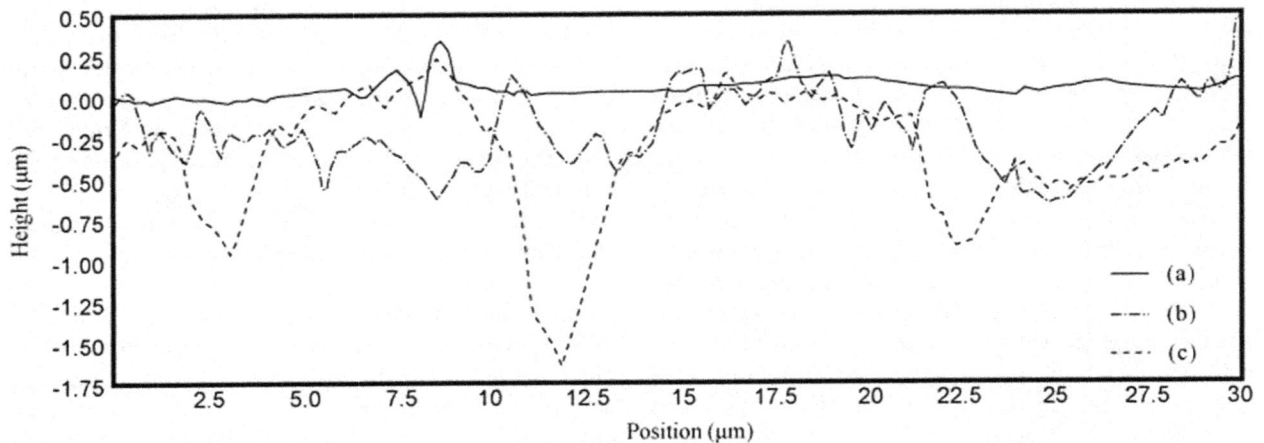

Fig. 4 The different depths of abrasions on the differently scraped needle surfaces were observed. The maximum depth were about 0.625 μm in lightly scraped and 1.625 μm in deeply scraped, respectively. The normal (solid line, a), lightly scraped (dash-dotted line, b) and deeply scraped (dashed line, c) needle surfaces

extracellular structures such as adipose tissue, connective tissue, hair follicle vein and artery were highly twisted and stretched (Fig. 6d).

Analgesic effect of twirling manipulation of scratched acupuncture needle in tail flick latency and formalin test

After confirming the proportional increase of grasp force depending on surface roughness of the acupuncture needle, we subsequently investigated whether the strength of needle grasp force can affect the analgesic effect of acupuncture manipulation using TFL and the rat paw formalin tests in the rats. We observed that the rougher the needle surface, the stronger the pain relieving effect although the difference of analgesic activity between deeply scraped and lightly scraped needles was not

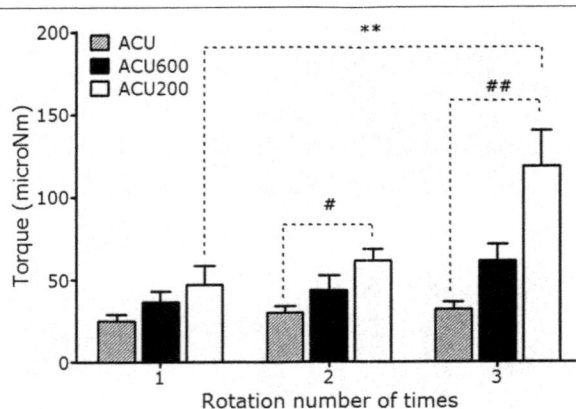

Fig. 5 Acupuncture needle torque developed by skin tissue resistance against uni-directional rotation of the needle (total three times of rotation) were measured by using Acusensor®. Manipulation of deeply scraped needle (ACU200) significantly increased the torque as the rotation number increased. **$p < 0.01$ versus one time of rotation; #$p < 0.05$, ##$p < 0.01$ versus ACU group

statistically significant 10 min after acupuncture treatment (Fig. 7). These results may indicate that the pain-relieving efficacy induced by twirling manipulation was gradually decreased after reaching its peak at 10 min whereas intraperitoneal administration of morphine as a positive control was gradually increase analgesic effect. Twirling plain needle did not increase TFL, as compared with non-treated normal group.

The analgesic effect of twirling manipulation with coarse surface needle was also verified in the rat formalin test. In the early phase, there was a trend of decrease in nociceptive behaviors in coarse surface acupuncture-treated groups although it was not statistically significant (Fig. 8). In the late phase, nociceptive behaviors were significantly decreased in deeply scraped acupuncture-treated group (ACU200 group) as compared with those in non-treated normal group (NOR group). However, there were little differences in nociceptive behaviors between plain (ACU group) and lightly scraped (ACU600 group) acupuncture-treated groups. Formalin-induced nociceptive behaviors were almost removed by morphine injection both in the early and late phases.

Discussion

In the present study, we investigated if the coarser needle surface of acupuncture induces the stronger needle grasp force by twirling manipulation and if anti-nociceptic effect of acupuncture becomes the more effective as the grater needle grasp force is occurred in distorted connective tissues. The main findings were that 1) acupuncture which has the deeper longitudinal scratches on the needle surface induced the grater needle grasp force in the skin tissue and that 2) the grater needle grasp force at acupoint ST36 showed the more effective anti-nociception.

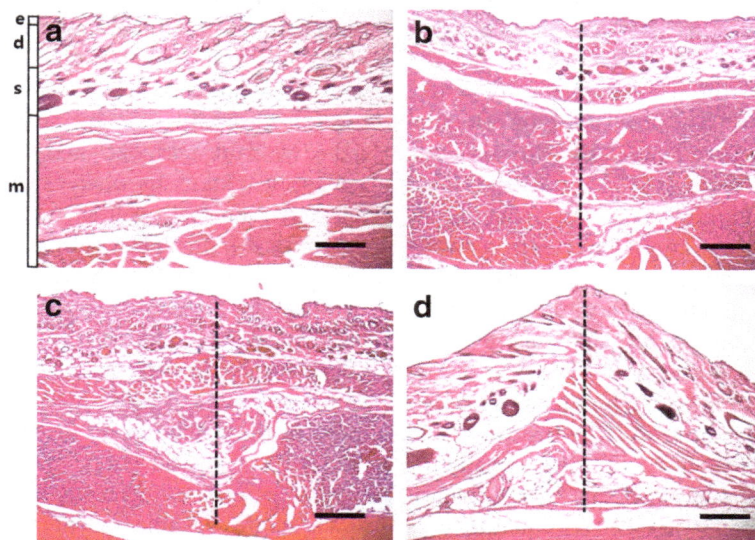

Fig. 6 The different intorsion shapes of dermal tissues induced by twirling manipulation with the differently scraped needles were observed by using hematoxylin-eosin (HE) staining of histological sections (40×) of abdominal skin tissues. Without manipulation-NOR (**a**) and after rotation manipulation of the needle with smooth surface-ACU (**b**), lightly scraped surface-ACU600 (**c**) and deeply scraped surface-ACU200 (**d**). Abdominal skin layers include epidermis (e), dermis (d), subcutaneous tissue (s) and abdominal muscle (m). The dotted line indicates the inserted trace of acupuncture needle. Scale bars, 100 μm

An important aspect of acupuncture treatment is that acupuncture needle must be manually manipulated to achieve the best outcome after inserted into the body [1, 5]. Therefore, most of physicians have always used various manipulation techniques during acupuncture treatment, such as twirling and rotating, lifting and thrusting, flicking and scraping, and shaking and vibrating to boost up stimulating effect of acupuncture on the acupoint in addition to pricking effect of acupuncture needle [5, 15]. Among them, twirling manipulation, a finger skill of sequential order in a clockwise-counterclockwise manner after insertion of needle into the acupoint, has been the most popular because it is optimal way to adjust the acupuncture stimulation to get the *de qi* response. However, the underlying mechanisms of acupuncture manipulation and the signaling initiators or mediators generated by needle pricking and manipulation at the acupuncture point have remained unresolved. To understand its mechanism, the initiation of signaling on the peripheral acupuncture point on the skin due

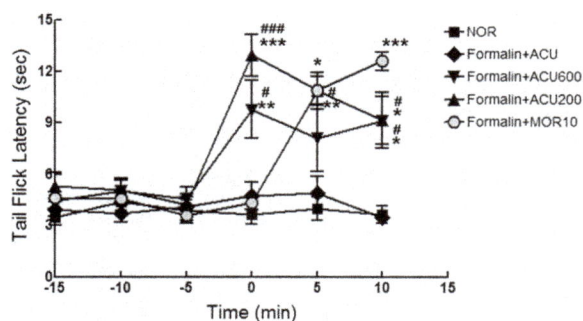

Fig. 7 Tail flick latency (TFL) in rats treated with acupuncture needle with different roughness. Time zero denotes the onset of acupuncture treatment with rotation manipulation. Morphine was used as a positive control. NOR: non-treated normal group, Formalin + ACU: plain needle group, Formalin + ACU600: lightly scraped needle group, Formalin + ACU200: deeply scraped needle group, Formalin + MOR10: morphine group. $^*p < 0.05$, $^{**}p < 0.01$, $^{***}p < 0.001$ versus NOR group; $^#p < 0.05$, $^{###}p < 0.001$ versus ACU group

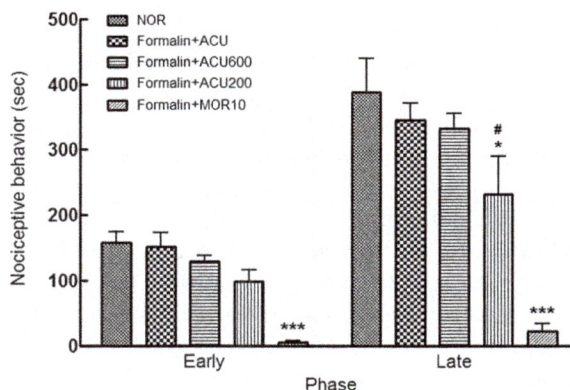

Fig. 8 Pain behavior after formalin injection roughness-dependently in early and late phase. NOR: non-treated normal group, ACU: plain needle group, Formalin + ACU600: lightly scraped needle group, Formalin + ACU200: deeply scraped needle group, Formalin + MOR10: morphine group. $^*p < 0.05$, $^{***}p < 0.001$ versus NOR group; $^#p < 0.05$ versus ACU group

to acupuncture pricking and manipulation, and its long distance conveyance to the cognate internal organs should be necessarily investigated.

Traditionally or even in the present, the *de qi* sensation between acupuncturist and patient is the essential to clinically succeed acupuncture therapy. However this sensation is necessarily dependent on the emotional states of individual patients and their environmental atmosphere, and therefore great efforts have been made to scientifically understand and establish the relationship between the degree of *de qi* and its clinical efficacy [16]. Among them, Langevin's group had assumed that the manipulation-associated acupuncturist's *de qi* was due to the needle grasp force attributed to the increased resistance between the twirled needle and the distorted skin tissue as the number of times being uni-directionally rotated was increased. They addressed this biomechanical component of *de qi* experienced by acupuncturist as "needle grasp force" and suggested as a plausible mechanism of acupuncture manipulation [17].

If the direction and number of twirling are fixed, the needle grasp force will definitely depend on friction between needle surface and adjacent tissues, cells or extracellular structures surrounding the needle. We therefore proposed a hypothesis that scratching the needle surface may increase the resistance in the twirling manipulation. If the twirling manipulation can reinforce acupuncture therapy, surface roughness of needle will be a crucial parameter influencing therapeutic efficacy of acupuncture. Taken together, we can readily assume that the coarser the acupuncture needle surface is, the more effective therapeutic efficacy of acupuncture manipulation is.

In the present study, we used two different silicon carbide sandpapers to make different levels of surface roughness on the acupuncture needles: sandpapers having the grit numbers of 200 (extra coarse, ACU200) and 600 (mild coarse, ACU600), and confirmed the longitudinal deeper scratches along the needle axis and even some splinters in the needle ground with extra coarse sandpaper (grit No. 200). We also confirmed the degree of needle surface roughness is closely associated with the twirling-induced torque and distortion in skin tissue, which indicates the frictional force between needle surface and adjacent tissues may be increased as the surface roughness becomes coarser. Although Langevin's group strongly formulated a grasp force hypothesis closely associated with winding of connective tissues as a biomechanical mechanism of twisting acupuncture manipulation, they have not suggested an experimental evidence proving that therapeutic effect of acupuncture manipulation is in accordance with the needle grasp force of skin tissues surrounding the inserted needle as of yet.

Thus, we investigated needle grasp force theory in nociceptive pain animal models, such as tail flick latency (TFL) test and the rat formalin test, to verify the analgesic activities of twirling manipulation using acupuncture needles with different surface roughness. TFL is a reflexive pain test designed to verify pain threshold against heat stimulus whereas the formalin test is a non-reflexive pain test, well-characterized tonic chemogenic pain model [18]. TFL was increased in proportion to the surface roughness of the acupuncture needles in the twirling of acupuncture. Acupuncture needle with rougher surface significantly exhibited larger analgesic effect during the late phases of the rat formalin test, as compared to that with smooth surface. These findings indicate the needle grasp force may be strongly associated with analgesic effect of twirling acupuncture manipulation against nociceptive pain.

We might be able to speculate the relationship between the needle grasp force and the analgesic effect from the review explaining the mechanistic and biological evidences of acupuncture manipulation. Acupuncture manipulation can induce the propagation of the acoustic wave and the response of calcium ion channel signaling, then the calcium ion channel-dependent peripheral secretion of endogenous opioids might subsequently follow, which might not show the addictive side effects [19]. Thus, it is possible that the increase in the dose of manipulation could get better analgesic effect because the stronger needle grasp force can induce the wider propagation of wave.

We could observe ACU200 showed anti-nociceptive effect in formalin test, nevertheless we did not figure out the reason that the ACU200 showed the effectiveness during the late phase only. The previous study showed manual acupuncture stimulation reversed nociceptive behavior during the late phase in the formalin test, which indicates acupuncture may be effective in relieving inflammatory pain rather than activation of peripheral nociceptors [20]. Moreover, the formalin response during the late phase is related to the CNS sensitization facilitated by the formalin-induced TRPA1 (Transient receptor potential cation channel, subfamily A, member 1) activation [21]. Taken together, we can guess ACU200 might be relieving inflammatory pain and modulating a part of TRPA1 signaling, which remains to be elucidated.

However, plain needle with twirling manipulation did now show significant analgesic effect in the present study. We previously reported formalin-induced pain was significantly alleviated by twirling acupuncture manipulation at acupoint ST36, but the number and total duration of manipulation cycle were ten times more than that in the present study [12]. This contradiction might be attributable to the reduced dose of manipulation. Because the discrepancy as four to five times in the torque induced by 3-cycle rotations between plain and extra coarse needle was found, we expected to get the grater stimulation from the coarser needle, which is the reason why we reduced the dose. In other words, we possibly get the *de qi* response with the much less quantity of manipulating coarser needle rather than plain needle.

The present study was designed to develop the optimal acupuncture device effective under the only manual stimulation for the shorter duration of manipulation. A lot of previous studies have shown the strong analgesic effect of electroacupuncture in the animal models of nociceptive pain, however electroacupuncture should be carefully considered by practitioners who take care of some patients (eg. unpleasant to electric stimuli, pacemaker user, etc.). Moreover, the best retaining-needle duration of manual acupuncture to get analgesic effect is suggested as 20 min [22], however the practitioners can experience the clinical case that they are not able to retain the acupuncture needle for such a long time. Therefore, we suggest the coarse needle surface acupuncture might be used to overcome those clinical difficulties. However, we recognize the limitations of the present study as the follows; 1) The scratches on the coarse needle surfaces of ACU200 and ACU600 were not even because we manually manufactured these needles as prototypes. This unevenness might occur the individual difference in the quantity of stimulation, so we need to find the way to improve quality control of the acupuncture needles. 2) Although we found the analgesic effect of the coarse acupuncture is comparable to the morphine, we did not unearth the specified mechanism which remains to be fully elucidated in the further study.

Conclusions
Taken together, the twirling manipulation using coarser surface acupuncture needle significantly improved tonic and phasic pain better than plain surface needle, and eventually exhibited the more effective anti-nociceptive activity in rats. These results strongly support Langevin group's mechanical signaling hypothesis of needle grasp force to elucidate the twirling acupuncture manipulation. Although we propose here a strategy for developing a novel acupuncture needle with coarser surface which probably produces stronger pain-relieving effect, a marked progress has not been achieved of yet and more investigations are required to be made in the future to elucidate molecular mechanism and all aspects of scientific mechanism of acupuncture therapy including manipulation.

Acknowledgements
We thank Prof. Park HK and Prof. Yin CS for their technical advice on atomic force microscope operation. We also thank Dr. Lee S and Prof Chae YB for technical assistance to make acupuncture needles having different surface roughness and to measure acupuncture needle torque using Acusensor®, respectively.

Funding
This research was supported by grants from the National Research Foundation of Korea funded by the Korean government (NRF-2015M3A9E3052338 & NRF- 2016R1D1A2B04933575).

Authors' contributions
Author contributions to the study and manuscript preparation are as the follows. Conception and design: SK, YL, HP and DH. Carried out the experiments: SK, YL and DH. Acquisition of data: SK, YL and DH. Analysis and interpretation: SK, YL, HP and DH. Drafting the article: SK, YL and DH. Statistical analysis: SK and YL and DH. Study supervision: HP and DH. All authors read and approved the final manuscript.

Authors' information
Not applicable.

Competing interests
The authors declare that they have no competing interests.

Author details
[1]Acupuncture and Meridian Science Research Center, College of Korean Medicine, Kyung Hee University, 26, Kyungheedae-ro, Dongdaemun-gu, Seoul 02447, Republic of Korea. [2]Department of Basic Science of Korean Medicine, Graduate School, Kyung Hee University, 26, Kyungheedae-ro, Dongdaemun-gu, Seoul 02447, Republic of Korea. [3]Department of Psychiatry and Behavioral Sciences, Northwestern University Feinberg School of Medicine, Chicago 60611, USA. [4]KM Fundamental Research Division, Korea Institute of Oriental Medicine, Daejeon 34054, Republic of Korea.

References
1. Yang J. The Golden Needle and Other Odes of Traditional Acupuncture., 1601.[Transl. by Bertschinger R. Edinburgh: Churchill Livingstone; 1991.
2. Gliedt JA, Daniels CJ, Wuollet A. Narrative Review of Perioperative Acupuncture for Clinicians. J Acupunct Meridian Stud. 2015;8(5):264–9.
3. Davis RT, Churchill DL, Badger GJ, Dunn J, Langevin HM. A new method for quantifying the needling component of acupuncture treatments. Acupuncture in medicine : journal of the British Medical Acupuncture Society. 2012;30(2):113–9.
4. Cheng X. Chinese acupuncture and moxibustion: Foreign Languages Press. In.: Beijing; 1987.
5. O'Connor J, Bensky D. Acupuncture: A Comprehensive Text.(9th Print) Shanghai College of Traditional Medicine. Seattle: Eastland Press; 1992.
6. Pomeranz B, Stux G, Berman B. Basics of acupuncture: Springer: Berlin; 2003.
7. Helms J. Acupuncture energetics: a clinical approach for physicians. 1995, Berkeley, Calif. USA: Medical Acpuncture Publishers; 1995. p. xxiii.
8. Gunn C, Milbrandt W. NEUROLOGICAL MECHANISM OF NEEDLE-GRASP IN ACUPUNCTURE. Am J Acupunct. 1977;5(2):115–20.

9. Shen E, Wu W, Du H, Wei J, Zhu D. Electromyographic activity produced locally by acupuncture manipulation. Chin Med J. 1973;9:532–5.
10. Langevin HM, Churchill DL, Cipolla MJ. Mechanical signaling through connective tissue: a mechanism for the therapeutic effect of acupuncture. FASEB journal : official publication of the Federation of American Societies for Experimental Biology. 2001;15(12):2275–82.
11. Langevin HM, Churchill DL, Fox JR, Badger GJ, Garra BS, Krag MH. Biomechanical response to acupuncture needling in humans. J Appl Physiol. 2001;91(6):2471–8.
12. Kim GH, Yeom M, Yin CS, Lee H, Shim I, Hong MS, Kim CJ, Hahm DH. Acupuncture manipulation enhances anti-nociceptive effect on formalin-induced pain in rats. Neurol Res. 2010;32 Suppl 1:92–5.
13. Gades NM, Danneman PJ, Wixson SK, Tolley EA. The magnitude and duration of the analgesic effect of morphine, butorphanol, and buprenorphine in rats and mice. Contemp Top Lab Anim Sci. 2000; 39(2):8–13.
14. Yin CS, Jeong HS, Park HJ, Baik Y, Yoon MH, Choi CB, Koh HG. A proposed transpositional acupoint system in a mouse and rat model. Res Vet Sci. 2008;84(2):159–65.
15. Cassidy C. A survey of six acupuncture clinics: demographic and satisfaction data. In: Proceedings of the Third Symposium of the Society for Acupuncture Research. 1995;1995:1–27.
16. Yang XY, Shi GX, Li QQ, Zhang ZH, Xu Q, Liu CZ. Characterization of deqi sensation and acupuncture effect. Evidence-based complementary and alternative medicine : eCAM. 2013;2013:319734.
17. Langevin HM, Churchill DL, Wu J, Badger GJ, Yandow JA, Fox JR, Krag MH. Evidence of connective tissue involvement in acupuncture. FASEB journal : official publication of the Federation of American Societies for Experimental Biology. 2002;16(8):872–4.
18. Gregory NS, Harris AL, Robinson CR, Dougherty PM, Fuchs PN, Sluka KA. An overview of animal models of pain: disease models and outcome measures. J Pain. 2013;14(11):1255–69.
19. Yang ES, Li PW, Nilius B, Li G. Ancient Chinese medicine and mechanistic evidence of acupuncture physiology. Pflugers Arch. 2011;462(5):645–53.
20. Chang KH, Bai SJ, Lee H, Lee BH. Effects of acupuncture stimulation at different acupoints on formalin-induced pain in rats. Korean J Physiol Pharmacol. 2014;18(2):121–7.
21. McNamara CR, Mandel-Brehm J, Bautista DM, Siemens J, Deranian KL, Zhao M, Hayward NJ, Chong JA, Julius D, Moran MM, et al. TRPA1 mediates formalin-induced pain. Proc Natl Acad Sci U S A. 2007;104(33): 13525–30.
22. Cui JM, Ma SX, Wu SJ, Yang XX, Qi F, Sun N. [Effect of needling "Housanli" (ST 36) with different retaining-needle time on the pain threshold of mice using the hot water tail-flick test]. Zhongguo Zhen Jiu. 2009;29(8):653–4.

6

Acupuncture for insomnia after stroke: a systematic review and meta-analysis

Sook-Hyun Lee and Sung Min Lim[*]

Abstract

Background: Insomnia is the common complaint among patients with stroke. Acupuncture has increasingly been used for insomnia relief after stroke.
The aim of the present study was to summarize and evaluate evidence on the effectiveness of acupuncture in relieving insomnia after stroke.

Methods: Seven databases were searched from inception through October 2014 without language restrictions. Randomized controlled trials (RCTs) were included if acupuncture was compared to placebo or other conventional therapy for treatment of insomnia after stroke. Assessments were performed using the Pittsburgh sleep quality index (PSQI), the insomnia severity index (ISI), the Athens insomnia scale (AIS), and the efficacy standards of Chinese medicine.

Results: A total of 165 studies were identified; 13 RCTs met our inclusion criteria. Meta-analysis showed that acupuncture appeared to be more effective than drugs for treatment of insomnia after stroke, as assessed by the PSQI (weighted mean difference, 4.31; 95 % confidence interval [CI], 1.67–6.95; $P = 0.001$) and by the efficacy standards of Chinese medicine (risk ratio, 1.25; 95 % CI, 1.12–1.40; $P < 0.001$). Intradermal acupuncture had significant effects compared with sham acupuncture, as assessed by the ISI (weighted mean difference, 4.44; 95 % CI, 2.75–6.13; $P < 0.001$) and the AIS (weighted mean difference, 3.64; 95 % CI, 2.28–5.00; $P < 0.001$).

Conclusions: Our results suggest that acupuncture could be effective for treating insomnia after stroke. However, further studies are needed to confirm the role of acupuncture in the treatment of this disorder.

Keywords: Acupuncture, Intradermal acupuncture, Stroke, Insomnia, Review

Background

Stroke is the second-leading global cause of death behind heart disease, accounting for 11.13 % of total deaths worldwide [1]. In addition, survivors often suffer from not only pain and various physical disabilities but also mood disorders such as depression [2]. Such physical and emotional consequences of stroke could have multiple effects on a patient's sleeping pattern. Previous studies have reported that the sleep-wake cycle is frequently disturbed after stroke [3, 4].

Insomnia is the most common sleep complaint, affecting approximately 40–60 % of stroke patients [3]. This frequency is higher than what observed in patients without a stroke (10–40 %) [5]. Insomnia after stroke is caused mainly by anxiety resulting from hyperactivity of the sympathetic nervous system [3–6]. In addition, post-stroke insomnia might be affected by damaged brain lesions resulted from the stroke, age, degree of disability after stroke, anxiety disorder, antipsychotic drugs, depression, and other comorbidities [6, 7]. During stroke recovery, psychological stress due to insomnia affects the effectiveness of therapy and the prognosis; it also affects quality of life, mental health, and rehabilitation [8–10].

Although effective pharmacological treatments are available, significant side effects have limited their clinical applications and long-term use [10]. Of the complementary treatment modalities, acupuncture has been one of the most popular and safest [11].

* Correspondence: limsm@outlook.kr
Department of Clinical Research on Rehabilitation, Korea National Rehabilitation Research Institute, 58 Samgaksan-ro, Gangbuk-gu, Seoul 142-070, Republic of Korea

Acupuncture has been widely used to treat a variety of clinical conditions, particularly those involving pathological changes in neuroendocrinology, such as menopause, depression, and insomnia [12]. Acupuncture is able to regulate the functioning of the heart and brain through stimulation of certain acupoints on the body. Many published clinical studies, including randomized controlled trials (RCTs), have explored acupuncture as a treatment for insomnia. Most reports have demonstrated positive clinical effects of acupuncture in the treatment of insomnia. Acupuncture treatment has also been reported to reduce sleep onset latency and increase sleep duration and sleep efficiency [13].

A few recent systematic reviews have examined the effectiveness of acupuncture in the treatment of insomnia [12, 14, 15]. However, none has focused on insomnia after stroke. Furthermore, the effectiveness of acupuncture in treating insomnia after stroke has not been fully determined. The aim of the present study was to summarize and evaluate evidence on the effectiveness of acupuncture for insomnia relief after stroke.

Methods
Search methods for identification of studies
The search was performed without restriction to language or year of publication. We searched Medline, EMBASE, and the Cochrane Central Register of Controlled Trials from database inception through October 2014. For Korean publications, we searched three Korean medical databases (Research Information Service System, National Discovery for Science Leaders, and OASIS). For Chinese articles, we searched the China National Knowledge Infrastructure (CNKI). The keywords used for the search were "stroke OR apoplexy OR cva OR cerebrovascular attack OR cerebrovascular accident OR cerebral infarction OR cerebral hemorrhage" AND "acupuncture OR acupoints OR electroacupuncture OR electro-acupuncture OR auriculotherapy OR auriculoacupuncture" AND "insomnia" in each database language. The search strategy was adjusted for each database (Appendix).

Inclusion/exclusion criteria
Relevant clinical trials were included if the following criteria were met: 1) they were randomized, controlled trials (RCTs); 2) they included patients diagnosed with insomnia after stroke; 3) stroke patients with insomnia at baseline were enrolled, and 4) they studied insomnia as an outcome measure. Trials were excluded if the study design did not allow evaluation of the effects of acupuncture on insomnia after stroke; that is, studies were excluded if they 1) compared different types of acupuncture, 2) adopted complex treatment without

examining the effects of acupuncture alone, or 3) reported insufficient information.

Data extraction
Two reviewers (L.S.H. and L.S.M.) independently extracted data using a standardized data extraction form and reached consensus on all items. Extracted data included authors, year of publication, sample size, interventions, main outcomes, and adverse events.

Instruments of the outcome measurements that were reported in the included studies were the Pittsburgh sleep quality index (PSQI), the efficacy standards of Chinese medicine, the Insomnia Severity Index (ISI), and the Athens insomnia scale (AIS).

The PSQI consists of 19 self-rated questions, which are grouped into seven component scores ranging from 0 to 3 each. The seven component scores are then summed to yield a global PSQI score, which has a range of 0 to 21, with higher scores indicating worse sleep quality. Specifically, a score of "0" indicates no difficulty, whereas a score of "21" indicates severe difficulties in all areas [16]. The ISI is a brief self-report instrument measuring a patient's perception of insomnia. The seven items are rated on a 0-to-4 scale, and the total score ranges from 0 to 28. A higher score indicates more severe insomnia [17]. The AIS is a self-administered psychometric instrument consisting of eight items. Each item of the AIS can be rated from 0 to 3 for a total score range of 0–24, with a score of "0" indicating no problem at all and a score of "24" indicating very serious problems in all areas [18]. We extracted data on the mean change from baseline measures (the "Mean", Fig. 3). The standard deviation of changes from baseline was determined using a correlation coefficient from a previously published study [19].

The efficacy standards of Chinese medicine is a measurement tool for the assessment of the states of the patients with complete improvement (recovery of normal sleep duration), partial improvement (increased sleep duration more than three hours), and no improvement after treatment [12]. Response rate was calculated based on proportion of the effective (complete or partial improvement) and not effective (no improvement) patients. We also considered measures of general safety reported for acupuncture as a treatment. We extracted data on the number of participants with improvement as an "Event" (Fig. 3).

Quality assessment
The two reviewers independently assessed the methodological quality and the risk of bias of the included studies by means of the risk of bias (ROB) tool in the Cochrane Handbook for Systematic Reviews of Interventions (Version 5.0.2). This instrument consists of 8

domains: random sequence generation; allocation concealment; blinding of patients, personnel, and outcome assessors; incomplete outcome data; selective outcome reporting; and other sources of bias. The tool ranks evidence from research studies as having "high," "low," or "unclear" levels of bias; it is also appropriate for evaluating the methodological quality of RCTs. In cases in which the reviewers' opinions differed, a joint opinion was reached through discussion.

Statistical analysis

All statistical analyses were performed with Reviewer Manager Software, version 5.3 (Cochrane Collaboration, Oxford, UK). Summary estimates of treatment effects were calculated using a random-effects model. The impact of acupuncture on dichotomous data was expressed as the risk ratio (RR); for continuous outcomes, the mean difference was calculated with a 95 % confidence interval (CI). The statistical heterogeneity in the subgroups was analyzed using the I^2 test and was considered to be significant when I^2 was greater than 50 %. Even when a low heterogeneity was detected, a random-effects model was applied, because the validity of tests of heterogeneity can be limited with a small number of component studies. Publication bias was detected using a funnel plot.

Results

Study description

We identified 165 publications; 13 met the eligibility criteria (Fig. 1). The articles included in the analysis are summarized in Table 1. The 13 articles were published from 2004 to 2012. Two originated in Korea [20, 21] and 11 were from China [8, 22–31]. The language of publication was English [20, 21] or Chinese [8, 22–31].

Study quality

The ROB results are shown in Table 2. With regards to random sequence generation and allocation concealment,

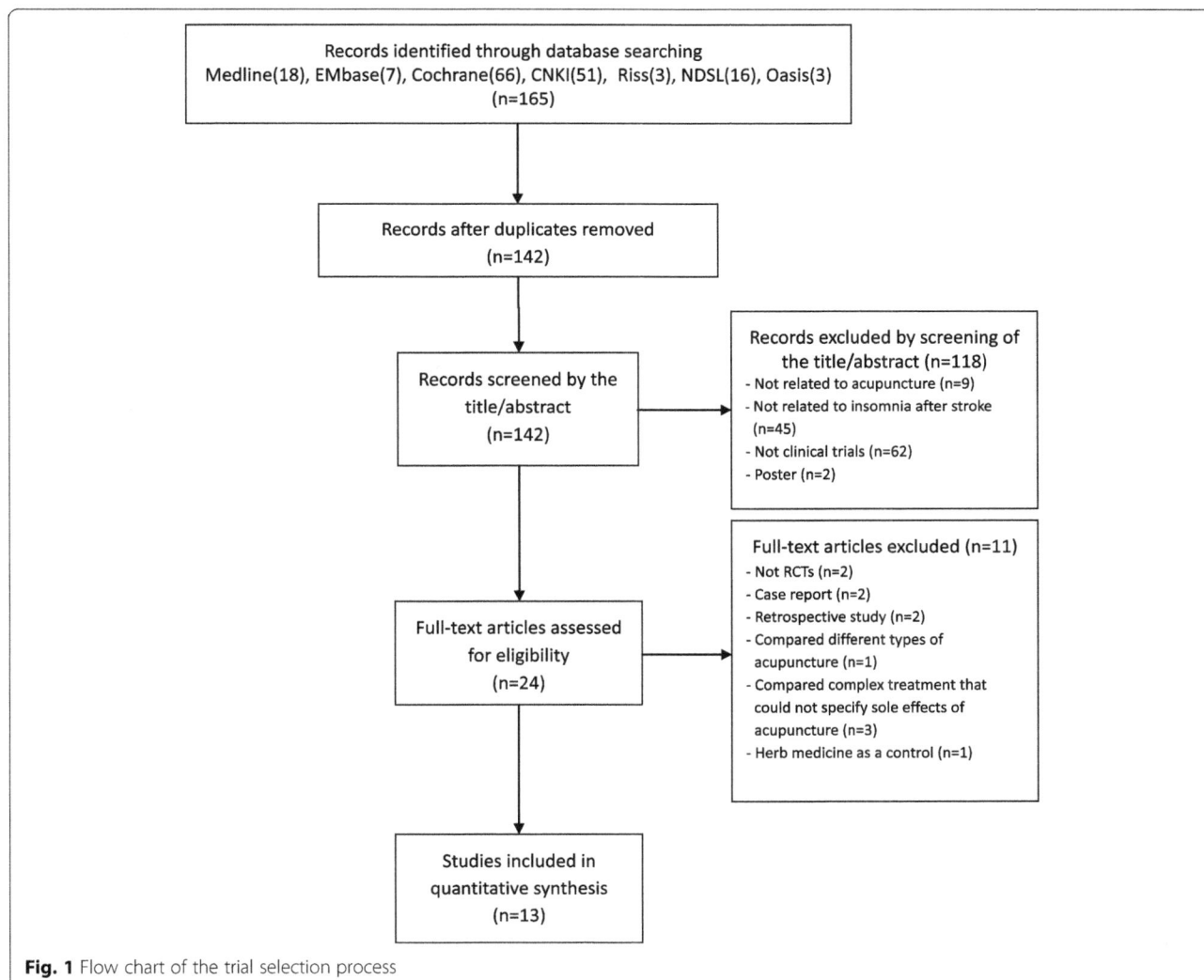

Fig. 1 Flow chart of the trial selection process

Table 1 Summary of randomized controlled trials of acupuncture for insomnia after stroke

Author (year) Country	Sample Size	Participants: Average age (years)	Sex (male/female)	Severity of insomnia	Time since stroke	Intervention Group Regimen	Control group regimen	Main outcomes	Results
Ye 2013 [22]	85	(a) 62.8 ± 7.2 (b) 67.3 ± 8.3	(a) 23/20 (b) 20/22	(a) n.r. (b) n.r.	(a) 15.9 ± 3.5 days (b) 14.17 ± 2.9 days	(a) AT (n = 43) (GV-20, EX-HN3, EX-HN1, HT-7, EX/ 5 times a week for 4 weeks, 30 min)	(b) Drugs (n = 42) (Alprazolam 0.4 mg once a day for 4 weeks)	(1) PSQI (2) Efficacy standards of Chinese medicine	(1) Significant differences in PSQI scores ($P < 0.05$) (2) Significant differences in Effective rates ($P < 0.01$)
Li 2012 [23]	300	(a) 49.2 (b) 51.3	(a) 79/71 (b) 77/73	(a) n.r. (b) n.r.	(a) n.r. (b) n.r.	(a) AT + Drugs (n = 150) (BL-62, KI-6, HT-7/ once a day for 10 days, 30 min)	(b) Drugs (n = 150) (Estazolam 0.5 mg once a day for 10 days)	(1) Efficacy standards of Chinese medicine	(1) Significant differences in Effective rates ($P < 0.05$)
Huang 2012 [24]	84	(a) n.r. (b) n.r.	(a) n.r. (b) n.r.	(a) n.r. (b) n.r.	(a) n.r. (b) n.r.	(a) AT (n = 42) (GV-20, EX-HN1, Auricular Shenmen, EX-HN3, EX, KI-6, BL-62/ 6 times a week for 2 weeks, 30 min)	(b) Drugs (n = 42) (Estazolam 2 mg 4–7 times a day for 2 weeks)	(1) Efficacy standards of Chinese medicine	(1) Significant differences in Effective rates ($P < 0.05$)
Wu 2012 [25]	80	(a) 67.6 ± 10.4 (b) 66.2 ± 9.6	(a) 20/20 (b) 18/22	(a) n.r. (b) n.r.	(a) n.r. (b) n.r.	(a) AA (n = 40) (Auricular Shenmen, heart, kidney, subcortex, internal ear/ 4–5 times a day for 10 days)	(b) Drugs (n = 40) (Estazolam 2 mg once a day for 10 days)	(1) Efficacy standards of Chinese medicine	(1) Significant differences in Effective rates ($P < 0.01$)
Huang 2011 [26]	60	(a) 66 (b) 67	(a) 11/19 (b) 13/17	(a) AIS > 6 (b) AIS > 6	(a) n.r. (b) n.r.	(a) AT + Drugs (n = 30) (GV-20, EX-HN1, SP-6, BL-23, HT-7, EX/ once a day for 14 days, 30 min)	(b) Drugs (n = 30) (Bailemianjiaonang 0.27 g × 4 capsules twice a day for 20 days)	(1) PSQI	(1) Significant differences in PSQI scores ($P < 0.01$)
Sun 2011 [27]	60	(a) 40 ± 15 (b) 40 ± 15	(a) 14/16 (b) 15/15	(a) PSQI 13.31 ± 2.4 (b) PSQI 12.09 ± 3.1	(a) 4.0 ± 2.6 years (b) 3.9 ± 2.8 years	(a) AT + AA (n = 30) (**AT**: GV-20, HT-7, SP-6, GB-20, EX-HN5, EX-HN1, EX/ once a day for 20 days, 30 min); **AA**: HT-7, sympathetic/ twice a day for 20 days, 15~20 min)	(b) Drugs (n = 30) (Estazolam 2 mg once a day for 20 days)	(1) PSQI (2) Efficacy standards of Chinese medicine	(1) Significant differences in PSQI scores ($P < 0.05$) (2) Significant differences in Effective rates ($P < 0.05$)
Ye 2010 [28]	60	(a) 61.5 ± 3.7 (b) 62.4 ± 4.9	(a) 16/14 (b) 17/13	(a) n.r. (b) n.r.	(a) n.r. (b) n.r.	(a) AT (n = 30) (GV-24, GV-20, GV-16, GV-11, EX-HN1/ 6 times a week for 4 weeks, 30 min)	(b) Drugs (n = 30) (Diazepam 5.0 mg once a day for 4 weeks)	(1) Efficacy standards of Chinese medicine	(1) Significant differences in Effective rates ($P < 0.01$)

Table 1 Summary of randomized controlled trials of acupuncture for insomnia after stroke (*Continued*)

Study	n	Age	Sex (M/F)	Baseline	Duration	Intervention (a)	Control (b)	Outcomes	Results
Lee 2009 [20]	52	(a) 66.7 ± 11.0 (b) 66.0 ± 9.6	(a) 12/15 (b) 12/13	(a) ISI 18.4 ± 2.7, AIS 15.8 ± 2.4 (b) ISI 18.1 ± 2.6, AIS 14.9 ± 2.2	(a) n.r. (b) n.r.	(a) IA (n = 27) (He7, EH6/ once a day for 3 days)	(b) Sham AT (n = 25)	(1) ISI (2) AIS	(1) Significant differences in ISI scores ($P < 0.01$) (2) Significant differences in AIS scores ($P < 0.01$)
Lu 2008 [29]	50	(a) 61.48 ± 3.72 (b) 62.40 ± 4.88	(a) 14/11 (b) 15/10	(a) PSQI 16.64 ± 2.3 (b) PSQI 17.28 ± 2	(a) 0.3 ~ 1 years (b) 0.3 ~ 1 years	(a) AT (n = 25) (GV-24, GV-20, GV-16, GV-11, BL-23, KI-3, HT-7, PC-6/ 6 days a week for 4 weeks, 30 min)	(b) Drugs (n = 25) (Diazepam 5.0 mg once a day for 4 weeks)	(1) PSQI	(1) Significant differences in PSQI scores ($P < 0.05$)
Li 2007 [8]	64	(a) 69.8 ± 7.1 (b) 67.3 ± 8.3	(a) 18/14 (b) 17/15	(a) n.r. (b) n.r.	(a) n.r. (b) n.r.	(a) AT + AA (n = 32) (**AT:** HT-7, SP-6, GV-24, EX-HN1, PC-6, LR-3, KI-3; **AA:** Auricular Shenmen/ 6 days a week for 4 weeks, 20–30 min)	(b) Drugs (n = 32) (Diazepam 2.5 mg or estazolam 1 mg once a day for 4 weeks)	(1) PSQI (2) Efficacy standards of Chinese medicine	(1) Significant differences in PSQI scores ($P < 0.05$) (2) Significant differences in Effective rates ($P < 0.05$)
Liu 2006 [30]	62	(a) 69.9 ± 6.9 (b) 67.5 ± 8.2	(a) 15/17 (b) 15/15	(a) n.r. (b) n.r.	(a) n.r. (b) n.r.	(a) AT (n = 32) (HT-7, SP-6, GV-24, EX-HN1, PC-6, LR-3, KI-3, ST-36/ 5 days a week for 4 weeks, 30 min)	(b) Drugs (n = 30) (Diazepam 2.5 mg or estazolam 1 mg once a day for 4 weeks)	(1) PSQI	(1) Significant differences in PSQI scores ($P < 0.05$)
Kim 2004 [21]	30	(a) 65.1 ± 9.0 (b) 68.3 ± 10.4	(a) 8/7 (b) 9/6	(a) ISI 21.9 ± 2.0, AIS 17.1 ± 1.6 (b) ISI 22.3 ± 2.1, AIS 17.7 ± 2.5	(a) n.r. (b) n.r.	(a) IA (n = 15) (He7, EH6/ once a day for 3 days)	(b) Sham AT (n = 15)	(1) ISI (2) AIS	(1) Significant differences in ISI scores ($P < 0.01$) (2) Significant differences in AIS scores ($P < 0.01$)
Wang 2004 [31]	64	(a) 42.5 ~ 70.5 (b) 41 ~ 70	(a) 22/12 (b) 17/13	(a) n.r. (b) n.r.	(a) n.r. (b) n.r.	(a) EA + AA (n = 34) (**EA:** HT-7, PC-6, CV-12, ST-36, KI-3; **AA:** Auricular Shenmen/ 5 times a week for 4 weeks, 20–30 min, 40 Hz)	(b) Drugs (n = 30) (Diazepam 2.5 mg or clozapine 25 mg once a day for 4 weeks)	(1) PSQI (2) Efficacy standards of Chinese medicine	(1) Significant differences in PSQI scores ($P < 0.01$) (2) Significant differences in Effective rates ($P < 0.01$)

Notes. AA auricular acupuncture, AIS Athens insomnia sale, AT acupuncture therapy, EA electro-acupuncture, IA intradermal acupuncture, ISI insomnia severity index, n.r. not reported, PSQI Pittsburgh sleep quality index. Adverse effects were not reported for any study

Table 2 Risk of bias of the studies included in the present review

	Ye 2013 [22]	Li 2012 [23]	Huang 2012 [24]	Wu 2012 [25]	Huang 2011 [26]	Sun 2011 [27]	Ye 2010 [28]	Lee 2009 [20]	Lu 2008 [29]	Li 2007 [8]	Liu 2006 [30]	Kim 2004 [21]	Wang 2004 [31]
1. Was the method of randomization adequate?	U	U	U	U	U	L	L	L	L	L	L	L	L
2. Was the treatment allocation concealed?	U	U	U	U	U	L	L	L	L	L	L	U	L
3. Was the patient blinded to the intervention?	U	U	U	U	U	U	U	L	U	U	U	U	U
4. Were the personnel blinded to the intervention?	U	U	U	U	U	U	U	U	U	U	U	U	U
5. Was the outcome assessor blinded to the intervention?	U	U	U	U	U	U	U	L	L	U	U	U	U
6. Were incomplete outcome data adequately addressed?	L	L	L	L	L	L	L	L	L	L	L	L	L
7. Are reports of the study free of suggestion of selective outcome reporting?	L	L	L	L	L	L	L	L	L	L	L	L	L
8. Was the study apparently free of other problems that could put it at a high risk of bias?	U	U	U	U	U	U	U	U	U	U	U	U	U

Notes. Based on the risk of bias assessment tool from the Cochrane handbook for systematic reviews of interventions, high risk of bias: H, low risk of bias: L, uncertain risk of bias: U

five studies had a low ROB [27–31] and eight studies had an unclear ROB [8, 20–26]. With regards to blinding of patients and outcome assessors, two studies had a low ROB [20, 21], and 11 studies had an unclear ROB [8, 22–31]. All RCTs had a low ROB in incomplete outcome data and selective outcome reporting [8, 20–31]. All RCTs had an unclear ROB in other sources of bias [8, 20–31].

Descriptions of acupuncture treatment

The majority of the included RCTs stated that the rationale for acupuncture point selection was drawn from Traditional Chinese Medicine theory. Two studies used intradermal acupuncture [20, 21], five used acupuncture alone [22, 24, 28–30], two used acupuncture and auricular acupuncture [8, 27], two used acupuncture and drugs [23, 26], one used auricular acupuncture [25], and one used electroacupuncture and auricular acupuncture [31]. A total of 33 acupuncture points (24 meridian points and nine auricular acupuncture points) were used for the treatment of insomnia. Acupoints used for insomnia treatment in most trials were Shenmen (HT-7) and Sishencong (EX-HN1) (Fig. 2). The number of acupoints used in each study ranged from two to 11.

Effects of acupuncture treatment according to PSQI assessment scales

We conducted a meta-analysis of the study results based on the insomnia assessment scales used (Fig. 3). In six studies that used the PSQI to assess treatment results, acupuncture appeared to be more effective than drugs for treatment of insomnia after stroke (weighted mean difference, 4.31; 95 % CI, 1.67–6.95; $P = 0.001$; $n = 385$, $I^2 = 91$ %).

Effects of acupuncture treatment according to the efficacy standards of Chinese medicine

In seven studies that used the efficacy standards of Chinese medicine to compare the effects of acupuncture with those of drugs, acupuncture was observed to have a significant difference in reducing insomnia after stroke (RR, 1.25; 95 % CI, 1.12–1.40; $P < 0.001$; n = 497, $I^2 = 54$ %).

Effects of intradermal acupuncture according to ISI or AIS assessment scales

Studies comparing the effects of intradermal acupuncture with those of sham acupuncture used the ISI or the AIS. In these studies, intradermal acupuncture had a significant difference on insomnia after stroke, as assessed both by the ISI (weighted mean difference, 4.44; 95 % CI, 2.75–6.13; $P < 0.001$; n = 82, $I^2 = 9$ %) and by the AIS (weighted mean difference, 3.64; 95 % CI, 2.28–5.00; $P < 0.001$; n = 82, $I^2 = 0$ %).

Publication bias

We assessed the publication bias using a funnel plot. However, it was difficult to determine any pattern indicative of publication bias based on the funnel plot's symmetry owing to the small sample size (fewer than 10 studies, Additional file 1: Figure S1).

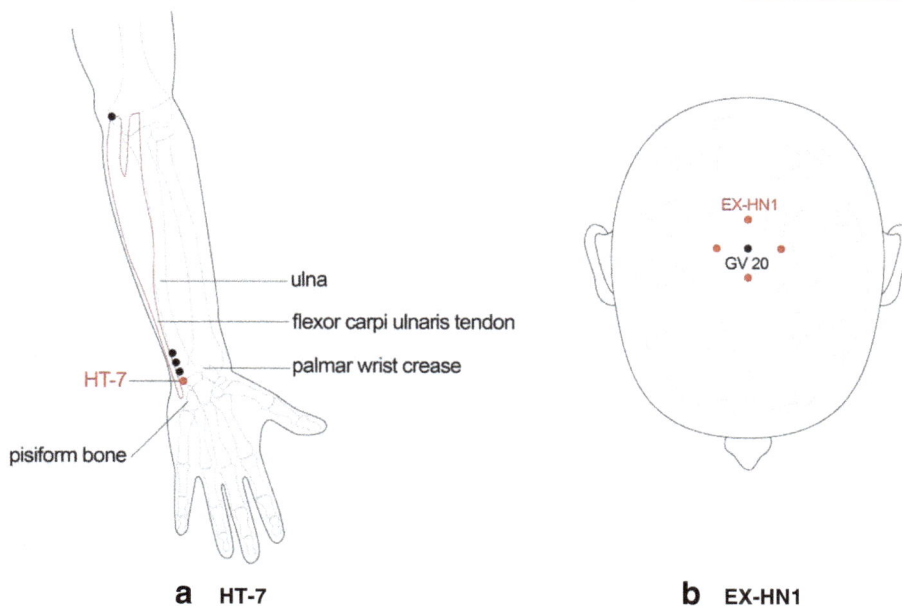

Fig. 2 Location of Shenmen (HT-7) and Sishenchong (EX-HN1) acupoints. HT-7 is located in the depression radial to the proximal border of the pisiform bone on the palmar wrist crease. EX-HN1 is a group of four acupoints on the vertex of the head located 1 cun posterior, anterior and lateral to GV 20

1. Pittsburgh sleep quality index

Study or Subgroup	AT Mean	SD	Total	Drugs Mean	SD	Total	Weight	Mean Difference IV, Random, 95% CI
Li(2007)	11.97	4.3	32	9.31	4.5	32	16.5%	2.66 [0.50, 4.82]
Liu(2006)	13.18	4.77	32	7.21	5.3	30	15.8%	5.97 [3.45, 8.49]
Lu(2008)	9.2	2.89	25	0.72	2.18	25	17.6%	8.48 [7.06, 9.90]
Sun(2011)	7.27	3.13	30	5.97	3.31	30	17.3%	1.30 [-0.33, 2.93]
Wang(2004)	13.42	4.73	34	7.94	5.74	30	15.7%	5.48 [2.88, 8.08]
Ye(2013)	6.67	4.33	43	4.62	3.5	42	17.2%	2.05 [0.38, 3.72]
Total (95% CI)			**196**			**189**	**100.0%**	**4.31 [1.67, 6.95]**

Heterogeneity: Tau² = 9.81; Chi² = 57.89, df = 5 (P < 0.00001); I² = 91%
Test for overall effect: Z = 3.20 (P = 0.001)

2. The efficacy standards of Chinese medicine

Study or Subgroup	AT Events	Total	Drugs Events	Total	Weight	Risk Ratio M-H, Random, 95% CI
Huang(2012)	40	42	38	42	21.2%	1.05 [0.93, 1.19]
Li(2007)	31	32	26	32	16.5%	1.19 [1.00, 1.42]
Sun(2011)	29	30	22	30	13.2%	1.32 [1.05, 1.65]
Wang(2004)	33	34	22	30	13.3%	1.32 [1.06, 1.66]
Wu(2012)	37	40	27	40	12.8%	1.37 [1.09, 1.73]
Ye(2010)	39	43	31	42	14.6%	1.23 [1.00, 1.51]
Ye(2013)	28	30	17	30	8.4%	1.65 [1.19, 2.28]
Total (95% CI)		**251**		**246**	**100.0%**	**1.25 [1.12, 1.40]**
Total events	237		183			

Heterogeneity: Tau² = 0.01; Chi² = 13.14, df = 6 (P = 0.04); I² = 54%
Test for overall effect: Z = 3.90 (P < 0.0001)

3. The Insomnia severity index and the Athens insomnia scale

Study or Subgroup	IA Mean	SD	Total	Sham AT Mean	SD	Total	Weight	Mean Difference IV, Random, 95% CI
ISI								
Lee(2009)	5.4	4	27	1.6	3.2	25	64.4%	3.80 [1.84, 5.76]
Kim(2004)	7	4.71	15	1.4	2.62	15	35.6%	5.60 [2.87, 8.33]
Subtotal (95% CI)			**42**			**40**	**100.0%**	**4.44 [2.75, 6.13]**

Heterogeneity: Tau² = 0.15; Chi² = 1.10, df = 1 (P = 0.29); I² = 9%
Test for overall effect: Z = 5.15 (P < 0.00001)

	IA Mean	SD	Total	Sham AT Mean	SD	Total	Weight	Mean Difference IV, Random, 95% CI
AIS								
Lee(2009)	4.6	3.3	27	1.2	2.4	25	76.2%	3.40 [1.84, 4.96]
Kim(2004)	6.5	4.46	15	2.1	3.26	15	23.8%	4.40 [1.60, 7.20]
Subtotal (95% CI)			**42**			**40**	**100.0%**	**3.64 [2.28, 5.00]**

Heterogeneity: Tau² = 0.00; Chi² = 0.37, df = 1 (P = 0.54); I² = 0%
Test for overall effect: Z = 5.23 (P < 0.00001)

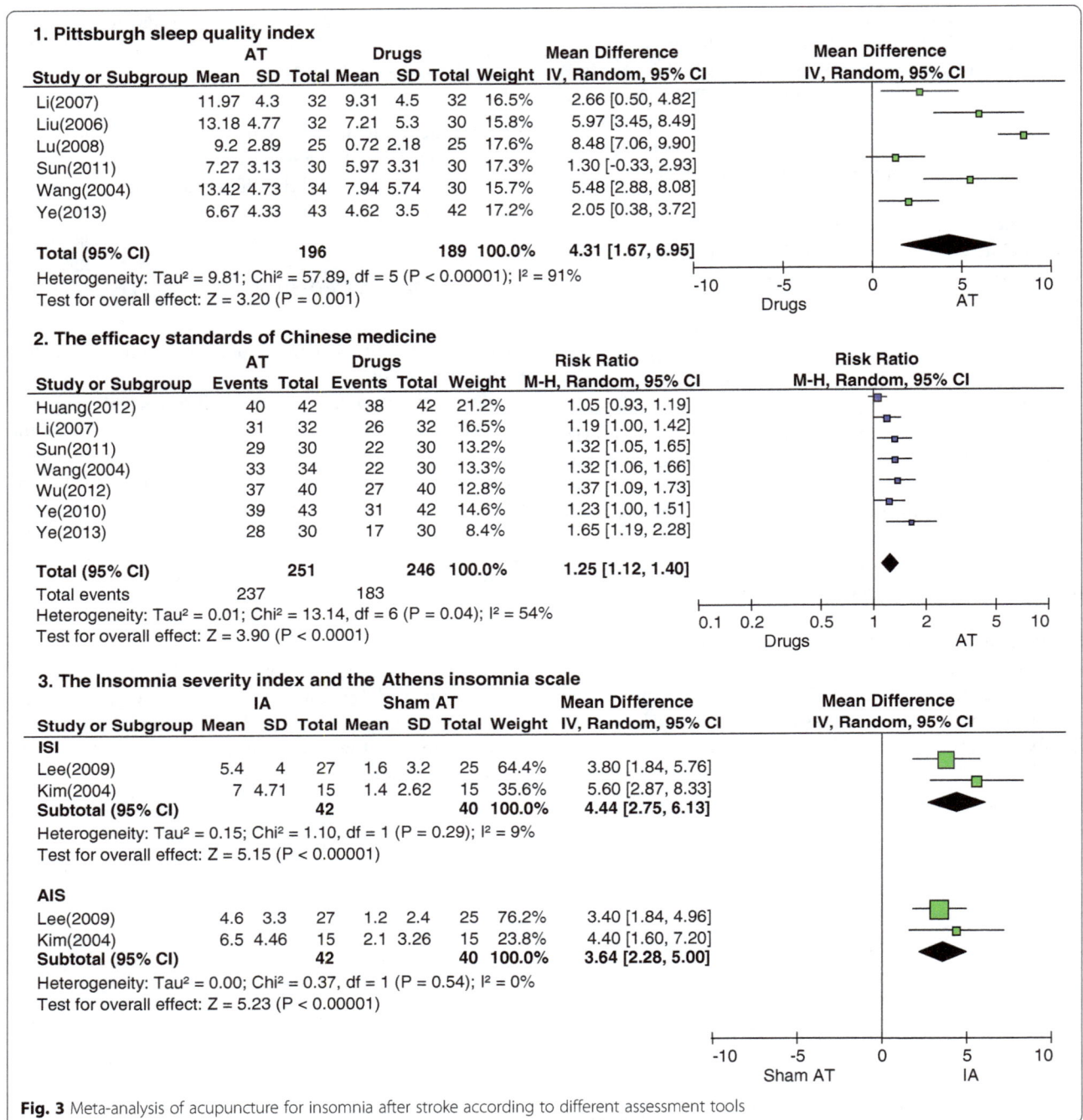

Fig. 3 Meta-analysis of acupuncture for insomnia after stroke according to different assessment tools

Discussion

The present review suggested that compared to drug treatment, acupuncture might be an effective treatment for insomnia after stroke, and that compared to sham treatment, intradermal acupuncture might have significant effects on insomnia after stroke.

Insomnia is a common complication following stroke, often interfering with activity, recovery, and rehabilitation [32]. Sleep problems have both immediate and long-term health effects. The immediate effects of sleep disturbances include well-being, daytime sleepiness, fatigue, and impaired performance, with their resulting impact on safety [33]. Long-term health effects include hypertension, inflammation, obesity, and glucose intolerance. These long-term effects can lead to chronic diseases and premature death [34]. Additionally, a strong relationship has been found between sleep disturbances and cognitive functioning, regulation of emotions, social problems, and substance abuse [35].

Zhao [12] documented that the clinical efficacy of acupuncture appeared to be supported by evidence obtained from basic neuroendocrinological studies. The evidence has suggested that the clinical efficacy of acupuncture in the treatment of insomnia is potentially mediated by a variety of neurotransmitters, including norepinephrine, melatonin, gamma-aminobutyric acid, and beta-endorphin. Huang [14] reviewed not only clinical trials but also case series and demonstrated that acupuncture is potentially beneficial for the treatment of insomnia. Cheuk [15] reported that acupuncture, when used as an adjunct to other treatments, improved sleep quality as compared with other treatments used alone in a population of patients with diverse medical conditions.

The current review offered significant perspectives. First, we aimed to identify all studies on this topic. There were no restrictions on the review publication language, and a large number of databases were searched. We are therefore confident that our search strategy located all relevant data on the subject. Second, the outcome measures including the PSQI, the efficacy standards of Chinese medicine, the ISI, and the AIS were widely used in practice for the measurements of sleep quality [36]. Significant differences were found between acupuncture treatment and drugs or sham treatment in all of the included assessment tools.

This review also had certain limitations. The scarcity of studies and the methodologically low to moderate quality of the primary data preclude us from drawing confirmative conclusions. The high I^2 values were probably because of substantial clinical and methodological variations. Most of the included studies had an unclear risk of bias for blinding, random sequence generation, and allocation concealment; therefore, a preponderance of positive results was observed. Although blinding of the therapists who perform acupuncture would be difficult, blinding of patients, other care providers, and outcome assessors should be attempted in order to minimize the performance and assessment bias of trials.

Therefore, we recommended that any future trial evaluating the effectiveness of acupuncture should have a well-designed protocol in place prior to the trial's initiation, which is appropriate to properly answer the research questions. Of the many important aspects of improving the quality of trial design, it is critical for any future studies to provide sufficient information about blinding, random sequence generation, and allocation concealment in order to clarify the risk of bias.

Future trials should address the methodological issues through rigorous trial designs, reasonable appraisals, and critical analyses to allow more robust conclusions regarding each treatment's effectiveness for relieving insomnia after stroke. Future researchers should follow not only the basic guidelines for reporting clinical trials,

such as the CONSORT statement, but also the STRICTA recommendations, which provide specific guidelines for reporting acupuncture trials [37, 38]. A large-scale study of multicenter trial is recommended. Long-term follow-up studies are needed to determine the efficacy and safety of treatments for insomnia after stroke and to assess their long-term effects. Moreover, a cost analysis should be considered.

Conclusions

The results of this study suggested that acupuncture could be effective in relieving insomnia after stroke. Further studies using large samples and a rigorous study design are needed to confirm the role of acupuncture in the treatment of insomnia after stroke.

Appendix
Search strings used for databases
MEDLINE

1. "stroke" OR "apoplexy" OR "cva" OR "cerebrovascular attack" OR "cerebrovascular accident" OR "cerebral infarction" OR "cerebral hemorrhage" 239,345
2. "acupunct" OR "acupress" OR "acupoints" OR "electroacupunct" OR "electro-acupunct" OR "auriculotherapy" OR "auriculoacupunct" 21,349
3. "insomnia" OR "sleep initiation and maintenance disorder" OR "sleep" OR "wakefulness" 142,430
4. 1 AND 2 AND 3 18

EMBASE

1. 'stroke'/exp OR stroke OR 'apoplexy'/exp OR apoplexy OR 'cva'/exp OR cva OR cerebrovascular AND attack OR cerebrovascular AND ('accident' /exp OR accident) OR cerebral AND ('infarction'/exp OR infarction) OR cerebral AND ('hemorrhage'/exp OR hemorrhage) 42,950
2. acupunct OR acupress OR acupoints OR electroacupunct OR 'electro acupunct' OR 'auriculotherapy' /exp OR auriculotherapy OR auriculoacupunct 36072
3. insomnia OR sleep AND initiation AND maintenance AND disorder OR sleep OR wakefulness 248,699
4. #1 AND #2 AND #3 7

Cochrane

1. stroke OR apoplexy OR cva OR cerebrovascular attack OR cerebrovascular accident OR cerebral infarction OR cerebral hemorrhage 36368
2. acupunct or acupress or acupoints or electroacupunct or electro-acupunct or auriculotherapy or auriculoacupunct 9101

3. insomnia or sleep initiation and maintenance disorder or sleep or wakefulness 17865
4. #1 AND #2 AND #3 66

CNKI

1. 脑卒中 AND 针 AND 失眠 4
2. 中风 AND 针 AND 失眠 10
3. 脑出血 AND 针 AND 失眠 1
4. stroke AND acupuncture AND insomnia 36

Korean data bases
RISS

1. stroke AND acupuncture AND insomnia 3
2. 뇌졸중 AND 침 AND 불면 0

NDSL

1. stroke AND acupuncture AND insomnia 16
2. 뇌졸중 AND 침 AND 불면 0

OASIS

1. stroke AND acupuncture AND insomnia 3
2. 뇌졸중 AND 침 AND 불면 1

Acknowledgements
This research was supported by a grant of the development of Korean medicine industry (Monitoring center for Korean medicine and Western medicine collaboration) by Ministry of Health & Welfare. Also this research was supported by a grant (12-D-02) from the Korea National Rehabilitation Center.

Authors' contributions
SHL and SML developed the study concept and design, performed data acquisition and analysis, and drafted the manuscript. Both authors read and approved the final manuscript for submission.

Competing interests
The authors declare that they have no competing interests.

References
1. Mozaffarian D, Benjamin EJ, Go AS, et al. Heart disease and stroke statistics-2015 update: a report from the American Heart Association. Circulation. 2015;131(4):e29–322.
2. Kim J, Choi KS. Poststroke depression and emotional incontinence: Correlation with lesion location. Neurology. 2000;54:1805–10.
3. Leppavuouri A, Pohjasvaara T, Kaste M, et al. Insomnia in ischemic stroke patients. Cerebrovasc Dis. 2002;14:90–7.
4. Pearce SC, Stolwyk RJ, New PW, et al. Sleep disturbance and deficits of sustained attention following stroke. J Clin Exp Neuropsychol. 2016;38(1):1–11.
5. Hohagen F, Rink K, Scharamm E, et al. Prevalence and treatment of insomnia in general practice. A longitudinal study. Eur Arch Psychiatry Clin Neurosci. 1993;242:329–36.
6. Palomaki HA, Berg E, Meririnne MK, et al. Complaints of post stroke insomnia and its treatment with Mianserin. Cerebrovasc Dis. 2003;15(1–2):56–62.
7. Hermann DM, Siccoli M, Brugger P, et al. Evolution of neurological, neuropsychological and sleep-wake disturbances after paramedian thalamic stroke. Stroke. 2008;39:62–8.
8. Li TB. Effect of Acupuncture on Poststroke Insomnia. Chin J Rehabil Theory Pract. 2007;13(7):656–7.
9. Schuiling WJ, Rinkel GJ, Walchenbach R, et al. Disorders of sleep and wake in patients after subarachoid hemorrhage. Stroke. 2005;3(6):578–82.
10. Jacob TC, Michels G, Silayeva L, et al. Benzodiazepine treatment induces subtype-specific changes in GABA(A) receptor trafficking and decreases synaptic inhibition. Proc Natl Acad Sci U S A. 2012;109(45):18595–600.
11. Shah SH, Engelhardt R, Ovbiagele B. Patterns of complementary and alternative medicine use among United States stroke survivors. J Neuro Sci. 2008;271:180–5.
12. Zhao KC. Acupuncture for the Treatment of Insomnia. Int Rev Neurobiol. 2013;111:217–34.
13. Yao HF, Zhang HF, Chen XL. Observation on therapeutic effect of scalpacupoint catgut embedding for 33 cases of insomnia patients. Zhen Ci Yan Jiu. 2012;37(5):394–7.
14. Huang W, Kutner N, Bliwise DL. A systematic review of the effects of acupuncture in treating insomnia. Sleep Med Rev. 2009;13:73–104.
15. Cheuk DKL, Yeung WF, Chung KF, et al. Acupuncture for insomnia (Review). Cochrane Libr. 2012;9:1–181.
16. Buysse DJ, Reynolds CF, Monk TH, et al. The Pittsburgh Sleep Quality Index: a new instrument for psychiatric practice and research. Psychiatry Res. 1989; 28(2):193–213.
17. Bastien CH, Vallières A, Morin CM. Validation of the Insomnia Severity Index as an outcome measure for insomnia research. Sleep Med. 2001;2(4):297–307.
18. Soldatos CR, Dikeos DG, Paparrigopoulos TJ. Athens Insomnia Scale: validation of an instrument based on ICD-10 criteria. J Psychosom Res. 2000; 48(6):555–60.
19. Higgins J, Green S, Cochrane Handbook for Systematic Reviews of Interventions [updated March 2008]. The Cochrane collaboration and John Wiley & Sons Ltd. 2008; 171–7, 485–8
20. Lee SY, Baek YH, Park SU, et al. Intradermal acupuncture on shen-men and nei-kuan acupoints improves insomnia in stroke patients by reducing the sympathetic nervous activity: a randomized clinical trial. Am J Chin Med. 2009;37(6):1013–21.
21. Kim YS, Lee SH, Jung WS, et al. Intradermal acupuncture on shen-men and nei-kuan acupoints in patients with insomnia after stroke. Am J Chin Med. 2004;32(5):771–8.
22. Ye CH, Ou CD, Xu ZJ, et al. Clinical observation on acupuncture treatment of post-stroke insomnia. Chinese J New Clin Med. 2013;6(7):665–7.
23. Li G, Zhang Y, Luo HQ. Effect of acupuncture combined with estazolam therapy of poststroke insomnia. Med J Nat Defending Forces SW Chin. 2012; 22(6):641–2.
24. Huang M, Gao SH. Effect of acupuncture on poststroke patients with sleep disorders. J Clin Acu mox. 2012;28(10):15–6.
25. Wu XL, Chen Q, Liu CX. Clinical effect of ear acupuncture in syndrome differentiation-based treatment of insomnia after stroke: an analysis of 40 cases. J Anhui Tradit Chin Med. 2012;31(5):45–6.
26. Huang JM, Wang KH. Clinical Effect of combined acupuncture with medicine on poststroke insomnia of 30 cases. Shaanxi J Tradit Chin Med. 2011;32(9):1227–8.
27. Sun YZ, Xia KP. Acupuncture plus auricular point sticking for treating post-stroke insomnia. Shanghai J Acu-mox. 2011;30(6):363–5.
28. Ye FW, Xu YL, Chen JW, et al. Clinical effect of Baihui acupuncture treatment on poststroke insomnia of 30 cases. Pract Clin J Inte Tradit Chin & W Med. 2010;10(5):21.
29. Lu YY, Li ZZ, Ye FW. Clinical observation on treatment of poststroke insomnia of 25 cases by kidney-reinforcing and Du channel-regulating acupuncture method. Jiangsu J Tradit Chin Med. 2008;40(7):59–61.
30. Liu JH, Huang JH, Chen XH. Effect of acupuncture on poststroke insomnia of 32 cases. Int Med Health Guid News. 2006;15:107–9.
31. Wang Y, Zhao ZF, Wu Y, et al. Clinical therapeutic effect of acupuncture on poststroke depression with insomnia. Chin Acu mox. 2004;24(9):603–6.
32. Ferrie JE, Kumari M, Salo P, et al. Sleep epidemiology-a rapidly growing field. Int J Epidemiol. 2011;40:1431 7.
33. Lillehei AS, Halcon LL. A systematic review of the effect of inhaled Essential oils on sleep. J Altern Complement Med. 2014;20(6):441–51.
34. Harvey RC, Bruce M. Sleep disorders and sleep deprivation. Committee on Sleep Medicine and Research. 2006. p. 75–9.
35. Bootzin RR, Epstein DR. Understanding and treating insomnia. Annu Rev Clin Psychol. 2011;7:435–58.
36. Sateia MJ, Daniel B. Insomnia: Diagnosis and Treatment. Informa healthcare. 2010. p. 90–2.
37. Begg C, Cho M, Eastwood S, et al. Improving the quality of reporting of randomized controlled trials. The CONSORT statement. JAMA. 1996;276(8): 637–9.

7

Change in the P300 index – a pilot randomized controlled trial of low-frequency electrical stimulation of acupuncture points in middle-aged men and women

Kwang-Ho Choi, O Sang Kwon, Seong Jin Cho, Sanghun Lee, Seok-Yun Kang and Yeon Hee Ryu[*]

Abstract

Background: The P300 is a major index used to evaluate improvements in brain function. Although a few studies have reported evaluating the effectiveness of manual acupuncture or electro-acupuncture by monitoring the P300, research in this field is not yet very active. The aim of this study was to investigate the effects of periodic low-frequency electrical stimulation applied to BL62 and KI6 on brain activity by analyzing the P300.

Method: The study was conducted as a randomized double-blind test of 55 subjects in their 50s, including 26 males and 29 females. Each subject received 12 sessions of stimulation over a one-month period. In each session, low-frequency electrical stimulation at an average of 24 μA and 2 Hz was applied to the acupuncture points BL62 and KI6, and event-related potentials (ERPs) were measured before the first session and after the last session of the electrical stimulation.

Results: The results of a chi-square test indicated that the double-blind test was conducted correctly. Compared to the Sham group, all the subjects in the Real stimulation group showed a tendency toward a decreasing P300 latency and increasing P300 amplitude after all 12 sessions of stimulation. In the women, the amplitude significantly increased at Fz, Fcz, Cz, Cpz, and Pz.

Conclusions: With this experiment, the low-frequency electrical stimulation of two acupuncture points (BL62 and K16) was confirmed to have a positive influence on the prevention of natural cerebral aging.

Trial registration: This study was registered at the Clinical Research Information Service (CRIS) of the National Research Institute of Health (https://cris.nih.go.kr/cris/search/search_result_st01_en.jsp?, Registration Number: KCT0001940). The date of registration was June 9, 2016.

Keywords: Low-frequency electrical stimulation, P300, BL62, KI6, Sex difference, Double-blind

Background

Event-related potentials (ERPs) are evoked potentials observed during electroencephalogram (EEG) measurements immediately after discontinuous sensory stimulation. From ERPs, we can obtain information related to brain activity, such as sensory, cognitive, and motor events. The brain activity information that can be obtained from ERPs includes sensory-evoked components (the P50 and N100) and cognitive-related components (the P300 and N400), one of which, the P300, is a positive potential that appears approximately 300 ms after auditory or visual stimulation [1]. This component was first observed in 1965 by Sutton et al. and was generated when a subject did not recognize the type of stimulation [2]. At present, the peak generated when a subject recognizes an auditory or visual stimulus is called the P3b, and the peak generated by an unexpected distracter is called the P3a. The distinction between the P3a and P3b remains

* Correspondence: yhryu@kiom.re.kr
KM Fundamental Research Division, Korea Institute of Oriental Medicine, 1672 Yuseong-daero, Yuseong-Gu, Daejeon 305-811, South Korea

controversial, and these components have been known to differ depending on task difficulty [3].

The P300 is an important index that is used in clinical fields to evaluate reductions in memory and other cognitive functions and has been known to show decreased amplitude and delayed latency with aging. A decreased amplitude and delayed latency of the P300 indicate a general slowing of cognitive processes due to neurodegeneration or other disease-related causes [4]. To study the mechanism that generates the P300, studies that track the signal source have been conducted, including studies in which information measured on the scalp is used to determine the site of signal generation [5] and those in which generation sites are directly identified by implanting electrodes within the brains of patients with epilepsy [6]. Lesion studies have shown that P300 generation is affected by damage to the temporo-parietal junction, and the inferior parietal lobe, supramarginal gyrus and hippocampus are already known to be very important in P300 induction. However, it is assumed that P300 induction is affected by complex influences in the brain; therefore, the identification of the source of the P300 is still controversial [7].

With the development of medical technology, society is aging. Aging is related to an increase in senile brain disorders, and this increase currently poses an unavoidable problem. According to recent reports, the number of patients with Alzheimer's dementia is expected to reach 13,500,000 by 2050 in the United States alone and will become a major problem around the world over time [8]. Efforts to improve the treatment and prevention of this affliction have been made for many years, and alternative medicine has recently been applied as a measure to supplement traditional treatments. Alternative medicine is widely used with patients suffering from diseases that are considered hopeless by current medical conventions or from chronic diseases that are seldom treated with conventional approaches [9, 10].

Electro-acupuncture (EA), used in alternative medicine, can be a good method to reduce the problem of senile brain disorders in an aging society because EA treatment can be implemented without surgery and is easy to access [11, 12]. Preliminary studies have shown that among the acupuncture points, BL62 and KI6 are effective for insomnia [13] and dementia [14]. Because insomnia is associated with brain disorders such as dementia [15] and cognitive impairment [16], BL62 and KI6 stimuli are likely to treat brain disorders in alternative medicine.

Therefore, this study evaluated the P300, a major index used to assess cognitive function, to investigate the effect of regular, non-invasive electrical stimulation of acupuncture points of the foot on cognitive function. Additionally, based on previous studies indicating that

cognitive function may be different according to gender, sex differences in the observed P300 changes were assessed to confirm the results regarding sex reported in previous ERP experiments [17, 18].

Methods

Subjects

Candidate subjects, who were healthy men and women in their 50s, were recruited through advertisements in the district of Jeonmin-dong, Daejeon-si, South Korea between January and June, 2012. Candidates were screened to ascertain their health status.

Candidates who met all of the following inclusion criteria were enrolled: 1) healthy males and females in their 50s or 60s; 2) individuals who agreed to voluntarily participate in the clinical trial and sign the consent form. Candidates who met any one of the following exclusion criteria were excluded: suffering from 1) an autoimmune disease; 2) an allergic skin disease; 3) a brain disorder; or 4) symptoms that could affect an electromyogram of the head or 5) the neck and face; 6) had major surgery or a critical illness within the past year; 7) had a metal prosthesis implanted in the body; 8) taking or planning to take medication; 9) unable to maintain a sitting position for one hour and thus unsuitable for electrical stimulation therapy; 10) unable to complete a legal document; or 11) unsuitable to participate in the study based on the investigator's judgment. A total of 57 subjects (27 male; 30 female) participated in the study, and the final results were analyzed with the data from 55 subjects (26 male; 29 female) after 2 subjects were excluded (1 male; 1 female). The data of these subjects were considered problematic due to the subject's sleepiness or to the malfunction of the machine (Fig. 1, Table 1).

Low-frequency electrical stimulation

A doctor who was licensed and certified in Korean Oriental Medicine applied non-invasive low-frequency electrical stimulation to the bilateral target acupuncture points BL62 and KI6 through a custom-built band (low-frequency electrical stimulation band, TrekSta, Korea) made of stainless steel, which was worn on the subject's ankle (Fig. 2). The stimulation was generated by a Pulse Generator (PG-306, SUZUKI IRYOKI, Japan) and was applied to each subject for 30 min at a frequency of 2 Hz based on the results of a prior study [14]. The electrical stimulation time was set at 15 min to 30 min for sufficient stimulation. The total amount of electrical stimulation was measured using a Precision Multi-meter (8846A, FLUKE, USA) and recorded (Table 1).

Randomized double-blind test

A total of 60 wires were prepared for the low-frequency electrical stimulation. Half of the wires were assigned to

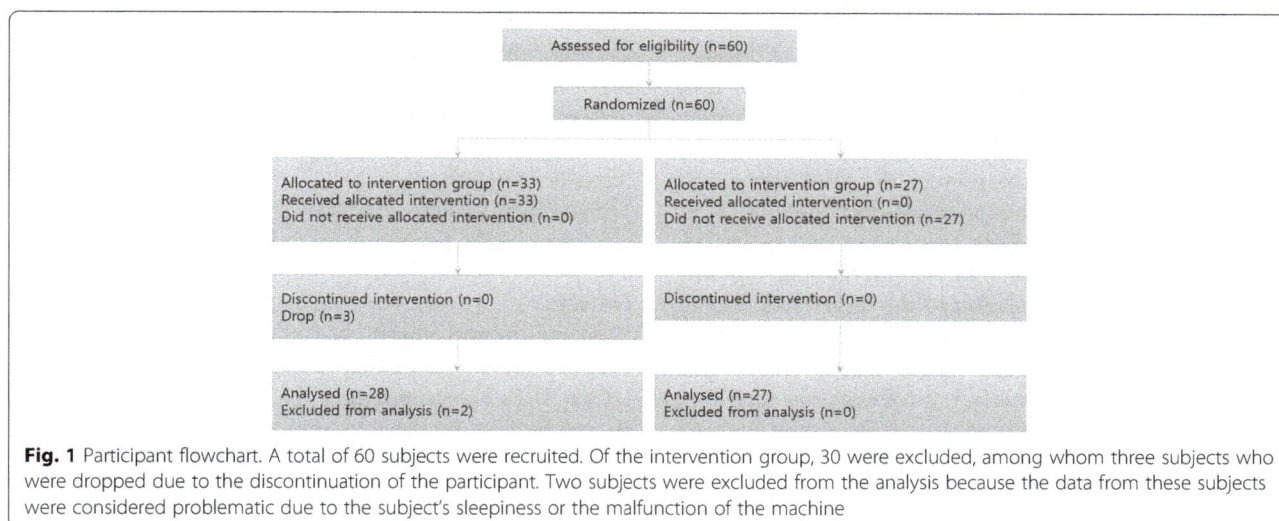

Fig. 1 Participant flowchart. A total of 60 subjects were recruited. Of the intervention group, 30 were excluded, among whom three subjects who were dropped due to the discontinuation of the participant. Two subjects were excluded from the analysis because the data from these subjects were considered problematic due to the subject's sleepiness or the malfunction of the machine

the male group, and the other half were assigned to the female group. Among the 30 wires for each group, 15 were cut prior to applying the same cover that was applied to the other 15 working wires; thus, the subjects could not see which type they were randomly assigned (Fig. 2). Furthermore, to prevent the subjects from feeling the electrical stimulation, the maximum current that could not be perceived by each subject was recorded before the study was initiated, and this maximum imperceptible current was applied to each subject on the predefined acupuncture points three times a week (for a total of 12 times over 4 weeks). Each stimulation lasted for 30 min and used the same current level. Therefore, the study was conducted under double-blind conditions, wherein neither the investigator nor the subject knew whether they gave or received electrical stimulation. The investigator also kept a record of whether the subject felt the electrical stimulation after each treatment.

Electroencephalogram measurement

The EEG was measured using a 32-channel encephalograph, WEEG-32 (LXE3232-RF, LAXTHA, Korea). The results were

collected at a sampling rate of 256 Hz, filtered from 0.7 ~ 47 Hz, and saved on a computer after 16-bit analog-to-digital (AD) conversion. Thirty-two electrodes were attached on the following locations: Fpz, Fp1, Fp2, F7, Ft7, T7, Tp7, P7, F3, Fc3, C3, Cp3, P3, F8, Ft8, T8, Tp8, P8, F4, Fc4, C4, Cp4, P4, Afz, Fz, Fcz, Cz, Cpz, Pz, O1, Oz, and O2 according to the international Modified Combinatorial Nomenclature

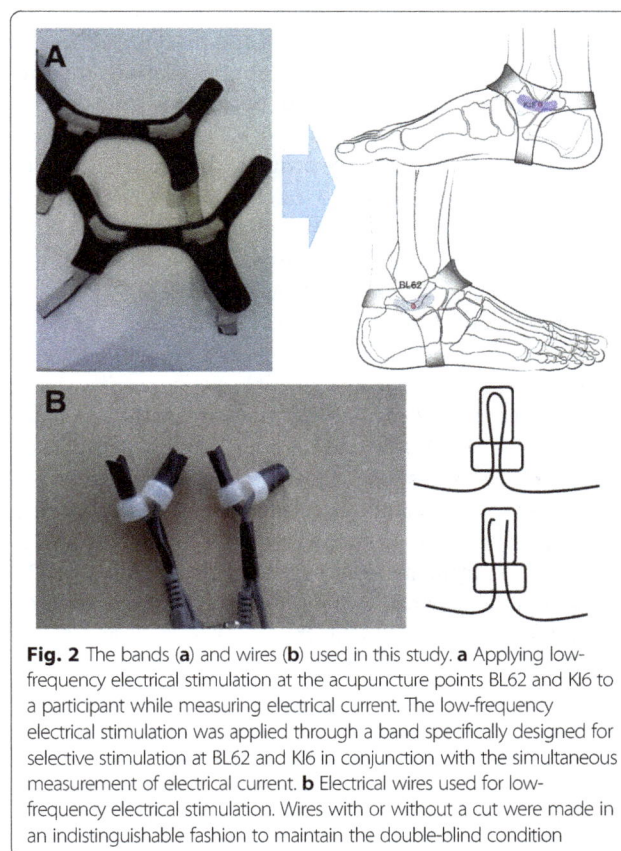

Fig. 2 The bands (**a**) and wires (**b**) used in this study. **a** Applying low-frequency electrical stimulation at the acupuncture points BL62 and KI6 to a participant while measuring electrical current. The low-frequency electrical stimulation was applied through a band specifically designed for selective stimulation at BL62 and KI6 in conjunction with the simultaneous measurement of electrical current. **b** Electrical wires used for low-frequency electrical stimulation. Wires with or without a cut were made in an indistinguishable fashion to maintain the double-blind condition

Table 1 Demographic characteristics of the participants and the average intensity of the electrical stimulation applied

Stimulus	Real		Sham	
Sex	Male	Female	Male	Female
Number of participants	14	14	12	15
Age (Years)	55.14 ± 2.74	53.77 ± 2.71	56.00 ± 2.09	53.73 ± 3.51
Height (Cm)	170.93 ± 5.34	158.64 ± 4.11	170.50 ± 5.02	158.40 ± 4.19
Weight (Kg)	71.79 ± 8.05	57.79 ± 6.99	70.08 ± 9.94	56.93 ± 6.50
Intensity of stimulus (μA)	27.00 ± 13.43	26.15 ± 11.74	21.18 ± 12.29	25.39 ± 11.43

(MCN) system. Control electrodes were placed behind the right ear, and the ground was placed at the back of the neck. The electrodes used in this study were dish-shaped disks covered with gold, and they were attached to the scalp using EEG glue. To make sure they were firmly secured to the surface of the scalp and to prevent the glue from drying quickly, gauze was placed on top of the electrodes.

Background EEG and ERPs were measured before the first treatment and after the last treatment of low-frequency electrical stimulation to the target acupuncture points. Prior to the EEG measurement, the subjects were given 30 min of resting time in a quiet environment where they sat on a chair any physical movement was restricted. First, background EEG was measured for 5 min with the subject's eyes closed. Then, after 10 min of resting time, ERPs were measured for 5 min. During the measurement of the ERPs, standard stimulation and target stimulation were applied at a 3:1 ratio in random order according to the oddball paradigm. The standard stimulation and target stimulation used 1000 Hz and 2000 Hz, respectively. A total of 600 auditory tones (57 dB SPL) were presented to the subjects through a speaker. To help the subjects perceive the target stimuli, the subjects were exposed to each sound prior to the ERP measurement and asked to count the target stimuli in their minds.

Sample size determination

This study was an investigation of the mechanism in the brain of low-frequency electrical stimulation on the ankle; therefore, this study did not follow the general method for calculating sample size. The current study was designed as a pilot to provide the initial data required to perform the power calculation necessary for a large-scale, randomized controlled trial. The sample size of 30 subjects in each group was chosen as the minimum sample size for statistical significance in a univariate analysis considering the subject attrition rate.

Outcomes

The recorded data were analyzed using an analysis program (Telescan, LAXTHA, Korea). From the recorded data of each subject, 30 sets of 2-s-long signals were randomly extracted from the signals without any noise to use for the background potential analysis. The mean power spectrum amplitude and the mean dominant frequency of the slow alpha waves (8–10 Hz) were computed. Among the ERP signals measured from 0.1 s before to 0.6 s after the stimulation, only the data with an amplitude difference of less than 100 were selected to calculate the mean values, and then the amplitude and latency of the P300 were analyzed. The P300 amplitude was defined as the difference between the highest peak value of the P300 and the mean value at 0.1 s before the target stimulation. The P300 latency was defined as the position at which the P300 value was obtained after the target stimulus was

applied. Only the channels Fz, Fcz, Cz, Cpz and Pz were selected for the data analysis. The primary outcomes were the P300 amplitude and latency, and the secondary outcomes were the slow alpha mean frequency and power.

Statistical analysis

For statistical analysis, ANCOVA was used to compare the groups using the SAS program (SAS 9.1.3, SAS Inc., USA).

Results

P300 latency and amplitude

When the changes in the P300 were measured by comparing ERPs before and after the low-frequency electrical stimulation, an increase in amplitude was observed at all of the analyzed channels in all subjects: Fz (F = 2.06, p = 0.158), Fcz (F = 1.93, p = 0.170) Cz (F = 1.91, p = 0.174), Cpz (F = 4.41, p = 0.041), and Pz (F = 3.79, p = 0.057). In particular, the change at the Cpz channel in the test group (Real) was found to be significant compared to that in the control group (Sham) (p = 0.041). Although the latency of the P300 tended to be shifted forward at channels Fz, Fcz, Cz, and Pz in the Real group, no significant differences were observed compared to the Sham group (Table 2).

The male group showed a tendency toward a reduced P300 latency at the Fz, Fcz, Cz, and Pz channels when comparing before and after stimulation. Although larger P300 amplitudes were detected at these channels, no significant differences were observed compared to the Sham group. In the female group, a shorter latency was observed at Fz, Fcz, and Cz, but no significant differences were detected compared to the Sham group. In contrast, in the Real group, the amplitude showed a significant increase at all the analyzed channels: Fz (F = 4.26, p = 0.049), Fcz (F = 5.23, p = 0.031), Cz (F = 4.63, p = 0.041), Cpz (F = 4.94, p = 0.035), and Pz (F = 6.49, p = 0.017)–compared to the corresponding values of the Sham group (Table 3).

According to the brain mapping analysis, the P300 amplitude was found to be increased in all subjects. Although the change in the P300 amplitude was small in the male group, a marked change was observed in the female group. The strongest change in the P300 amplitude was observed in the frontal and parietal lobe areas. In particular, a noticeable increase in the P300 amplitude was detected in the female group (Fig. 3).

Slow alpha wave power spectrum

The slow alpha waves of the background potential were analyzed separately for the male and female groups, and no significant changes in the mean frequency were observed in either group. However, the mean power decreased at all the analyzed channels in the male group: Fz (F = 0.77, p = 0.384), Fcz (F = 1.15, 0.293), Cz (F = 1.54, p = 0.227),

Table 2 Mean and standard error of the P300 latency and amplitude obtained from all subjects

| | | Total (n = 55) | | | | | | Group difference (AS-NS) | p-value |
| | | Sham (n = 27) | | | Real (n = 28) | | | | |
		Before	After	Difference	Before	After	Difference		
Latency of P300 (sec)	Fz	0.31 ± 0.06	0.31 ± 0.07	0.00	0.32 ± 0.07	0.30 ± 0.07	−0.02	−0.02	0.39
	Fcz	0.30 ± 0.07	0.29 ± 0.06	−0.01	0.32 ± 0.07	0.30 ± .007	−0.02	−0.01	0.69
	Cz	0.30 ± 0.06	0.28 ± 0.05	−0.02	0.32 ± 0.07	0.30 ± 0.07	−0.02	0.00	0.35
	Cpz	0.30 ± 0.06	0.27 ± 0.07	−0.03	0.31 ± 0.08	0.31 ± 0.07	0.00	0.03	0.13
	Pz	0.31 ± 0.07	0.28 ± 0.08	−0.03	0.31 ± 0.09	0.30 ± 0.08	−0.01	0.02	0.05
Amplitude of P300 (μV)	Fz	3.49 ± 1.35	3.37 ± 1.91	−0.12	3.76 ± 2.24	4.28 ± 2.53	0.52	0.64	0.16
	Fcz	3.28 ± 1.40	3.46 ± 1.90	0.18	3.59 ± 2.05	4.41 ± 2.56	0.82	0.64	0.17
	Cz	3.09 ± 1.23	3.35 ± 1.98	0.26	3.28 ± 1.87	4.17 ± 2.27	0.89	0.63	0.17
	Cpz	2.92 ± 1.23	2.78 ± 1.79	−0.14	3.11 ± 1.93	3.80 ± 2.03	0.69	0.83	*0.04*
	Pz	2.70 ± 1.24	2.51 ± 1.53	−0.19	2.81 ± 1.70	3.32 ± 1.81	0.51	0.70	0.06

The differences between the groups were calculated by subtracting the change from before and after the stimulation of the Sham group from that of the Real group, which shows the extent of the changes in the Real group compared with those in the Sham group. Compared to the Sham group, the Real group showed a tendency toward an increase in the P300 amplitude, particularly in channel Cpz (F = 4.41, p = 0.04)
Italicized data: A significant increase in P300 amplitude

Cpz (F = 2.52, p = 0.126), and Pz (F = 1.78, p = 0.195). In contrast, in the female group, the mean power increased at all the analyzed channels: Fz (F = 4.19, p = 0.051), Fcz (F = 4.41, p = 0.46), Cz (F = 2.30, p = 0.141), Cpz (F = 356, p = 0.070), and Pz (F = 4.52, p = 0.043). In particular, a significant increase was observed at the Fcz, and Pz channels (Table 4).

Double-blind index
According to the results of subject survey administered immediately following the experiment, 11 subjects thought they had received stimulation, 4 thought they had not, and 13 answered that it was hard to tell in the Real group. In the Sham group, 12, 7, and 8 subjects

were in each category, respectively. The presence of actual stimulation and the subject's perception of the presence of stimulation were tested by a chi-square test and a p-value of 0.68 was obtained, indicating that this study was successfully conducted as double-blind (Table 5).

Discussion
Based on previous studies, the physiological significance of the amplitude and latency of the P300 can be summarized as follows: The amplitude of the P300 represents contextual updating of attentional allocation and working memory resources and is proportional to the resource allocation for a specific task or stimulus. The latency represents cognitive processing and classification speed

Table 3 Mean and standard error of the P300 latency and amplitude in the female group

| | | Female (n = 29) | | | | | | Group difference (AS-NS) | p-value |
| | | Sham (n = 15) | | | Real (n = 14) | | | | |
		Before	After	Difference	Before	After	Difference		
Latency of P300 (sec)	Fz	0.31 ± 0.06	0.32 ± 0.07	0.01	0.32 ± 0.07	0.31 ± 0.07	−0.01	−0.02	0.39
	Fcz	0.29 ± 0.07	0.29 ± 0.06	0.00	0.32 ± 0.07	0.31 ± 0.07	−0.01	−0.01	0.69
	Cz	0.29 ± 0.06	0.28 ± 0.05	−0.01	0.32 ± 0.07	0.32 ± 0.06	0.00	0.01	0.35
	Cpz	0.29 ± 0.06	0.28 ± 0.07	−0.01	0.31 ± 0.09	0.32 ± 0.07	0.01	0.02	0.13
	Pz	0.32 ± 0.07	0.28 ± 0.07	−0.04	0.31 ± 0.08	0.33 ± 0.07	0.02	0.06	0.05
Amplitude of P300 (μV)	Fz	3.75 ± 1.66	3.34 ± 1.66	−0.41	4.06 ± 2.57	4.83 ± 3.15	0.77	1.18	*0.05*
	Fcz	3.48 ± 1.80	3.17 ± 1.49	−0.31	3.93 ± 2.35	5.09 ± 3.24	1.16	1.47	*0.03*
	Cz	3.30 ± 1.58	3.14 ± 1.56	−0.16	3.64 ± 2.15	4.74 ± 2.86	1.10	1.26	*0.04*
	Cpz	3.14 ± 1.56	2.91 ± 1.62	−0.23	3.49 ± 2.25	4.42 ± 2.51	0.93	1.16	*0.04*
	Pz	2.96 ± 1.53	2.59 ± 1.48	−0.37	3.08 ± 2.02	3.95 ± 2.18	0.87	1.24	*0.02*

In the female group, the Real group exhibited a significant increase at all five analyzed channels around the parietal lobe: Fz (F = 4.26, p = 0.049), Fcz (F = 5.23 p = 0.031), Cz (F = 4.63, p = 0.041), Cpz (F = 4.94 p = 0.035), and Pz (F = 6.49 p = 0.017) compared with the corresponding values of the Sham group
Italicized data: A significant increase in P300 amplitude

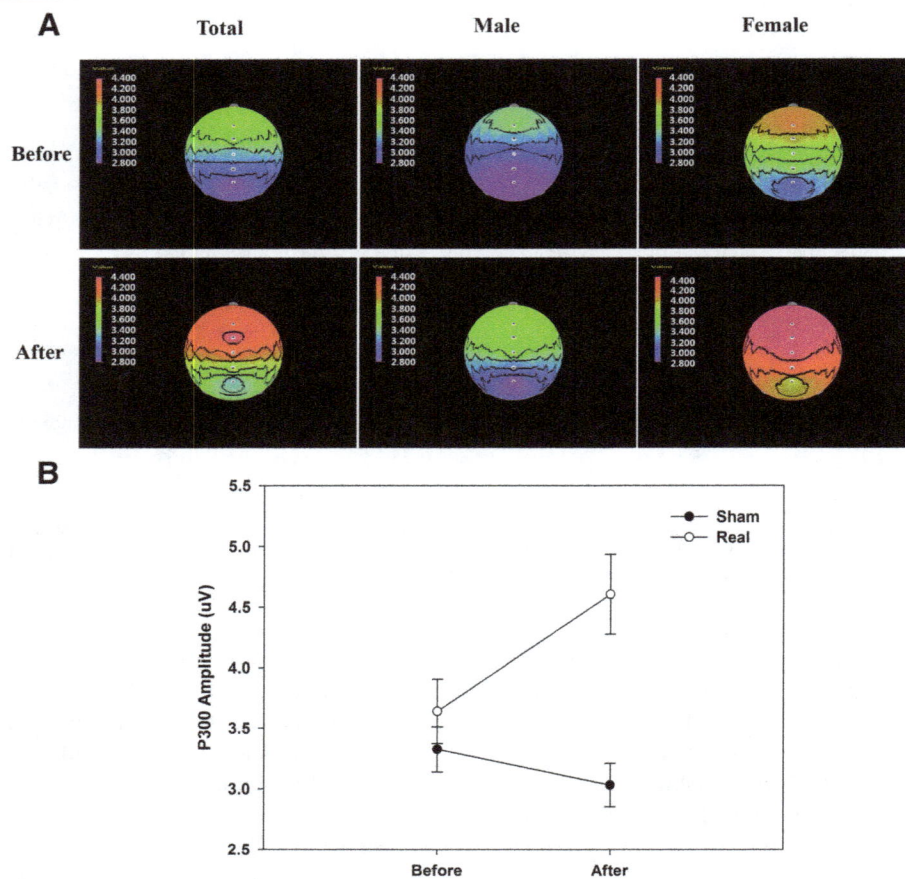

Fig. 3 P300 amplitude change after electrical stimulation. **a** ERP topographical maps showing (the differences in) the P300 amplitude obtained from the male and female subjects before and after electrical stimulation. Power was found to increase around the parietal lobe after stimulation in both the female and male groups. In particular, changes around the frontal lobe and parietal lobe were more significant in the female group than in the male group. **b** Total P300 amplitude difference in the females. The results from five channels were averaged, demonstrating the differences in the P300 amplitude before and after the low-frequency electrical stimulation. In the Real group, the amplitude was significantly increased compared to that of the Sham group

Table 4 Mean power and frequency of the slow alpha waves in the female group

| | | Female (n = 29) | | | | | | Group difference (AS-NS) | p-value |
| | | Sham (n = 15) | | | Real (n = 14) | | | | |
		Before	After	Difference	Before	After	Difference		
Slow alpha mean frequency (Hz)	Fz	9.31 ± 0.23	9.34 ± 0.19	0.03	9.35 ± 0.23	9.35 ± 0.23	0.00	−0.03	0.94
	Fcz	9.32 ± 0.24	9.33 ± 0.22	0.01	9.37 ± 0.21	9.34 ± 0.22	−0.03	−0.04	0.65
	Cz	9.34 ± 0.23	9.35 ± 0.21	0.01	9.37 ± 0.22	9.35 ± 0.22	−0.02	−0.03	0.50
	Cpz	9.34 ± 0.22	9.36 ± 0.19	0.02	9.39 ± 0.22	9.38 ± 0.22	−0.01	−0.03	0.44
	Pz	9.36 ± 0.23	9.39 ± 0.17	0.03	9.42 ± 0.23	9.40 ± 0.23	−0.02	−0.05	0.61
Slow alpha mean power	Fz	61.11 ± 53.13	41.91 ± 29.97	−19.20	45.34 ± 46.20	45.88 ± 45.65	0.54	19.74	0.05
	Fcz	64.42 ± 54.31	45.89 ± 35.54	−18.53	49.82 ± 52.09	50.84 ± 51.38	1.02	19.55	*0.05*
	Cz	64.43 ± 59.39	51.44 ± 58.03	−12.99	51.91 ± 57.46	52.62 ± 56.64	0.71	13.70	0.14
	Cpz	75.47 ± 99.73	62.11 ± 98.03	−13.36	54.37 ± 62.78	55.64 ± 64.53	1.27	14.63	0.07
	Pz	81.83 ± 124.38	63.86 ± 102.47	−17.97	53.70 ± 64.64	56.12 ± 69.15	2.42	20.39	*0.04*

Similar to the results in the male group, in the female group, there was no significant change in the mean frequency of the slow alpha waves. Unlike in the male group, however, the mean power tended to increase at all the analyzed channels, and significant changes were observed at three channels: Fcz (F = 4.41, p = 0.046), and Pz (F = 4.52, p = 0.043)
Italicized data: A significant increase in the slow alpha mean power

Table 5 Double-blind index

	Real (n(%))	Sham (n(%))	Unknown (n(%))	Total (n(%))	p-value
Real	11 (20.00%)	4 (7.27%)	13 (23.64%)	28 (50.91%)	**0.68**
Sham	12 (21.82%)	7 (12.73%)	8 (14.54%)	27 (49.09%)	
Total	23()	11()	21()	55()	

The chi-square test results indicate that the blinding was well-maintained, with a p-value of 0.68

Bold data: No placebo effect (p > 0.05)

and is inversely proportional to cognitive capability and attentional allocation. In this study, changes in the amplitude and latency of the P300 were used to evaluate the effect of electrical stimulation of the foot on the reduced cognitive function that can develop with aging.

BL62 and KI6 are acupuncture points effective in the treatment of mind-related diseases in oriental medicine. They are known to stabilize mental conditions and to clear the mind, and they have recently been found to be effective in cases of insomnia. Studies of the acupuncture stimulation of acupuncture points have shown that continuous stimulation at BL62 reduced the speed of nerve reactions and that the stimulation of several acupuncture points, including KI6, was effective in treating postmenopausal hot flashes. Few studies of BL62 and KI6 stimulation have been conducted with regard to responses to stimulation or treatment effects, but such studies should be considered because this stimulation has been shown to be effective in the treatment and prevention of insomnia, hypersomnia, and brain disorders.

In this study, low-frequency electrical stimulation of BL62 and KI6, which is easily applied to human patients and is inexpensive and safe, with few adverse reactions, was performed to determine its effect on cognitive function by measuring and analyzing background EEG and ERPs. Using low-frequency electrical stimulation, a double-blind test was performed to prevent any placebo effects, and the objectivity of the study results were confirmed by a chi-square test.

Studies of the P300 generally use closely related channels such as Fz, Cz, and Pz for analysis, but in this study, in addition to those 3, 2 more channels, Fcz and Cpz, were selected among the 32 channels to increase the resolution. For statistical analysis, ANCOVA was performed to compare changes before and after stimulation because brain waves vary greatly in amplitude from individual to individual. Additionally, the stimulation group and the Sham group did not contain the same individuals, and the number of subjects in each group differed; thus, the pre-stimulation values were different.

The latency of the P300 tended to increase at 4 of the channels (Fz, Fcz, Cz, and Pz) in all the subjects, but the differences between the stimulation and non-stimulation groups were not significant. However, the amplitude was

increased at all 5 the analyzed channels after stimulation, with particularly significant changes at Cpz.

The results of the male and female subjects were compared in the analysis. In the males, the latency and amplitude did not differ between the stimulation group and the non-stimulation group, but in the females, the amplitude was significantly increased at the channels Fz, Fcz, Cz, Cpz, and Pz in the stimulation group compared to the non-stimulation group. Brain mapping confirmed that the amplitude of the P300 was greatly enhanced in the frontal and parietal lobes in the females.

Studies have long shown prolongation of the latency and diminution of the amplitude of the P300 with increasing age, which suggests that cognitive functions decline, with reduced responsiveness and brain function due to a reduction in brain cell capacity and to neurodegeneration, as an individual ages. The increase in P300 latency and amplitude with low-frequency electrical stimulation of BL62 and KI6 suggests the possibility of delaying these age-related phenomena.

Intriligator et al. [19] reported a relationship between background EEG and the P300, in which the latency of the P300 and the slow alpha mean frequency were both increased, whereas the amplitude of the P300 and the slow alpha mean power were both decreased. Hillman et al. [20] confirmed that vigorous cardiovascular exercise not only increased alpha activity but also increased the amplitude and decreased the latency of the P300. In our study, the analysis of the mean frequency and power of the slow alpha waves showed that in the women, the frequency increased and the mean power tended to increase at all 5 channels after stimulation most significantly at Fcz, and Pz. This result may be related to the increased P300 amplitude at all the channels.

Polich and Criado [3] reported that long-term alcohol intake can reduce the amplitude of the P300, and Kalmijn et al. [21] reported that smoking and alcohol consumption can lead to greater reductions in cognitive function in males than in females. In this study, through an additional survey, it was confirmed that among those subjects who received the stimulus, the males were exposed to more alcohol and engaged in more smoking than the women (Table 6); this may have acted as a negative factor for the improvement of the P300 amplitude.

The results described above confirmed that the two dimensions of the P300 (latency and amplitude) were

Table 6 Subject ratings of each gender group with respect to drinking, smoking during the study period

	Drinking	Smoking
Male	30.77%	15.38%
Female	23.08%	0%

The male subjects drank and smoked more than the female subjects

improved by long-term, low-frequency electrical stimulation, with a particularly significant increase in the amplitude of the P300. Changes in the amplitude of the P300 are known to be related to the regions responsible for attention and working memory. Thus, it is possible that low-frequency electrical stimulation of Bl62 and KI6 has a positive effect on memory function in middle-aged women and thus may prevent brain aging due to a reduction in brain cell capacity and to neurodegeneration, thereby reducing risk for dementia. However, because this study was performed on subjects in their 50s, additional studies are needed to determine the effects on different age groups and also to assess the stimulation effect in men by minimizing distracting factors. In addition, the pathways by which the stimulation of acupuncture points affects the brain neurologically and the mechanisms that change the two dimensions of the P300 should be further explored through animal experiments.

Conclusion

This study confirmed that the amplitude of the P300 is increased in middle-aged women by low-frequency electrical stimulation at BL62 and KI6. Thus, the results of this study may serve as a foundation for the treatment of dementia and various brain disorders due to brain aging and impaired cognition. However, because the results of this study are limited to middle-aged women, further studies are necessary to determine the therapeutic effects in different age groups as well as in men and to discover the neurological mechanisms underlying the positive influence of low-frequency electrical stimulation on the brain.

Acknowledgments
The authors are grateful to the residents who participated in this study.

Funding
This research was supported by a grant to study the peripheral-spinal-cerebral signaling pathway of acupuncture stimulus (No. K17070) from the Korea Institute of Oriental Medicine, Korea.

Authors' contributions
KHC, OSK, SJC, SHL, and YHR conceived of and designed the study. KHC, OSK, and SHL conducted the fieldwork. KHC and SJC performed the data analysis. KHC, OSK, SYK, and YHR drafted the paper. All the authors read and approved the final paper. KHC acted as joint first author to this paper.

Competing interests
The authors have no actual or potential conflicts of interest.

References

1. van der Stelt O, Belger A. Application of electroencephalography to the study of cognitive and brain functions in schizophrenia. Schizophr Bull. 2007;33(4):955–70.
2. Sutton S, Braren M, Zubin J, John ER. Evoked-potential correlates of stimulus uncertainty. Science. 1965;150(3700):1187–8.
3. Polich J, Criado JR. Neuropsychology and neuropharmacology of P3a and P3b. Int J Psychophysiol. 2006;60(2):172–85.
4. Knight RT. Aging decreases auditory event-related potentials to unexpected stimuli in humans. Neurobiol Aging. 1987;8(2):109–13.
5. Pae JS, Kwon JS, Youn T, Park HJ, Kim MS, Lee B, Park KS. LORETA imaging of P300 in schizophrenia with individual MRI and 128-channel EEG. NeuroImage. 2003;20(3):1552–60.
6. McCarthy G, Wood CC, Williamson PD, Spencer DD. Task-dependent field potentials in human hippocampal formation. J Neurosci. 1989;9(12):4253–68.
7. Linden DEJ. The P300: where in the brain is it produced and what does it tell us? Neuroscientist. 2005;11(6):563–76.
8. Sperling RA, Aisen PS, Beckett LA, Bennett DA, Craft S, Fagan AM, Iwatsubo T, Jack CR Jr, Kaye J, Montine TJ, et al. Toward defining the preclinical stages of Alzheimer's disease: recommendations from the National Institute on Aging-Alzheimer's Association workgroups on diagnostic guidelines for Alzheimer's disease. Alzheimers Dement. 2011;7(3):280–92.
9. Franconi G, Manni L, Schroder S, Marchetti P, Robinson N. A systematic review of experimental and clinical acupuncture in chemotherapy-induced peripheral neuropathy. Evidence-based complementary and alternative medicine : eCAM. 2013;2013:516916.
10. Kaptchuk TJ. Acupuncture: theory, efficacy, and practice. Ann Intern Med. 2002;136(5):374–83.
11. Wu SB, He GY, Zhou MQ. Effects of electroacupuncture on the apoptosis of brain tissue cells and the expression of caspase-3 in the rats with cerebral-cardiac syndrome. Zhongguo Zhong Xi Yi Jie He Za Zhi. 2012;32(5):639–42.
12. Toosizadeh N, Lei H, Schwenk M, Sherman SJ, Sternberg E, Mohler J, Najafi B. Does integrative medicine enhance balance in aging adults? Proof of concept for the benefit of Electroacupuncture therapy in Parkinson's disease. Gerontology. 2015;61(1):3–14.
13. Han KH, Kim SY, Chung SY. Effect of acupuncture on patients with insomnia: study protocol for a randomized controlled trial. Trials. 2014;15:403.
14. Park W-S, Lee T-Y, Kim S-Y, Leem K-G, Yuk S-W, Lee C-H, Lee S-R. The immediate effect of electroacupuncture at the B62(Shinmaek) K6(Chohae) on the EEG of vascular dementia. J Korean Acupunct Moxibustion Soc. 2001;18(2):67–78.
15. de Almondes KM, Costa MV, Malloy-Diniz LF, Diniz BS. Insomnia and risk of dementia in older adults: systematic review and meta-analysis. J Psychiatr Res. 2016;77:109–15.
16. Joo EY, Kim H, Suh S, Hong SB. Hippocampal substructural vulnerability to sleep disturbance and cognitive impairment in patients with chronic primary insomnia: magnetic resonance imaging morphometry. Sleep. 2014; 37(7):1189–98.
17. Olofsson JK, Nordin S. Gender differences in chemosensory perception and event-related potentials. Chem Senses. 2004;29(7):629–37.
18. Slewa-Younan S, Gordon E, Harris AW, Haig AR, Brown KJ, Flor-Henry P, Williams LM. Sex differences in functional connectivity in first-episode and chronic schizophrenia patients. Am J Psychiatry. 2004;161(9):1595–602.
19. Intriligator J, Polich J. On the relationship between background EEG and the P300 event-related potential. Biol Psychol. 1994;37(3):207–18.
20. Hillman CH, Snook EM, Jerome GJ. Acute cardiovascular exercise and executive control function. Int J Psychophysiol. 2003;48(3):307–14.
21. Kalmijn S, van Boxtel MP, Verschuren MW, Jolles J, Launer LJ. Cigarette smoking and alcohol consumption in relation to cognitive performance in middle age. Am J Epidemiol. 2002;156(10):936–44.

8

Predicting adherence to acupuncture appointments for low back pain

Felicity L. Bishop[1][*], Lucy Yardley[1], Cyrus Cooper[2], Paul Little[3] and George Lewith[3]

Abstract

Background: Acupuncture is a popular form of complementary and alternative medicine (CAM), but it is not clear why patients do (or do not) follow acupuncturists' treatment recommendations. This study aimed to investigate theoretically-derived predictors of adherence to acupuncture.

Methods: In a prospective study, adults receiving acupuncture for low back pain completed validated questionnaires at baseline, 2 weeks, 3 months, and 6 months. Patients and acupuncturists reported attendance. Logistic regression tested whether illness perceptions, treatment beliefs, and treatment appraisals measured at 2 weeks predicted attendance at all recommended acupuncture appointments.

Results: Three hundred twenty-four people participated (aged 18–89 years, M = 55.9, SD = 14.4; 70% female). 165 (51%) attended all recommended acupuncture appointments. Adherence was predicted by appraising acupuncture as credible, appraising the acupuncturist positively, appraising practicalities of treatment positively, and holding pro-acupuncture treatment beliefs. A multivariable logistic regression model including demographic, clinical, and psychological predictors, fit the data well (x^2 (21) = 52.723, $p < .001$), explained 20% of the variance, and correctly classified 65.4% of participants as adherent/non-adherent.

Conclusions: The results partially support the dynamic extended common-sense model for CAM use. As hypothesised, attending all recommended acupuncture appointments was predicted by illness perceptions, treatment beliefs, and treatment appraisals. However, experiencing early changes in symptoms did not predict attendance. Acupuncturists could make small changes to consultations and service organisation to encourage attendance at recommended appointments and thus potentially improve patient outcomes.

Keywords: Acupuncture, Adherence, Back pain, Health knowledge, Attitudes, Practice, Illness perceptions, Treatment beliefs

Background

The inclusion of acupuncture in clinical practice guidelines for chronic back pain encourages increased integration of acupuncture into mainstream healthcare systems [1, 2]. As more acupuncture is funded by and accessed through public health care systems, acupuncture research needs to expand beyond questions of efficacy and incorporate a focus on questions related to health services and healthcare delivery. Poor attendance at appointments contributes to wasted resources throughout health care [3, 4] and could reduce the effectiveness of acupuncture. This study therefore investigated the predictors of full attendance at recommended acupuncture treatments in a cohort of patients with low back pain (LBP), a common reason for using acupuncture [5, 6].

Attendance for a course of treatments can be conceptualised as a form of adherence – the extent to which patients follow specific recommendations that have been agreed with a health care practitioner [7]. Research on acupuncture has rarely focused explicitly on adherence. However, good adherence predicts better outcomes in other therapies, including among patients taking placebos

* Correspondence: F.L.Bishop@soton.ac.uk
[1]Psychology, Faculty of Social and Human Sciences, University of Southampton, Building 44 Highfield Campus, Southampton SO17 1BJ, UK
Full list of author information is available at the end of the article

[8]. This suggests that good adherence might also predict better outcomes in acupuncture. One research letter reported that only 13 of 32 participants in a small clinical study completed all ten acupuncture treatments, suggesting that attendance can be poor [9]. Major trials of individualised acupuncture for back pain have reported the number of appointments attended but not compared this to recommendations, making it difficult to ascertain adherence [10–12]. Qualitative studies suggest that after initiating treatment, patients particularly value aspects of the relationship with the acupuncturist (e.g. individualised holistic caring consultations; egalitarian or collaborative relationships; length of time with the acupuncturist; seeing the same acupuncturist) and immediate and longer-term health benefits (e.g. the treatment itself being relaxing and enjoyable; improvements in symptoms, wellbeing, and function; gaining new insights into one's health and/or treatment) [13–18]. In one study patients valued more mundane practicalities of treatment (e.g. clinics running to time) [19]. Patients' reasons for stopping acupuncture can include financial considerations (although some patients make sacrifices elsewhere to enable on-going access) and perceived lack of effect [13, 18]. In the NHS in particular, patients are dissatisfied with inflexible appointment times and fixed (short) courses of treatment [13, 16, 20] which could lead to poor attendance.

Research on adherence to other forms of complementary and alternative medicine (CAM) suggests that patients evaluate CAMs against multiple criteria including: congruence with health-related beliefs; impact on and insight into symptoms, wellbeing, and energy levels; the quality of the therapeutic relationship; and practicalities such as financial cost [21–25]. Quantitative studies suggest that continued or committed use of CAMs might be higher in people with greater on-going medical need [26] health worries [27] and pro-CAM attitudes such as holistic models of health [28]. In surveys, respondents describe stopping CAM because it is too expensive, has not had the desired effects, or has been completely effective [29, 30]. Different personality traits predict adherence to CAM in different studies, including absorption [31], agreeableness [32], and low neuroticism [33]. Dissatisfaction with biomedicine can trigger initial CAM use but appears to be less relevant to decisions about ongoing CAM use [21, 26, 28].

An extended Common-Sense Model (CSM) provides a comprehensive and testable framework within which to study adherence to treatment [34–36]. According to this model, patients hold abstract beliefs about illness ('illness perceptions') and treatments ('treatment beliefs') which inform decisions to initiate treatment. Studies confirm that illness perceptions and treatment beliefs are indeed associated with CAM use [37–39]. Having initiated treatment, patients then continue or discontinue it based on a combination of abstract beliefs and concrete experiences such as improvements in symptoms or side-effects [40–42]. The CSM further specifies that relationships between concrete experiences and abstract beliefs are bidirectional [43]. One implication of this is that experiencing early improvements during treatment should not only predict adherence but should also strengthen the illness perceptions and treatment beliefs that originally led to treatment uptake. Adherence research within this framework has focused mainly on illness perceptions and treatment beliefs in long-term medication regimes for chronic illness and has shown that illness perceptions are only weakly associated with adherence [44] while treatment beliefs are stronger, more proximal determinants of adherence [34, 45]. Patients with chronic illness are more adherent to prescribed medication when beliefs about personal need for the medicine outweigh any concerns about it [46].

We have previously adapted the extended CSM to study adherence to CAM by suggesting that patients appraise four particular aspects of CAM therapies: the therapy itself, the therapist, practicalities (e.g. convenience, cost), and symptom improvements early in treatment [28]. Qualitative data suggest relationships between these factors; for example, lack of improvement early in treatment might not deter patients if they are encouraged to continue treatment by their therapist [21, 42]. Appraisals of the therapy itself may be less important for adherence than appraisals of other aspects: in a longitudinal study adherence to CAM was predicted by positive appraisals of the therapist and practicalities but not the therapy [28]. More trusting and patient-centered therapeutic relationships have also been shown to increase adherence to biomedical treatments [47–49]. The dynamic extended CSM for CAM is shown in Fig. 1.

This study used the dynamic extended CSM for CAM to investigate adherence to acupuncture. The aim was to identify the predictors of full attendance at recommended acupuncture treatments in a cohort of patients with LBP. Specifically, we hypothesised that full attendance would be predicted by appraising the acupuncturist positively, appraising practicalities of treatment positively, experiencing early improvements in symptoms, holding pro-acupuncture treatment beliefs, and having positive perceptions of one's LBP. We also hypothesised that experiencing early improvements in symptoms and appraising the acupuncturist positively would predict pro-acupuncture treatment beliefs and positive perceptions of LBP.

Methods
Design
The data for this analysis are drawn from a larger prospective observational cohort of patients with LBP receiving acupuncture [50]. Participants completed paper-based

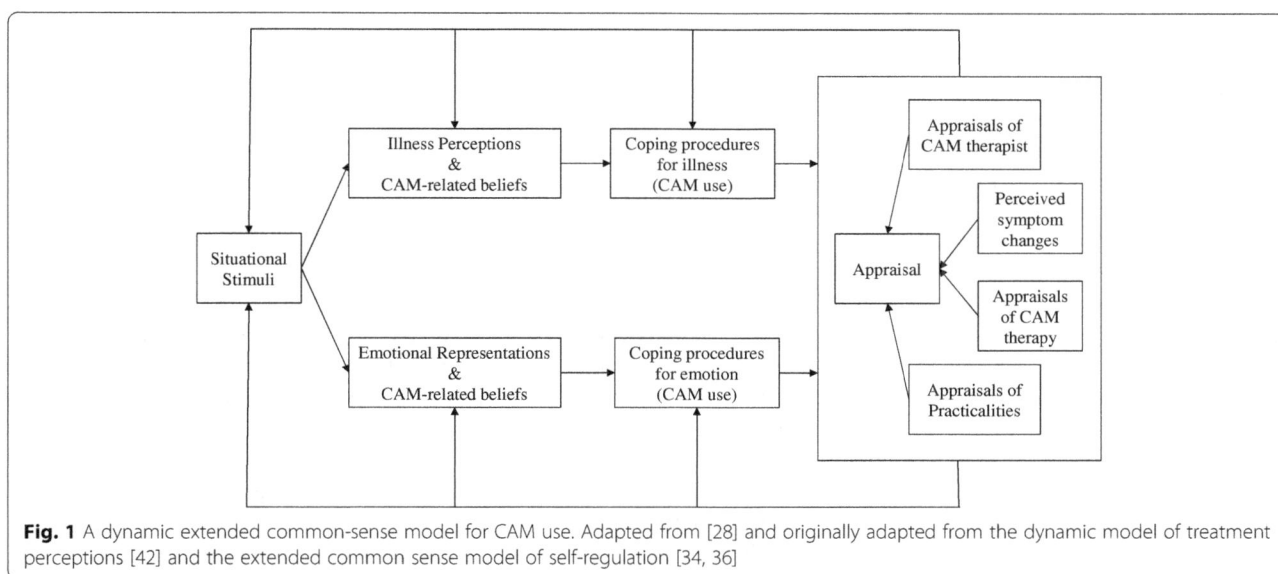

Fig. 1 A dynamic extended common-sense model for CAM use. Adapted from [28] and originally adapted from the dynamic model of treatment perceptions [42] and the extended common sense model of self-regulation [34, 36]

questionnaire measures of health and psychological variables four times – before starting treatment, 2 weeks, 3 months (when most courses of acupuncture for LBP have been completed), and 6 months later. Hypothesised predictors of adherence derived from the extended common-sense model were illness perceptions, treatment beliefs, and appraisals. This analysis used the 2-week measures of predictors unless otherwise specified (as pre-treatment beliefs should predict treatment initiation but not necessarily maintenance). The primary outcome was adherence at 3 months. The protocol was approved by Southampton and South West Hampshire Research Ethics Committee (A) (08/H0502/92) and data collection occurred between November 2008 and October 2010.

Measures

All questionnaires were chosen for their theoretical relevance, psychometric properties, and brevity.

Predictors

Illness perceptions were measured using the validated and reliable 8-item Brief Illness Perceptions Questionnaire [51] worded specifically to assess perceptions of LBP. Eight single items assess perceptions of LBP as having severe consequences (consequences), lasting a long time (timeline), being controllable by the patient (personal control), being treatable (treatment control), causing many severe symptoms (identity), being worrying (concerns), being understandable (coherence), and having emotional effects (emotional). An open-ended question asks participants to identify three causes of their own LBP. All named causes were reviewed and inductively categorised, creating five separate binary variables. Fear avoidance beliefs and catastrophising can be conceptualised as illness perceptions

specifically relevant to pain and were also included. Fear avoidance beliefs about physical activity and work were measured using the validated and reliable four and seven-item subscales from the Fear Avoidance Beliefs Questionnaire [52] (Cronbach's α in this sample = 0.78 and 0.90 respectively). Catastrophising was measured using the validated and reliable 6-item subscale from the Coping Strategies Questionnaire [53] (α = 0.90).

Four dimensions of treatment beliefs were measured using the validated and reliable Complementary and Alternative Medicine Beliefs Inventory (CAMBI) [54] and Credibility Expectancy Questionnaire (CEQ) [55]. On the CAMBI, six items assessed holistic health beliefs (α = 0.67), six items assessed beliefs that treatments should be 'natural' or non-toxic (α = 0.83), and five items assessed belief that patients should actively participate in treatment (α = 0.63). On the CEQ, three items assessed expectations that acupuncture is an effective treatment for LBP (α = 0.94).

Four aspects of appraisals were measured. Appraisals of the acupuncturist were measured using the validated and reliable 10-item perceptions of therapist subscale from the Treatment Appraisal Questionnaire (TAQ) [28] (α = 0.91). Appraisals of the credibility of acupuncture for LBP were measured using the three item credibility subscale from the CEQ (α = 0.88). Appraisals of practicalities were measured using five single-items from the TAQ which were highly skewed and so negatively phrased items were reverse-scored and then all items dichotomised into "strongly agree" vs all other responses. Thus participants were classified according to whether they appraised their acupuncture as: value for money, not difficult to travel to, convenient appointments, not too much effort to attend, and not too expensive. Three dimensions of appraisals of early symptom changes were measured: back-related disability, using the 24-item Roland Morris Disability Questionnaire [56]; pain, using an 11-item numerical rating scale [57]; and wellbeing, using the single-item (100 mm visual analogue scale) Arizona Integrative Outcomes Scale [58]. Early symptom changes were assessed by calculating change scores on these three measures of health status, subtracting pre-treatment scores from 2-week scores. Continuous measures of health changes were used in the analyses of relationships among appraisals, illness perceptions and treatment beliefs, because linear relationships were hypothesised among these variables. For the analyses of predictors of adherence, participants were classified into five groups on each of the change variables (moderate improvement, small improvement, no change, small deterioration, moderate deterioration – see Table 1 for cut-offs). This classification facilitated investigation of non-linear relationships between health changes and adherence, e.g. any deterioration might discourage attendance, small improvements might encourage attendance, while large improvements might lead to early discontinuation.

Outcome

The duration of acupuncture treatment is often evaluated on an on-going basis and negotiated between patient and acupuncturist, resulting in individualised recommendations for the number of treatments (although this is less common in the NHS than the private sector [59]). Adherence was therefore operationalised as the extent to which patients attended all appointments as recommended by/agreed with their acupuncturist. Participants reported this on a 7-point likert scale. Acupuncturists reported, for each patient, the number of appointments recommended and the number attended. Acupuncturists' recommendations were made based on usual clinical practice. A dichotomous measure of adherence (complete attendance vs incomplete attendance) was computed based on a combination of acupuncturists' and participants' reports – for a patient to be categorised as adherent both the patient and their acupuncturist had to report complete attendance.

Procedure and participants

Eighty three acupuncturists (24 male, 59 female) were recruited from CAM clinics, general practice, pain clinics, and physiotherapy departments across Great Britain and Northern Ireland. They distributed baseline questionnaire packs (including information leaflets and consent forms) to consecutive eligible patients (aged over 18, scoring at least four on the Roland Morris Disability Questionnaire [56], no malignant pain). Patients returned questionnaires and consent forms to the researchers in Freepost envelopes. Subsequent questionnaires were mailed directly to patients. Gift vouchers and personalised and repeated follow-ups were used to enhance recruitment and retention [60, 61]. Four hundred and eighty five patients were recruited, of whom 324 provided attendance data and were included in this analysis.

Statistical analyses

Missing values analysis in SPSS showed the proportion of missing data was low and Missing at Random, thus missing values were imputed using EM [62]. Analysis in MLWin confirmed that there was no significant effect on adherence of clustering of patients within clinics and so no adjustments for clustering were required.

To test hypotheses concerning predictors of adherence, SPSS was used to compute a series of univariable logistic regressions. Significant predictors (at $p < .10$) were entered into multivariable hierarchical logistic regression to identify independent predictors of adherence and to assess whether psychological variables predict adherence after controlling for demographic and clinical characteristics. Clinical and demographic variables were entered in Block 1, psychological variables were entered in Block 2. Variables were forced to enter the model within each block. The appropriateness of the data for logistic regression was tested. The Box-Tidwell procedure confirmed the data satisfied the assumption of linearity of the logit [63]. A linear regression was run and collinearity diagnostics examined; this confirmed there was no multicollinearity: all tolerance values > 0.1, all VIF < 10, no evidence of dependence in the variance

Table 1 Cut points for health change categories

Category	Change scores in category		
	Disability (RMDQ)[a]	Pain (NRS)[b]	Wellbeing (AIOS)[c]
Small deterioration	1 to 4	1	−7 to 2
Moderate deterioration	>= 4	>= 2	<= − 7
No change	0	0	2–11
Small improvement	−1 to −4	−1	11 to 24
Moderate improvement	<= − 4	<= − 2	>= 24

Notes. [a] 4-point change on Roland Morris Disability Questionnaire is clinically/statistically meaningful [75]. [b] Patients view 2 point reduction on Numerical Rating Scale as moderately meaningful [76]. [c] No guidance available for Arizona Integrative Outcome Scale so quintile split used

of the regression co-efficients [64]. To test hypotheses concerning relationships among treatment appraisals, treatment beliefs and illness perceptions, partial correlations were conducted between continuous measures of these variables (controlling for baseline treatment beliefs and illness perceptions).

Results

Demographic and clinical characteristics and adherence

Table 2 summarises participants' characteristics and presents the results of univariable logistic regressions to predict adherence. A slight majority of participants (51%, $n = 165$) attended all their recommended appointments. Participants were aged between 18 and 89 years old (M = 55.9, SD = 14.4). The majority were female, had chronic LBP, had not had acupuncture before, were receiving acupuncture in the public sector and were having other treatment(s) alongside acupuncture. Patients who were more likely to attend all their acupuncture appointments were older, had previous experience of acupuncture, were receiving additional treatments, were receiving acupuncture in the NHS, and were receiving acupuncture in a physiotherapy, GP, or pain clinic. Characteristics that were not significantly associated with attendance were: gender, duration of LBP, having a comorbid condition, and economic factors (see Table 2).

Psychological variables and adherence

Table 3 summarises scores on the psychological variables and presents the results of univariable logistic regressions to predict adherence. One illness perception dimension predicted adherence: the odds of attending all appointments decreased with perceptions that one's LBP causes many severe symptoms (illness identity). Two dimensions of treatment beliefs predicted adherence: the odds of attending all appointments increased with higher expectations of effectiveness and stronger preferences for participating in treatment. Five dimensions of appraisals predicted adherence: the odds of attending all appointments increased with more positive appraisals of the acupuncturist, appraisals of acupuncture as credible, and appraising appointments as convenient, not too much effort to attend, and affordable. Changes in disability, wellbeing, or pain scores in the first 2 weeks of treatment did not predict adherence.

Table 4 presents the results of the hierarchical multivariable logistic regressions to predict adherence. Demographic and clinical characteristics were entered in Block 1 and this model was a good fit to the data (χ^2 (11) = 25.899, p = .007), but explained only approximately 10% of the variance in attendance (Nagelkerke's R^2 = 0.102), and resulted in 62.7% of participants being correctly classified as adherent/non-adherent. Adding psychological variables in Block 2 significantly improved model

fit (χ^2 (10) = 26.824, p = .003). The final model including demographic, clinical, and psychological variables was a good fit to the data (χ^2 (21) = 52.723, $p < .001$), explained approximately 20% of the variance in attendance (Nagelkerke's R^2 = 0.200), and resulted in 65.4% of participants being correctly classified as adherent/non-adherent. Two variables remained as a significant independent predictor of adherence: the odds of attending all appointments were 1.23 times lower for every 1-unit increase in illness identity (perceptions that LBP causes many severe symptoms) and 2.09 times higher for participants who strongly disagreed that "seeing my therapist can be too much effort".

Appraisals, illness perceptions, and treatment beliefs

Table 5 summarises the partial correlations between appraisals and illness perceptions and treatment beliefs. After controlling for baseline beliefs, appraising acupuncture as credible, appraising the acupuncturist positively, and experiencing early health improvements were all associated with positive treatment beliefs and illness perceptions 2 weeks into treatment. In particular, positive appraisals were associated with higher expectations of acupuncture's effectiveness, perceiving higher levels of personal and treatment-related control over LBP, and perceiving one has a good understanding of LBP. Out of the four dimensions of appraisals, experiencing early health improvements were the most strongly and consistently associated with treatment beliefs and illness perceptions 2 weeks into treatment. Appraisals of practicalities of treatment were only weakly associated with illness perceptions and treatment beliefs. Positive appraisals were not associated with more general CAM-related beliefs.

Discussion

Data from a longitudinal prospective cohort study were used to investigate the predictors of complete attendance for a course of acupuncture for LBP. As hypothesised, adherence to appointments was predicted by appraising acupuncture as credible, appraising the acupuncturist positively, appraising practicalities of treatment positively, and holding pro-acupuncture treatment beliefs. Contrary to predictions, experiencing early changes in symptoms did not predict attendance, which makes it likely that our findings are not conflated by treatment effects. Experiencing early symptom improvements and appraising acupuncture and the acupuncturist positively were all associated with higher expectations of acupuncture's effectiveness and perceptions of LBP as more controllable and comprehensible.

In the univariable models, patients who had higher odds of attending all of their acupuncture appointments were older, had previous experience of acupuncture, were receiving additional treatments, were receiving

Table 2 Descriptive statistics and simple logistic regression analyses of demographic and clinical characteristics predicting attendance ($n = 324$)

Characteristic	Descriptive statistics		Regression results			
	f	%	Odds Ratio	95% Confidence Interval		p
				Lower	Upper	
Personal characteristics						
Age	—	—	1.02*	1.00	1.04	.012
Gender						
Female	228	70.4	1.51	0.93	2.43	.094
Education						.743
Left school aged <16 years [a]	38	11.7				
Educated to 16	136	42	1.04	0.51	2.14	.909
Educated to 18	80	24.7	0.90	0.42	1.95	.789
Post-school education	70	21.6	0.76	0.34	1.67	.492
Economic factors						
Compensation claim pending	30	9.3	0.96	0.45	2.04	.915
Receiving back-related benefits	58	17.9	1.34	0.76	2.38	.316
Employment						.259
Employed at usual work [a]	109	33.6				
On restricted duties	72	22.2	1.12	0.61	2.03	.718
Unpaid work (house work, student, retired)	143	44.1	1.50	0.91	2.47	.114
Clinical factors						
Prior acupuncture	133	41	1.61*	1.03	2.52	.037
Comorbidity	156	48.1	1.32	0.85	2.04	.217
Co-treatment	256	79	1.78*	1.03	3.06	.039
LBP duration						.429
Acute (<6 weeks) [a]	41	12.7				
Persistent (6–52 weeks)	103	31.8	0.72	0.35	1.50	.385
Chronic (>52 weeks)	180	55.6	0.99	0.50	1.95	.970
Clinic characteristics						
Sector						
Private	111	34.3	0.50*	0.31	0.80	.004
Acupuncture style						.059
Unclear [a]	60	18.5				
Western	164	50.6	0.97	0.54	1.76	.922
Traditional or TCM	85	26.2	0.52	0.27	1.01	.055
Mixed	15	4.6	1.64	0.50	5.37	.416
Clinic type						.070
CAM or acupuncture/TCM [a]	96	29.6				
Physiotherapy	83	25.6	1.90*	1.05	3.44	.035
Pain clinic	95	29.3	1.85*	1.04	3.28	.037
GP	50	15.4	2.11*	1.05	4.22	.035

Notes. *$p < .05$. **$p < .01$. [a] Reference category

acupuncture in the NHS, and were receiving acupuncture in physiotherapy, GP, or pain clinics (compared to acupuncture or CAM clinics). This suggests that previous acupuncture users are more committed to treatment than patients new to acupuncture, probably because the former are returning for a treatment they previously found effective. Receiving additional treatments might indicate worse overall health which could increase

Table 3 Descriptive statistics and univariable logistic regression analyses of adherence on psychological variables ($n = 324$)

	Descriptive statistics				Regression results			
	f	%	M	SD	Odds Ratio	95% C.I.		p
						Lower	Upper	
Illness perceptions								
LBP as threatening	—	—	47.63	10.73	0.99	0.97	1.01	.173
Consequences			6.82	2.11	1.00	0.91	1.11	.935
Timeline			7.78	2.18	0.97	0.88	1.07	.514
Personal control			4.54	2.33	1.03	0.94	1.13	.580
Treatment control			6.62	2.18	1.10	1.00	1.22	.058
Identity			6.95	1.86	0.89	0.79	1.00	.050
Concerns			7.86	1.96	0.99	0.88	1.10	.792
Comprehensible			6.83	2.57	1.08	0.99	1.18	.085
Emotional			6.21	2.46	1.01	0.93	1.11	.800
Caused by activities of daily living	120	37.0	—	—	0.89	0.57	1.40	.627
Caused by work	140	43.2	—	—	0.85	0.55	1.32	.460
Caused by accident/injury	123	38.0	—	—	0.83	0.53	1.29	.405
Caused by aging/genes	92	28.4	—	—	1.07	0.66	1.74	.777
Caused by disease	102	31.5	—	—	1.06	0.66	1.70	.801
Fear avoidance– physical activity			14.54	5.52	0.98	0.94	1.02	.301
Fear avoidance– work			15.17	13.11	0.97	0.98	1.01	.599
Catastrophising			2.45	1.43	0.93	0.80	1.08	.351
Treatment beliefs								
Expectancy	—	—	0.08	2.79	1.11*	1.02	1.21	.014
Holistic health	—	—	30.38	5.54	0.99	0.96	1.03	.785
Natural treatments	—	—	31.86	6.60	1.00	0.97	1.03	.988
Participation in treatment	—	—	26.85	4.88	1.05*	1.01	1.10	.030
Appraisals								
Credibility of acupuncture	—	—	0.11	2.64	1.08*	1.00	1.17	.046
Acupuncturist	—	—	60.31	8.86	1.03*	1.00	1.06	.028
Change in disability								.112
No change [a]	49	15.1	—	—				
Small deterioration	78	24.1	—	—	1.28	0.63	2.62	.500
Moderate deterioration	16	4.9	—	—	2.29	0.69	7.58	.174
Small improvement	108	33.3	—	—	0.74	0.38	1.47	.393
Moderate improvement	73	22.5	—	—	1.41	0.68	2.92	.353
Change in pain								.777
No change [a]	74	22.8	—	—				
Small deterioration	50	15.4	—	—	0.92	0.45	1.89	.827
Moderate deterioration	31	9.6	—	—	1.07	0.46	2.47	.880
Small improvement	75	23.1	—	—	1.34	0.70	2.56	.370
Moderate improvement	94	29.0	—	—	0.92	0.50	1.69	.784
Change in Wellbeing								
No change [a]	67	20.7	—	—				.637
Small deterioration	64	19.8	—	—	1.50	0.75	2.99	.250
Moderate deterioration	69	21.3	—	—	1.00	0.51	1.97	.994

Table 3 Descriptive statistics and univariable logistic regression analyses of adherence on psychological variables (*n* = 324) (*Continued*)

Small improvement	62	19.1	—	—	1.33	0.66	2.66	.422
Moderate improvement	62	19.1	—	—	0.96	0.48	1.92	.911
Value for money	92	28.4	—	—	1.55	0.95	2.52	.079
Not difficult to travel	184	56.8	—	—	1.12	0.72	1.74	.607
Convenient appointments	106	32.7	—	—	1.67*	1.04	2.67	.033
Not effortful to attend	219	67.6	—	—	2.29**	1.42	3.70	.001
Not too expensive	118	36.4	—	—	1.90**	1.20	3.01	.006

Notes. *p < .05. **p < .01. [a] Reference category

Table 4 Multiple logistic regression analysis of predictors of attendance (*n* = 324)

	Odds ratio	95% C.I.		*p*
		Lower	Upper	
Demographic/Clinical characteristics				
Gender				
Female	1.40	0.81	2.41	.223
Age	1.01	0.99	1.03	.240
Prior acupuncture	1.55	0.93	2.59	.094
Co-treatment	1.46	0.78	2.76	.240
Sector				
Private	0.33	0.09	1.19	.089
Clinic type				
CAM or acupuncture/TCM [a]				.820
Physiotherapy	0.93	0.24	3.64	.921
Pain clinic	0.74	0.16	3.56	.710
GP	0.63	0.13	3.11	.566
Acupuncture style				.660
Unclear [a]				
Western	0.79	0.39	1.61	.520
Traditional or TCM	0.69	0.31	1.55	.368
Mixed	1.32	0.37	4.79	.671
Psychological variables				
Illness perceptions				
Treatment control	0.99	0.83	1.17	.869
Identity	0.81**	0.90	0.94	.006
Comprehensible	1.04	0.93	1.15	.521
Treatment beliefs				
Expectancy	1.10	0.94	1.28	.259
Participation in treatment	1.05	1.00	1.11	.072
Appraisals				
Credibility of acupuncture	0.96	0.81	1.14	.663
Acupuncturist	1.00	0.97	1.03	.850
Convenient appointments	1.40	0.79	2.45	.254
Not effortful to attend	2.09*	1.18	3.73	.012
Not too expensive	1.23	0.72	2.08	.454

Notes. *p < .05. **p < .01. [a] Reference category

motivation for acupuncture. Acupuncture users in the NHS might be more likely than those in the private sector to adhere to appointments because they are grateful for free access to acupuncture [13] and/or because they are more likely to have shorter treatment courses of fixed duration [59]. Physiotherapy, GP and pain clinics are more likely to be in the NHS than are CAM clinics, which might explain increased adherence in the former settings. The impact of age was small - for each additional year of age the odds of attending all appointments were 1.02 times higher – and may indicate increasing commitment to health in general with increasing age. A recent large-scale study of adherence to medications in chronic illness found that older adults were also more likely to adhere to medications [65].

Odds of attending all acupuncture appointments increased with: weak perceptions that LBP causes many severe symptoms; high expectations of effectiveness and strong preferences for participating in treatment; and positive appraisals of the acupuncturist, appraisals of acupuncture as credible, and appraisals of acupuncture appointments as convenient, affordable, and not effortful to attend. Patients who do not associate lots of severe symptoms with their LBP might be more able physically to attend acupuncture appointments, which would lead to increased adherence (although LBP severity was not associated with adherence). Alternatively, patients who associate lots of severe symptoms with their LBP might feel they need a comprehensive multidisciplinary treatment to address these symptoms. While traditional acupuncture typically addresses the patient as a whole rather than focusing on a single symptom or condition, non-traditional acupuncture (e.g. Western styles) may be more symptom-focussed [66] and only approximately 25% of patients in this study were receiving traditional acupuncture. It is worth noting however that acupuncture style did not in itself predict adherence in this study.

People who expected acupuncture to be effective and believed it is important to participate in treatment were more likely to attend all their appointments, which can be understood as demonstrating the tendency towards common-sense coherence between treatment beliefs and

Table 5 Partial correlations between appraisals, illness perceptions and treatment beliefs

	Appraisals									
	Credibility of Acupuncture	Acupuncturist	Disability change	Pain change	Wellbeing change	Value for money	Not difficult to travel	Convenient appointments	Not effortful to attend	Not too expensive
Illness perceptions										
Consequences	-.10	-.06	.34**	.34**	-.29**	.04	.02	.05	.03	-.05
Timeline	-.16**	-.05	.25**	.26**	-.22**	-.05	-.02	-.02	.01	-.09
Personal control	.19**	.14*	-.23**	-.13*	.17**	.09	.10	.03	.11	.06
Treatment Control	.62**	.28**	-.20**	-.26**	.24**	.16**	.07	.16**	.11*	.06
Identity	-.10	.03	.34**	.30**	-.16**	.04	.01	.01	.06	-.12*
Concerns	-.14*	-.08	.26**	.26**	-.18**	-.03	-.02	-.06	-.10	-.12*
Comprehensible	.36**	.19**	-.17**	-.14*	.18**	.18**	.04	.07	.08	.04
Emotional	-.13*	-.01	.25**	.24**	-.15**	-.04	-.07	-.10	-.10	-.10
Treatment beliefs										
Expectancy	.70**	.28**	-.22**	-.33**	.27**	.16**	.11	.08	.08	.03
Holistic health	.06	.15**	-.02	-.04	.08	.05	-.05	.01	-.02	-.06
Natural treatments	.01	.11*	-.07	-.08	.06	-.01	-.03	.01	-.09	-.10
Participation in treatment	.03	.05	.02	.03	-.13*	.09	.07	.01	.07	.08

Notes. Each partial correlation controls for the baseline score on the relevant illness perception/treatment belief. $*p < .05$. $**p < .01$

adherence suggested by the extended common-sense model [34–36]. That participants apparently appraised multiple aspects of treatment when deciding whether to continue attending appointments is consistent with qualitative research in which patients evaluated multiple aspects of CAM when deciding whether to continue treatment [21]. This finding also supports the explication of multiple dimensions of appraisal in the dynamic extended common sense model for CAM [28]. Experiencing early changes in symptoms did not predict attendance, which can be explained if participants, like other CAM users [21], preferred to delay judging the effectiveness of therapy or if acupuncturists, like chiropractors [42] and rehabilitation therapists [67], reassured patients and helped them to interpret early changes (or lack thereof) positively.

In the final logistic regression model, a combination of demographic, clinical and psychological variables accounted for 20% of the variance in complete attendance. Psychological and other variables contributed similar amounts, confirming that attendance is dependent on multiple factors of different types. However, only two variables emerged as significant predictors of attendance (perceiving that one's LBP causes many severe symptoms and perceiving acupuncture appointments as not too much effort to attend) which suggests shared variance among the predictors and possible mediation effects. A large proportion of variance in attendance (80%) remained unaccounted for by our predictors. This is broadly comparable to our previous study of adherence to diverse CAM therapies in which illness perceptions, treatment beliefs and treatment appraisals explained 25% of the variance in attendance, 19% of the variance in adherence to lifestyle recommendations and 39% of the variance in adherence to remedies [28]. These findings strongly suggest that additional variables to the illness perceptions, treatment beliefs, and treatment appraisals measured in this study are needed to understand and predict complete attendance for acupuncture and other CAM treatments. Such variables might include not only other beliefs, such as perceived need for and concerns about treatment [46, 68], health locus of control (previously associated with acupuncture use [69]), and health-related self-perceptions (previously predicted CAM use [70]), but also social constructs such as social network characteristics (associated with CAM use [71]) and social support (associated with adherence to biomedical therapies [72]). Alternative measures of some constructs might have been more appropriate. For example, self-rated health changes may be more strongly related to adherence than researcher-computed health changes; other measures related to the therapeutic relationship such as working alliance [73] might better capture the impact of therapist-patient communication on adherence [42].

Strengths of this study include its prospective design, use of reliable and previously validated measures of multiple predictors of adherence derived from an established theoretical framework, and the comparatively large sample of acupuncture patients drawn from diverse clinics across the UK. The lack of an objective measure of attendance is a limitation, although the possible bias introduced by self-report measures of adherence is somewhat mitigated by the combined use of patient and practitioner reports. It is possible that acupuncture patients who volunteer to participate in research are more likely to adhere to treatment than patients who do not volunteer, and if this were the case then this study may have overestimated adherence rates. We could locate no comparable published data on adherence in practice to test this possibility.

The results suggest several ways in which acupuncturists could encourage patients to attend all recommended appointments and thus probably improve patient outcomes. Patients who associated lots of severe symptoms with their LBP were less likely to adhere, so acupuncturists from all traditions could ensure they discuss and address diverse symptoms and comorbidities with patients. Patients who appraised their acupuncturist positively - finding them to be trustworthy and good communicators - were more likely to attend than other patients. This is consistent with previous studies in CAM [28] and biomedicine [74], and reinforces the importance of good communication and relationship-building skills for encouraging adherence to treatment recommendations. Acupuncturists may also be able to structure their services to facilitate adherence and minimise the practical barriers that were associated with incomplete attendance in this study. This would entail offering more convenient and affordable appointments that patients can easily fit into their lives and attend with minimal effort. Acupuncturists could consider asking patients to complete the five practical items from the TAQ [28] early in treatment to identify patients most at risk of early discontinuation and open up a discussion with them about ways to ease the burden of attending appointments.

Conclusions

In conclusion, the results broadly supported the dynamic extended CSM for CAM use. Adherence to acupuncture was predicted by patients' perceptions of their LBP, their expectations of acupuncture, and their appraisals of their early experiences of their acupuncturist, the credibility of acupuncture, and the practicalities of attending appointments. Contrary to predictions, experiencing early changes in symptoms did not predict attendance. We have suggested several ways in which acupuncturists could encourage patients to attend all recommended appointments. Future research should explore additional variables to improve our understanding of adherence to acupuncture.

Acknowledgements

We are grateful to the Primary Care Research Network, the Acupuncture Association of Chartered Physiotherapists, and British Acupuncture Council, and the British Medical Acupuncture Society for help recruiting acupuncturists. We are grateful to the acupuncturists for recruiting our participants and to the participants for completing the questionnaires. We thank Jane Cousins, Naomi Guppy and Gemma Fitzsimmons for administrative support.

Funding

This study was funded by Arthritis Research UK (Career Development Fellowship 18099 to FLB). GTL's post is supported by a grant from the Rufford Maurice Laing Foundation. The funding bodies had no role in the design, collection, analysis and interpretation of the data, or in the writing of the manuscript or in the decision to submit the manuscript for publication.

Authors' contributions

FLB conceived of the study, led its design, data acquisition, analysis and interpretation, and drafted the manuscript for publication. GTL, LY, PL and CC contributed to study conception and design and revised the article critically for important intellectual content. All authors have given final approval of the version to be published.

Competing interests

The authors declare that they have no competing interests.

Author details

[1]Psychology, Faculty of Social and Human Sciences, University of Southampton, Building 44 Highfield Campus, Southampton SO17 1BJ, UK. [2]MRC Lifecourse Epidemiology Unit, University of Southampton, Southampton General Hospital, Tremona Road, Southampton SO16 6YD, UK. [3]Primary Care and Population Sciences, Aldermoor Health Centre, University of Southampton, Southampton SO16 5ST, UK.

References

1. Chou R, Qaseem A, Snow V, Casey D, Cross Jr JT, Shekelle P, Owens DK, for the Clinical Efficacy Assessment Subcommittee of the American College of P, the American College of Physicians/American Pain Society Low Back Pain Guidelines P. Diagnosis and treatment of low back pain: a joint clinical practice guideline from the American College of Physicians and the American Pain Society. Ann Intern Med. 2007;147(7):478–91.
2. Savigny P, Kuntze S, Watson P, Underwood M, Ritchie G, Cotterell M, Hill D, Browne N, Buchanan E, Coffey P, et al. Low back pain. Early management of persistent non-specific low back pain. In: NICE clinical guideline 88. London: National Collaborating Centre for Primary Care and Royal College of General Practitioners; 2009. www.nice.org.uk/CG88.
3. Guy R, Hocking J, Wand H, Stott S, Ali H, Kaldor J. How effective are short message service reminders at increasing clinic attendance? A meta-analysis and systematic review. Health Serv Res. 2012;47(2):614–32.
4. Hasvold PE, Wootton R. Use of telephone and SMS reminders to improve attendance at hospital appointments: a systematic review. J Telemed Telecare. 2011;17(7):358–64.
5. Hopton AK, Curnoe S, Kanaan M, MacPherson H. Acupuncture in practice: mapping the providers, the patients and the settings in a national cross-sectional survey. BMJ Open. 2012; 2(1): e000456. doi:10.1136/bmjopen-2011-000456.
6. Murthy V, Sibbritt DW, Adams J. An integrative review of complementary and alternative medicine use for back pain: a focus on prevalence, reasons

for use, influential factors, self-perceived effectiveness, and communication. Spine J. 2015;15(8):1870–83.

7. Horne R. Compliance, adherence, and concordance*. Chest. 2006;130(1 suppl):65S–72S.

8. Granger BB, Swedberg K, Ekman I, Granger CB, Olofsson B, McMurray JJV, Yusuf S, Michelson EL, Pfeffer MA. Adherence to candesartan and placebo and outcomes in chronic heart failure in the CHARM programme: double-blind, randomised, controlled clinical trial. Lancet. 2005;366(9502):2005–11.

9. Moroz A, Spivack S, Lee MHM. Adherence to acupuncture treatment for chronic pain. J Altern Complement Med. 2004;10(5):739–40.

10. Cherkin DC, Eisenberg D, Sherman KJ, Barlow W, Kaptchuk TJ, Street J, Deyo RA. Randomized trial comparing traditional chinese medical acupuncture, therapeutic massage, and self-care education for chronic low back pain. Arch Intern Med. 2001;161(8):1081–8.

11. Haake M, Muller HH, Schade-Brittinger C, Basler HD, Schafer H, Maier C, Endres HG, Trampisch HJ, Molsberger A. German acupuncture trials (GERAC) for chronic low back pain. Randomized, multicenter, blinded, parallel-group trial with 3 groups. Arch Intern Med. 2007;167(17):1892–8.

12. Witt CM, Jena S, Selim D, Brinkhaus B, Reinhold T, Wruck K, Liecker B, Linde K, Wegscheider K, Willich SN. Pragmatic randomized trial evaluating the clinical and economic effectiveness of acupuncture for chronic low back pain. Am J Epidemiol. 2006;164(5):487–96.

13. Bishop FL, Barlow F, Coghlan B, Lee P, Lewith GT. Patients as healthcare consumers in the public and private sectors: a qualitative study of acupuncture in the UK. BMC Health Serv Res. 2011;11(129). doi:10.1186/1472-6963-11-129. https://bmchealthservres.biomedcentral.com/articles/10.1186/1472-6963-11-129.

14. Cassidy CM. Chinese medicine users in the United States - Part II: preferred aspects of care. J Altern Complement Med. 1998;4(2):189–202.

15. Gould A, MacPherson H. Patient perspectives on outcomes after treatment with acupuncture. J Altern Complement Med. 2001;7(3):261–8.

16. Hughes JG. "When I first started going I was going in on my knees, but I came out and I was skipping": Exploring rheumatoid arthritis patients' perceptions of receiving treatment with acupuncture. Complement Ther Med. 2009;17(5):269–73.

17. Paterson C, Britten N. Acupuncture as a complex intervention: a holistic model. J Altern Complement Med. 2004;10(5):791–801.

18. Rugg S, Paterson C, Britten N, Bridges J, Griffiths P. Traditional acupuncture for people with medically unexplained symptoms: a longitudinal qualitative study of patients' experiences. Br J Gen Pract. 2011;61:e306–15.

19. Frank R, Stollberg G. Medical acupuncture in Germany: patterns of consumerism among physicians and patients. Sociol Health Illn. 2004;26:351–72.

20. Cheshire A, Polley M, Peters D, Ridge D. Is it feasible and effective to provide osteopathy and acupuncture for patients with musculoskeletal problems in a GP setting? A service evaluation. BMC Fam Pract. 2011; 12(1):49.

21. Bishop FL, Yardley L, Lewith GT. Why consumers maintain complementary and alternative medicine use: a qualitative study. J Altern Complement Med. 2010;16(2):175–82.

22. Cartwright T, Torr R. Making sense of illness: the experiences of users of complementary medicine. J Health Psychol. 2005;10(4):559–72.

23. Caspi O, Koithan M, Criddle MW. Alternative medicine or "alternative" patients: a qualitative study of patient-oriented decision-making processes with respect to complementary and alternative medicine. Med Decis Making. 2004;24(1):64–79.

24. Mercer SW, Reilly D. A qualitative study of patient's views on the consultation at the Glasgow Homoeopathic Hospital, an NHS integrative complementary and orthodox medical care unit. Patient Educ Couns. 2004;53(1):13–8.

25. Thorne S, Paterson B, Russell C, Schultz A. Complementary/alternative medicine in chronic illness as informed self-care decision making. Int J Nurs Stud. 2002;39(7):671–83.

26. Sirois FM, Gick ML. An investigation of the health beliefs and motivations of complementary medicine clients. Soc Sci Med. 2002;55(6):1025–37.

27. Furnham A. Are modern health worries, personality and attitudes to science associated with the use of complementary and alternative medicine? Br J Health Psychol. 2007;12:229–43.

28. Bishop FL, Yardley L, Lewith GT. Treatment appraisals and beliefs predict adherence to complementary therapies: a prospective study using a dynamic extended self-regulation model. Br J Health Psychol. 2008;13(4):701–18.

29. Endrizzi C, Rossi E. Patient compliance with homeopathic therapy. Homeopathy. 2006;95:206–14.

30. Rao JK, Kroenke K, Mihaliak KA, Grambow SC, Weinberger M. Rheumatology patients' use of complementary therapies: results from a one-year longitudinal study. Arthritis Care Res. 2003;49(5):619–25.

31. Owens JE, Taylor AG, Degood D. Complementary and alternative medicine and psychologic factors: toward an individual differences model of complementary and alternative medicine use and outcomes. J Altern Complement Med. 1999;5(6):529–41.

32. Sirois FM, Purc-Stephenson RJ. Personality and consultations with complementary and alternative medicine practitioners: a five-factor model investigation of the degree of use and motives. J Altern Complement Med. 2008;14(9):1151–8.

33. Jerant A, Chapman B, Duberstein P, Robbins J, Franks P. Personality and medication non-adherence among older adults enrolled in a six-year trial. Br J Health Psychol. 2011;16(1):151–69.

34. Horne R, Weinman J. Self-regulation and self-management in asthma: exploring the role of illness perceptions and treatment beliefs in explaining non-adherence to preventer medication. Psychol Health. 2002;17(1):17–32.

35. Horne R. Representations of medication and treatment: advances in theory and measurement. In: Petrie KJ, Weinman JA, editors. Perceptions of Health and Illness. Amsterdam: Harwood Academic Publishers; 1997. p. 155–88.

36. Leventhal HA, Brissette I, Leventhal EA. The common-sense model of self-regulation of health and illness. In: Cameron LD, Leventhal H, editors. The self-regulation of health and illness behaviour. London: Routledge; 2003. p. 42–65.

37. Olchowska-Kotala A. Illness representations in individuals with rheumatoid arthritis and the willingness to undergo acupuncture treatment. Eur J Integr Med. 2013;5(4):347–51.

38. Bishop FL, Yardley L, Lewith GT. Why do people use different forms of complementary medicine? Multivariate associations between treatment and illness beliefs and complementary medicine use. Psychol Health. 2006;21:683–98.

39. Porter MC, Diefenbach MA. Pushed and pulled: the role of affect and cognition in shaping CAM attitudes and behavior among men treated for prostate cancer. J Health Psychol. 2009;14(2):288–96.

40. Pound P, Britten N, Morgan M, Yardley L, Pope C, Daker-White G, Campbell R. Resisting medicines: a synthesis of qualitative studies of medicine taking. Soc Sci Med. 2005;61:133–55.

41. Vermeire E, Hearnshaw H, Van Royen P, Denekens J. Patient adherence to treatment: three decades of research. A comprehensive review. J Clin Pharm Ther. 2001;26:331–42.

42. Yardley L, Sharples K, Beech S, Lewith G. Developing a dynamic model of treatment perceptions. J Health Psychol. 2001;6(3):269–82.

43. Diefenbach MA, Leventhal H. The common-sense model of illness representation: theoretical and practical considerations. J Soc Distress Homeless. 1996;5(1):11–38.

44. Brandes K, Mullan B. Can the common-sense model predict adherence in chronically ill patients? A meta-analysis. Health Psychol Rev. 2014;8(2):129–53.

45. Nicklas LB, Dunbar M, Wild M. Adherence to pharmacological treatment of non-malignant chronic pain: the role of illness perceptions and medication beliefs. Psychol Health. 2009;25(5):601–15.

46. Horne R, Chapman SCE, Parham R, Freemantle N, Forbes A, Cooper V. Understanding patients' adherence-related beliefs about medicines prescribed for long-term conditions: a meta-analytic review of the necessity-concerns framework. PLoS One. 2013;8(12), e80633.

47. Arbuthnott A, Sharpe D. The effect of physician-patient collaboration on patient adherence in non-psychiatric medicine. Patient Educ Couns. 2009; 77(1):60–7.

48. Julius RJ, Novitsky MAJ, Dubin WR. Medication adherence: a review of the literature and implications for clinical practice. J Psychiatr Pract. 2009;15(1):34–44. doi:10.1097/01.pra.0000344917.43780.77.

49. Safran DG, Taira DA, Rogers WH, Kosinski M, Ware JE, Tarlov AR. Linking primary care performance to outcomes of care. J Fam Pract. 1998;47(3):213–20.

50. Bishop FL, Yardley L, Prescott P, Cooper C, Little P, Lewith GT. Psychological covariates of longitudinal changes in back-related disability in patients undergoing acupuncture. Clin J Pain. 2015;31(3):254–64.

51. Broadbent E, Petrie KJ, Main J, Weinman J. The brief illness perception questionnaire. J Psychosom Res. 2006;60:631–7.

52. Waddell G, Newton M, Henderson I, Somerville D, Main C. A fear-avoidance beliefs questionnaire (FABQ) and the role of fear-avoidance beliefs in chronic low back pain and disability. Pain. 1993;52:157–68.

53. Rosentiel AK, Keefe FJ. The use of coping strategies in chronic low back pain patients: relationship to patient characteristics and current adjustment. Pain. 1983;17:33–44.

54. Bishop FL, Yardley L, Lewith G. Developing a measure of treatment beliefs: the complementary and alternative medicine beliefs inventory. Complement Ther Med. 2005;13:144–9.
55. Devilly GJ, Borkovec TD. Psychometric properties of the credibility/expectancy questionnaire. J Behav Ther Exp Psychiatry. 2000;31:73–86.
56. Roland M, Morris R. A study of the natural history of back pain. Part I: development of a reliable and sensitive measure of disability in low-back pain. Spine. 1983;8(2):141–4.
57. Dworkin RH, Turk DC, Farrar JT, Haythornthwaite JA, Jensen MP, Katz NP, Kerns RD, Stucki G, Allen RR, Bellamy N. Core outcome measures for chronic pain clinical trials: IMMPACT recommendations. Pain. 2005;113(1–2):9–19.
58. Bell IR, Cunningham V, Caspi O, Meek P, Ferro L. Development and validation of a new global well-being outcomes rating scale for integrative medicine research. BMC Complement Altern Med. 2004;4:1. doi:10.1186/1472-6882-1184-1181.
59. Bishop FL, Amos N, Yu H, Lewith GT. Health-care sector and complementary medicine: practitioners' experiences of delivering acupuncture in the public and private sectors. Prim Health Care Res Dev. 2012;13(03):269–78.
60. Edwards P, Cooper R, Roberts I, Frost C. Meta-analysis of randomised trials of monetary incentives and response to mailed questionnaires. J Epidemiol Community Health. 2005;59:987–99.
61. Edwards P, Roberts I, Clarke M, DiGuiseppi C, Pratap S, Wentz R, Kwan I. Increasing response rates to postal questionnaires: systematic review. Br Med J. 2002;324:1183–93.
62. Tabachnick BG, Fidell LS. Using multivariate statistics, vol. 4. Boston: Allyn and Bacon; 2001.
63. Box GEP, Tidwell PW. Transformation of the independent variables. Technometrics. 1962;4(4):531–50.
64. Field A. Discovering statistics using SPSS for windows. London: Sage; 2000.
65. Rolnick SJ, Pawloski PA, Hedblom BD, Asche SE, Bruzek RJ. Patient characteristics associated with medication adherence. Clin Med Res. 2013; 11(2):54–65. doi:10.3121/cmr.2013.1113.
66. White A, the editorial board of Acupuncture in M. Western medical acupuncture: a definition. Acupunct Med. 2009;27(1):33–5.
67. Muller I, Kirby S, Yardley L. The therapeutic relationship in telephone-delivered support for people undertaking rehabilitation: a mixed-methods interaction analysis. Disabil Rehabil. 2015;37(12):1060–5.
68. Hök J, Falkenberg T, Tishelman C. Lay perspectives on the use of biologically based therapies in the context of cancer: a qualitative study from Sweden. J Clin Pharm Ther. 2011;36(3):367–75.
69. Cramer H, Chung VCH, Lauche R, Zhang Y, Zhang A, Langhorst J, Dobos G. Characteristics of acupuncture users among internal medicine patients in Germany. Complement Ther Med. 2015;23(3):423–9.
70. Sirois FM. Health-related self-perceptions over time and provider-based Complementary and Alternative Medicine (CAM) use in people with inflammatory bowel disease or arthritis. Complement Ther Med. 2014;22(4):701–9.
71. Goldman AW, Cornwell B. Social network bridging potential and the use of complementary and alternative medicine in later life. Soc Sci Med. 2015;140:69–80.
72. DiMatteo MR. Social support and patient adherence to medical treatment: a meta-analysis. Health Psychol. 2004;23(2):207–18.
73. Fuertes JN, Mislowack A, Bennett J, Paul L, Gilbert TC, Fontan G, Boylan LS. The physician-patient working alliance. Patient Educ Couns. 2007;66(1):29–36.
74. Zolnierek KB, DiMatteo MR. Physician communication and patient adherence to treatment: a meta-analysis. Med Care. 2009;47(8):826–34. doi:10.1097/MLR.0b013e31819a5acc.
75. Maughan EF, Lewis JS. Outcome measures in chronic low back pain. Eur Spine J. 2010;19(9):1484–94.
76. Dworkin RH, Turk DC, Wyrwich KW, Beaton D, Cleeland CS, Farrar JT, Haythornthwaite JA, Jensen MP, Kerns RD, Ader DN, et al. Interpreting the clinical importance of treatment outcomes in chronic pain clinical trials: IMMPACT recommendations. J Pain. 2008;9(2):105–21.

9

Electroacupuncture at LI11 promotes jejunal motility via the parasympathetic pathway

Xuanming Hu, Mengqian Yuan, Yin Yin, Yidan Wang, Yuqin Li, Na Zhang, Xueyi Sun, Zhi Yu[*] and Bin Xu[*]

Abstract

Background: Gastrointestinal motility disorder has been demonstrated to be regulated by acupuncture treatment. The mechanisms underlying the effects of acupuncture stimulation of abdominal and lower limb acupoints on gastrointestinal motility have been thoroughly studied; however, the physiology underlying the effects of acupuncture on the forelimbs to mediate gastrointestinal motility requires further exploration. The aim of this study was to determine whether electroacupuncture (EA) at LI11 promotes jejunal motility, whether the parasympathetic pathway participates in this effect, and if so, which somatic afferent nerve fibres are involved.

Methods: A manometric balloon was used to observe jejunal motility. The effects and mechanisms of EA at LI11 were explored in male Sprague-Dawley rats with or without drug administration (propranolol, clenbuterol, acetylcholine, and atropine) and with or without vagotomy. Three types of male mice ($\beta_1\beta_2$ receptor-knockout [$\beta_1\beta_2^{-/-}$] mice, M_2M_3 receptor-knockout [$M_2M_3^{-/-}$] mice and wild-type [WT] mice) were also studied by using different EA intensities (1, 2, 4, 6, and 8 mA). A total of 72 rats and 56 mice were included in the study.

Results: EA at LI11 increased the contractile amplitude of jejunal motility in the majority of both rats and mice. However, EA at LI11 did not enhance jejunal motility in rats administered atropine, rats that underwent vagotomy, and $M_2M_3^{-/-}$ mice (at all intensities). In WT mice, EA at LI11 significantly increased jejunal motility at all intensities except 1 mA, and a plateau was reached at intensities greater than 4 mA.

Conclusion: Our results suggest that EA at LI11 promotes jejunal motility primarily by exciting the parasympathetic pathway, and that Aδ-fibres and C-fibres may play important roles in the process.

Keywords: Electroacupuncture (EA), LI11, Jejunal motility, Parasympathetic pathway, Sympathetic pathway

Background

Gastrointestinal motility disorder consists of multiple clinical symptoms and occurs in numerous diseases, including diarrhoea, constipation and irritable bowel syndrome (IBS) [1, 2]. Functional bowel disorders have become a common research focus in recent decades, owing to the rapid advances in neurogastroenterology and the development of many new methods to study gastrointestinal motility [3].

An important role of the somatic-autonomic reflex in gastrointestinal motility has been demonstrated, whereas the autonomic nervous system has been reported to be highly involved in modulating visceral organ function [4–8]. Further studies have shown that small bowel contractile activity is under nervous system control via parasympathetic excitatory and sympathetic inhibitory nerve fibres directly act on smooth muscle cells [9, 10].

Many studies have provided reliable evidence of the effectiveness of acupuncture therapy for treating gastrointestinal motility disorder, primarily through autonomic nerve reflexes [4, 11, 12]. In animal models, acupuncture stimulation of abdominal skin inhibits gastrointestinal motility primarily by exciting sympathetic pathways [13], whereas acupuncture at hind paws enhances gastric motility mainly via parasympathetic pathways [14, 15]. Electroacupuncture (EA) is a variant of manual acupuncture (MA) in which electrical stimulation is applied through

* Correspondence: mickey28282@sina.com; xuuuux@sina.com
Key Laboratory of Integrated Acupuncture and Drugs Constructed, Nanjing University of Chinese Medicine, Ministry of Education, Nanjing 210023, China

needles. Owing to the ease of modulating its stimulation frequency and intensity, EA is recognized as a quantifiable treatment and is widely used in clinical and experimental research [16]. For this reason, we chose EA as the stimulation method in this study.

Previous research has focused on stimulation of the abdomen or the hind paws, whereas few studies have used the forepaws. LI11 (Quchi), located at the midpoint between the lateral end of the transverse cubital crease and the lateral humeral epicondyle [14], is traditionally used to regulate gastrointestinal motility, because there sufficient supporting clinical and experimental evidence of its efficacy [17–26]. However, in contrast to other acupoints for regulating gastrointestinal motility, such as ST36 (Zusanli) and ST25 (Tianshu), the more evidence from basic research regarding the use of LI11 in acupuncture is needed.

We hypothesized that the immediate effect of EA stimulation at LI11 would be promoting jejunal motility, primarily by exciting parasympathetic pathways and inhibiting sympathetic pathways.

Methods
Animals
Male Sprague-Dawley rats (180–230 g; Model Animal Research Center of Nanjing Medical University, China) and male mice (22–28 g), including $\beta_1\beta_2^{-/-}$ mice (B6.129X1-$\beta_1\beta_2^{tm1Jul/NJU}$, J003810; donated by the Jackson Laboratory, USA), $M_2M_3^{-/-}$ mice (B6.129X1-$M_2M_3^{tm1Jul/NJU}$, D0407; from Kumamoto University, Japan), and wild-type counterparts (WT mice; purchased from the Model Animal Research Center of Nanjing University, China) were used in this study. Gene knockout in mice ($\beta_1\beta_2^{-/-}$ mice and $M_2M_3^{-/-}$ mice) was verified with PCR, and their genetic background is shown in the Additional file 1.

The animals were housed under a temperature of 22 °C and a relative humidity of 40%–60% at the SPF Experimental Animal Center, Nanjing University of TCM. They were housed under a 12 h/12 h light/dark cycle and were given free access to food and water. Animals underwent an adaptation period for seven days before inclusion in experiments. All experimental manipulations were undertaken in accordance with the Principles of Laboratory Animal Care and the Guide for the Care and Use of Laboratory Animals, published by the National Science Council, China.

Drugs
All animals in the study were anaesthetized with urethane (U2500; Sigma, St. Louis, MO, USA). The beta adrenoceptor agonist clenbuterol hydrochloride (clen; C5423; Sigma, St. Louis, MO, USA) and the beta adrenoceptor antagonist propranolol hydrochloride (prop; P0084; Sigma) were administered to the rats. Next, the muscarinic receptor

antagonist atropine hydrochloride (atropine; A6625; Sigma) and the agonist acetylcholine hydrochloride (ACh; A0132; Sigma) were administered. Penicillin antibiotic (B151226; Shandong Lukang Pharmaceutical Co., Ltd., Jining, China) was administered after surgery. The concentration, doses, and administration methods were 1) urethane: 20%, 8 mL/kg for rats and 5 mL/kg for mice, I.P.; 2) clenbuterol: 0.2%, maintenance dose of 80 μL/kg/min, intravenous (I.V.); 3) propranolol: 0.4%, initial dose of 1.0 mL/kg and maintenance dose of 40 μL/kg/min, I.V.; 4) acetylcholine: 0.1%, maintenance dose of 20 μL/kg/min, I.V.; 5) atropine: 0.2%, initial dose of 0.8 mL/kg and maintenance dose of 40 μL/kg/min, I.V.; and 6) penicillin: 8×10^5 IU dissolved in 2 mL saline, 0.4 mL/d per rat, intramuscular (I.M.).

Recording of the jejunal motility
All animals in the study were fasted for 12 h and given free access to water prior to anaesthetization with urethane. After supplementary anaesthesia, the rats in the drug-administered groups underwent endotracheal intubation to maintain the respiratory tract unobstructed and the left internal jugular venous catheter accessible for drug administration. A small incision (length: 5–8 mm in rats, 2–3 mm in mice) was made below the xiphoid, and a small balloon (diameter: approximately 2 mm) made of flexible rubber was inserted into the jejunum to approximately 3–5 cm (rats) or 0.8–1.2 cm (mice) distal to the duodenal suspensory ligament. The balloon, which was connected to a polyethylene tube (length: 10 cm), was then filled with 0.05–0.1 mL warm water to maintain the jejunal baseline pressure at approximately 0.3 kPa. The jejunal pressure was recorded with a transducer (YPJ01; Chengdu Instrument Factory, China) through the balloon and tube. The signal was collected with a biological signal-sampling system (RM6240; Chengdu Instrument Factory) for further analysis. The baseline pressure was maintained at 0.28–0.32 kPa. During the experiment, an electric heating board was used to maintain the temperature of the animals at 37 ± 0.5 °C.

EA stimulation
LI11 (Quchi) is located midway between the lateral end of the transverse cubital crease and the lateral humeral epicondyle. A pair of stainless steel acupuncture needles (diameter: 0.3 mm) were inserted to a depth of 3 mm into the muscle layer at the right LI11. The needles were connected to a Han EA therapeutic stimulator (LH402A; Beijing Huawei Industrial Development Corporation, China). The frequency of EA was set at 2/15 Hz for each stimulation.

Vagotomy
The animals were anaesthetized with urethane, and a small incision was made in the midline of the abdomen.

Animals then underwent bilateral vagotomy by dissection of the ventral and dorsal branches of the vagus nerve. The animals in the sham control group underwent the same procedure but without vagus nerve dissection. After suturing, the animals received penicillin antibiotic shots (0.2 mL each rat per day, I.M.) and were allowed three days to recover before the experimental session. Control group animals did not undergo any treatment before experiments. Twenty-four rats were used in this experiment.

Study design

To verify our hypothesis, we sought to 1) demonstrate whether EA at LI11 could promote jejunal motility; 2) explore the effects of EA at LI11 on the sympathetic pathway and the parasympathetic pathway, and 3) explore which somatic afferent nerve fibres participate in the stimulation process associated with EA at LI11.

In the first experiment, we divided animals into four groups (rats with EA, rats without EA, mice with EA and mice without EA) and then recorded the jejunal pressure to describe the characteristics of jejunal motility.

In the second experiment, we first used drugs to excite or inhibit a specific pathway before EA stimulation. Then, we cut the gastro-vagal nerves of the rats to evaluate the role of the parasympathetic pathway. Lastly, $\beta_1\beta_2$ adrenoceptor double-knockout ($\beta_1\beta_2^{-/-}$) mice, M_2M_3 muscarinic double-knockout ($M_2M_3^{-/-}$) mice, and wild-type mice were used to further verify the results.

In the last experiment, we divided animals into three groups (WT group, $\beta_1\beta_2^{-/-}$ group and $M_2M_3^{-/-}$ group) and used different intensities of EA to explore the mechanism by which somatic afferent nerve fibres participate in the stimulation process associated with EA at LI11. The procedure and details of the experiments are shown in Fig. 1. There were 8 animals per group in all experiments.

Assessment

Jejunal pressure during EA (dur-EA) was compared with the jejunal pressure before EA was performed (pre-EA)

[27]. The response was identified as being enhanced if the dur-EA pressure was >105% of the pre-EA pressure. The formula used to calculate the percentage change is given below (1).

$$\text{Percentage change} = \frac{\text{dur-EA}}{\text{pre-EA}} \times 100\% \tag{1}$$

Statistical analysis

Results are expressed as the mean ± SEM (standard error of the mean). Data were analysed using SPSS 19.0 (IBM, Armonk, NY, USA) and GraphPad Prism 5.0 (GraphPad Software, La Jolla, CA, USA) software programs. Paired-sample t tests (within the group) and one-way ANOVA (between groups) were used for statistical analyses. $P < 0.05$ was considered statistically significant. The data curves for different intensities were fitted with eq. (2) (X: log of intensity; Y: response, increasing as X increases. Top and bottom: plateaus in the same units as Y. LogEC50: same log units as X).

$$Y = \text{Bottom} + \frac{(\text{Top-Bottom})}{1 + 10^{\text{X-LogEC50}}} \tag{2}$$

Results

Characteristics of jejunal motility of normal animals with or without EA at LI11

After the injection of warm water into the balloon and stabilization of jejunal motility, we observed that the jejunal pressure was maintained in rats at approximately 0.8–1.0 kPa (Fig. 2a) and in mice at approximately 0.4–0.5 kPa, after injecting 0.05 mL warm water into the balloon (Fig. 2c). EA at LI11 induced increases in the contractile amplitude of jejunal motility in both mice and rats. In mice, the amplitude increased by approximately 0.05–0.3 kPa, and for rats, it increased by approximately 0.01–0.05 kPa (see Fig. 2b and d). The results suggested that EA at LI11 promotes jejunal motility.

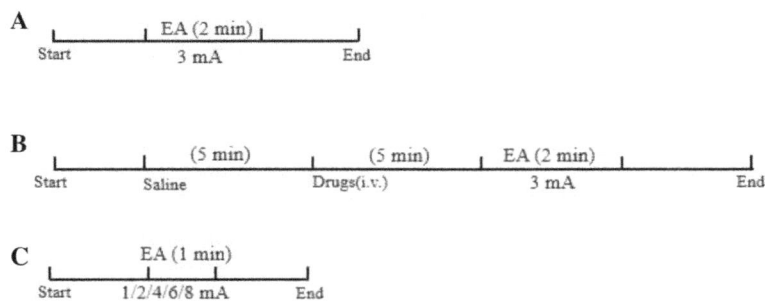

Fig. 1 The experimental procedure. **a** Intervention timeline in rats stimulated by ordinary EA. **b** Intervention timeline in rats with drug (clenbuterol, propranolol, acetylcholine or atropine) administration. **c** Intervention timeline in three kinds of mice (wild-type, $\beta_1\beta_2^{-/-}$, $M_2M_3^{-/-}$) with different intensities of electroacupuncture (1, 2, 4, 6, and 8 mA)

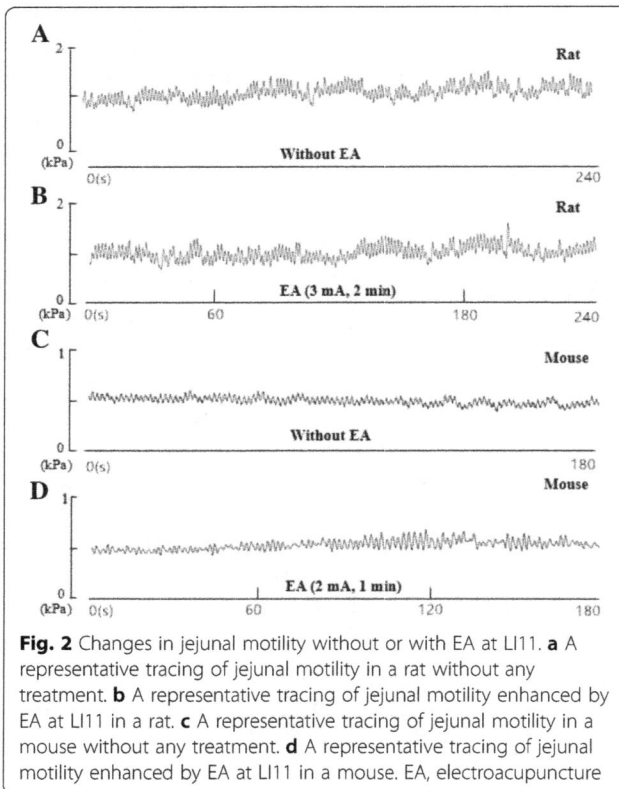

Fig. 2 Changes in jejunal motility without or with EA at LI11. **a** A representative tracing of jejunal motility in a rat without any treatment. **b** A representative tracing of jejunal motility enhanced by EA at LI11 in a rat. **c** A representative tracing of jejunal motility in a mouse without any treatment. **d** A representative tracing of jejunal motility enhanced by EA at LI11 in a mouse. EA, electroacupuncture

The role of the sympathetic pathway in the effect of EA at LI11

We used the beta adrenoceptor agonist clenbuterol and antagonist propranolol in rats and then performed EA at LI11 at an intensity of 3 mA. We divided rats into three groups: a control group (no administration), a clenbuterol group and a propranolol group (8 rats per group). Jejunum movement was markedly inhibited by the beta receptor agonist but was excited by propranolol.

As shown in Fig. 3Ab and Ac, we found that EA induced excitement of jejunum movement in animals in all groups, corresponding to changes greater than 105%, whereas no significant differences were observed among groups. To further substantiate whether the sympathetic pathway was involved in the effect of EA at LI11, we applied EA stimulation of 2 mA to the LI11 of $\beta_1\beta_2^{-/-}$ mice and found no significant differences between WT and $\beta_1\beta_2^{-/-}$ mice (8 mice per group, Fig. 3Bb and Bc). These data suggested that the sympathetic pathway may not play a key role in the effect of EA at LI11.

The role of the parasympathetic pathway in the effect of EA at LI11

Next, to determine whether the parasympathetic pathway was involved in the effect of EA at LI11 in regulating jejunal motility, we used the muscarinic receptor agonist ACh and antagonist atropine. We divided rats

into three groups (control group, Ach group and atropine group) with 8 rats per group.

The jejunal motility of the animals increased after Ach administration but decreased with atropine administration. We found that the internal pressure of the jejunum of rats in the Ach and control groups increased after EA stimulation. However, there were no obvious differences in jejunal motility between pre-EA and dur-EA after administration of atropine (from 0.24 ± 0.04 to 0.25 ± 0.04 in 8 rats, $P > 0.05$); hence, EA at LI11 did not enhance jejunal motility in the presence of atropine (Fig. 4Ab and Ac).

We then used rats with gastric vagotomy. We divided rats into three groups including a control group (no administration), a sham control group (subjected to the same procedure as the vagotomy group except for vagus nerve dissection) and a vagotomy group (8 rats per group). The experiment was performed three days after surgery. The results (see Fig. 4Ba, Bb and Bc) showed that movement of the jejunum was markedly inhibited and was not excited by EA stimulation when the bilateral gastro-vagal nerves were cut. The rats in the sham control group still exhibited enhanced jejunal motility after EA, as did the control group.

Furthermore, we used $M_2M_3^{-/-}$ mice to determine the role of the parasympathetic pathway in the effect of EA at LI11. There were 8 mice in the WT group and in the $M_2M_3^{-/-}$ group. The $M_2M_3^{-/-}$ group also did not exhibit enhanced jejunal motility, thus further suggesting that the parasympathetic pathway may mediate the effect of EA at LI11 (see Fig. 4Cb and Cc). Together, these results demonstrated that the parasympathetic pathway plays an important role in the promotion effect of EA at LI11.

Effects of EA at LI11 of different intensities on jejunal motility in mice

To gain further insight into the mechanism through which somatic afferent nerve fibres participate in the stimulation process associated with EA at LI11, different intensities of EA (1, 2, 4, 6, and 8 mA) were applied to three groups of mice ($\beta_1\beta_2^{-/-}$, $M_2M_3^{-/-}$ and WT mice). In the WT group, we observed that the promotion of jejunal motility by EA at LI11 with different intensities exceeded 105%, except for 1 mA stimulation (Fig. 5a and d). The $logEC_{50}$ value of EA stimulation in WT mice was 1.71 ± 0.59 mA, and the promotion of jejunal motility increased in response to increasing EA intensity up to 4 mA. When the intensity exceeded 4 mA, a plateau in jejunal motility was reached (Fig. 5d).

The $logEC_{50}$ value of EA stimulation in $\beta_1\beta_2^{-/-}$ mice was 4.60 ± 0.41 mA, and the value in $M_2M_3^{-/-}$ mice was 1.24 ± 1.77 mA. Compared with WT mice, the rate of change of jejunal pressure caused by EA at LI11 was significantly lower with intensities of 4 mA to 8 mA in M_2 $M_3^{-/-}$ mice, and a similar trend was observed for

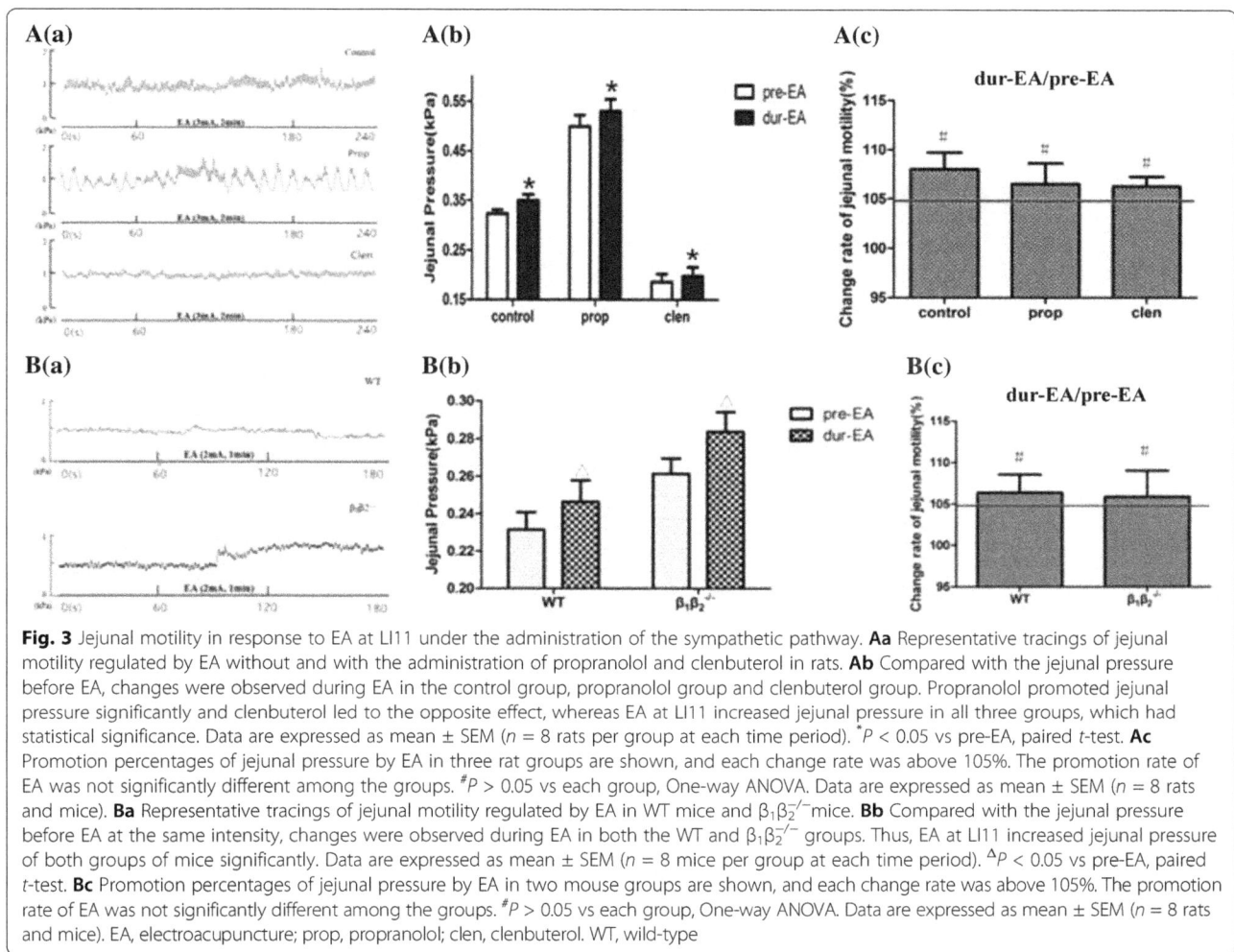

Fig. 3 Jejunal motility in response to EA at LI11 under the administration of the sympathetic pathway. **Aa** Representative tracings of jejunal motility regulated by EA without and with the administration of propranolol and clenbuterol in rats. **Ab** Compared with the jejunal pressure before EA, changes were observed during EA in the control group, propranolol group and clenbuterol group. Propranolol promoted jejunal pressure significantly and clenbuterol led to the opposite effect, whereas EA at LI11 increased jejunal pressure in all three groups, which had statistical significance. Data are expressed as mean ± SEM (n = 8 rats per group at each time period). $^*P < 0.05$ vs pre-EA, paired t-test. **Ac** Promotion percentages of jejunal pressure by EA in three rat groups are shown, and each change rate was above 105%. The promotion rate of EA was not significantly different among the groups. $^\#P > 0.05$ vs each group, One-way ANOVA. Data are expressed as mean ± SEM (n = 8 rats and mice). **Ba** Representative tracings of jejunal motility regulated by EA in WT mice and $\beta_1\beta_2^{-/-}$ mice. **Bb** Compared with the jejunal pressure before EA at the same intensity, changes were observed during EA in both the WT and $\beta_1\beta_2^{-/-}$ groups. Thus, EA at LI11 increased jejunal pressure of both groups of mice significantly. Data are expressed as mean ± SEM (n = 8 mice per group at each time period). $^\Delta P < 0.05$ vs pre-EA, paired t-test. **Bc** Promotion percentages of jejunal pressure by EA in two mouse groups are shown, and each change rate was above 105%. The promotion rate of EA was not significantly different among the groups. $^\#P > 0.05$ vs each group, One-way ANOVA. Data are expressed as mean ± SEM (n = 8 rats and mice). EA, electroacupuncture; prop, propranolol; clen, clenbuterol. WT, wild-type

2 mA. However, the $M_2M_3^{-/-}$ mice showed markedly different results as compared with those for other groups of mice subjected to EA of the same intensity, because EA at any intensity did not alter jejunal motility of these mice (Fig. 5c and f). No differences in the effects of EA were found between WT and $\beta_1\beta_2^{-/-}$ mice stimulated at intensities of 1, 2, or 4 mA.

There was a sudden increase in the rate of change of jejunal motility when the EA intensity was increased to 4 mA. However, the motility subsequently reached a plateau and did not further change when the EA intensity was increased to 6 mA.

In general, these data further demonstrated that the parasympathetic pathway plays an important role in the jejunal mobility promotion effect of EA at LI11.

Discussion

Gastrointestinal motility disorders occur in many gastrointestinal and other systemic diseases. Current drug therapy is not particularly effective at controlling the symptoms, and people with the disorder require long-term drug therapy. This therapy increases patients' economic burden and is associated with increased risks of possible drug side effects [28–31]. Acupuncture has been reported to be an effective method of complementary and alternative medicine for the treatment of gastrointestinal motility disorders in numerous clinical studies [32–35]. LI11 (Quchi) is a useful acupoint on the arm that is often used to treat gastrointestinal diseases. It has been studied primarily for mediating gastrointestinal motility [17–26].

Along the gastrointestinal tract, normal peristalsis and homeostatic sensory and motor mechanisms are under the control of extrinsic parasympathetic and sympathetic pathways. By exploring the response to vagal stimulation of the jejunum and ileum in cats, Kewenter has found clear evidence that splanchnic sympathetic fibres exert an inhibitory effect on the ileum at the intramural ganglionic, but not directly on smooth muscle cells [36]. Although Sato et al. have found that abdominal stimulation inhibits gastrointestinal motility, stimulation of the hind paw enhances gastrointestinal motility in rats [4–6]. On the basis

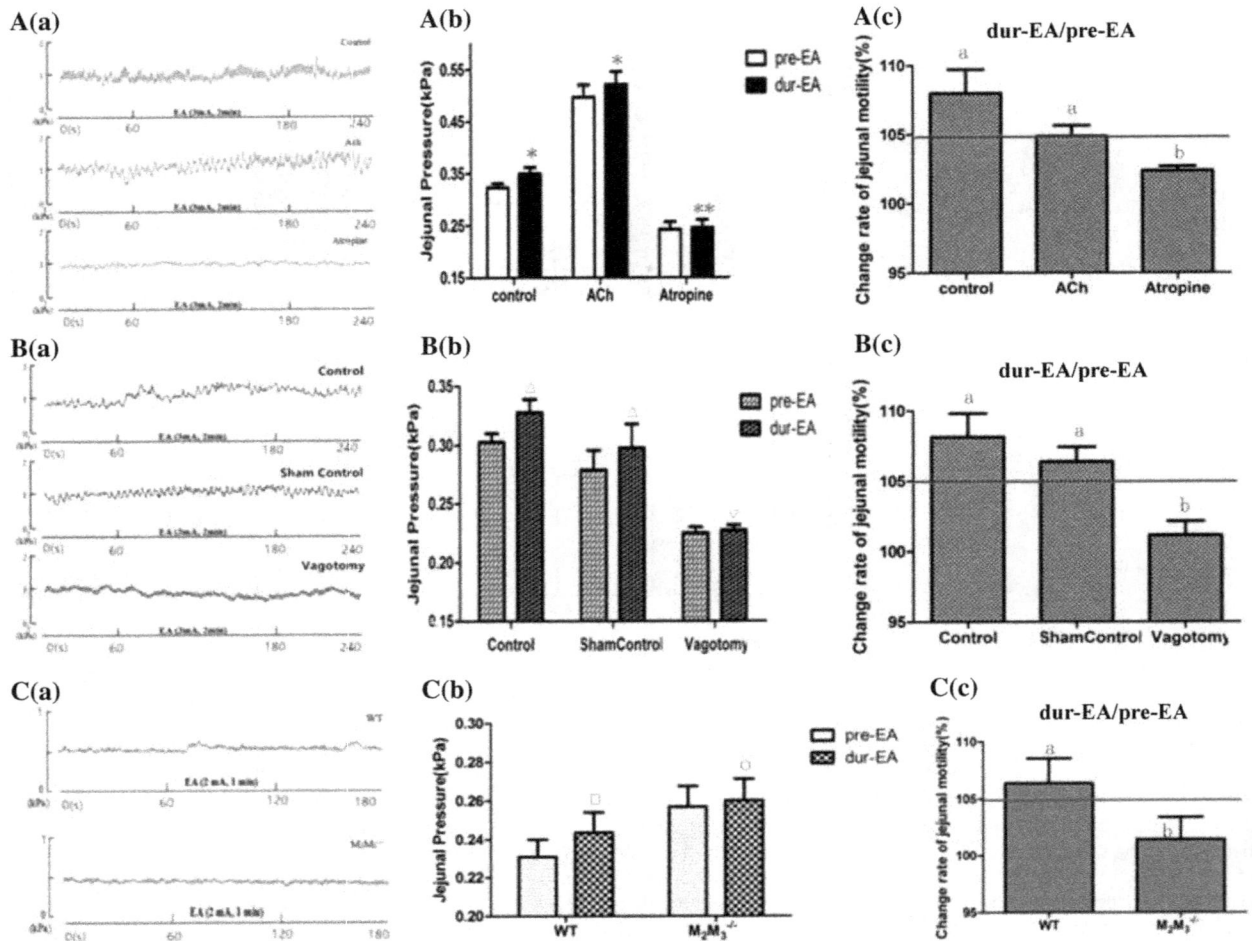

Fig. 4 Jejunal motility in response to EA at LI11 under the administration of the parasympathetic pathway. **Aa** Representative tracings of jejunal motility regulated by EA, EA with the administration of ACh and atropine in rats. **Ab** Compared with the jejunal pressure before EA, changes were observed during EA in the control group and ACh group, but EA at LI11 failed to enhance jejunal pressure in the atropine group. Data are expressed as mean ± SEM ($n = 8$ rats per group at each period). [a]$P < 0.05$ vs pre-EA, [#]$P > 0.05$ vs pre-EA, paired t-test. **Ac** Promotion percentages of jejunal pressure from EA in the atropine group was below 105%, and were significantly lower than the other two groups. Data are expressed as mean ± SEM ($n = 8$ rats/mice). [a]$P < 0.05$ vs control group, Ach group, [b]$P > 0.05$ vs control group, Ach group, One-way ANOVA. **Ba** Representative tracings of jejunal motility regulated by EA, EA with the vagotomy, sham operation in rats. **Bb** Compared with the jejunal pressure before EA, changes were observed during EA in the control group and sham control group, but EA at LI11 failed to enhance jejunal pressure in the vagotomy group. Data are expressed as mean ± SEM ($n = 8$ rats per group at each period). Δ$P < 0.05$ vs pre-EA, ▽$P > 0.05$ vs pre-EA, paired t-test. **Bc** Promotion percentages of jejunal pressure from EA in the vagotomy group was below 105%, and were significantly lower than the other two groups. Data are expressed as mean ± SEM ($n = 8$ rats/mice). [a]$P < 0.05$ vs control group, Ach group, [b]$P > 0.05$ vs control group, Ach group, One-way ANOVA. **Ca** Representative tracings of jejunal motility regulated by EA in WT mice and $M_2M_3^{-/-}$ mice. **Cb** Compared with the jejunal pressure before EA at the same intensity, the jejunal pressure in the WT group was enhanced with EA at LI11, but no impact was demonstrated in the $M_2M_3^{-/-}$ group. Data are expressed as mean ± SEM ($n = 8$ mice per group at each period). [*]$P < 0.05$ vs pre-EA, [o]$P > 0.05$ vs pre-EA, paired t-test. **Cc** Promotion percentages of jejunal pressure from EA in the $M_2M_3^{-/-}$ group were below 105%, and was significantly lower than the WT group. Data are expressed as mean ± SEM ($n = 8$ rats/mice). [a]$P < 0.05$ vs WT group, [b]$P > 0.05$ vs WT group, One-way ANOVA. EA, electroacupuncture; ACh, acetylcholine; WT, wild-type

of these discoveries, Zhu Bing et al. [14, 15, 37–39] have studied the effects of acupuncture stimulation and its physiological mechanisms and have demonstrated that acupuncture stimulation at abdominal points inhibits gastrointestinal motility but that acupuncture at hind paw points enhances gastrointestinal motility. These authors have also defined "homotopic" and "heterotopic"

acupoints as part of a new theoretical approach to interpret acupuncture effects and mechanisms. According to this approach, afferent innervation of a homotopic acupoint is in the same spinal cord segment from which the efferent branch innervates visceral organs, whereas afferent innervation is in a different segment for heterotopic acupoints. Acupuncture stimulation at homotopic points

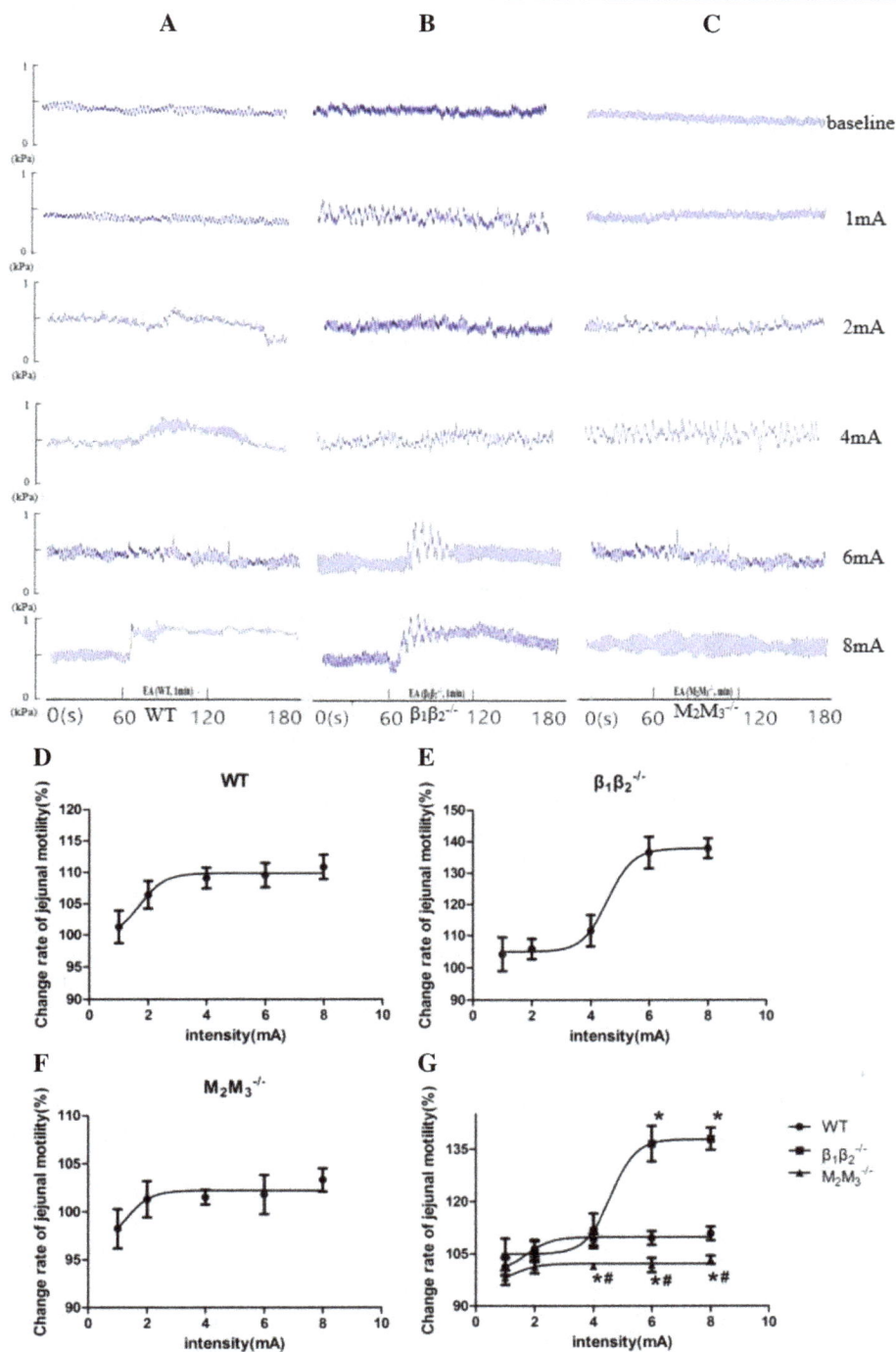

Fig. 5 The effect of different intensities of EA at LI11 on jejunal motility in WT, $\beta_1\beta_2^{-/-}$ and $M_2M_3^{-/-}$ mice. **a-c** Representative tracings of jejunal motility with different intensities of EA in WT, $\beta_1\beta_2^{-/-}$ and $M_2M_3^{-/-}$ mice, respectively. **d-f** The fitting curves of the EA effect with different intensities on jejunal motility in WT, $\beta_1\beta_2^{-/-}$ and $M_2M_3^{-/-}$ mice, respectively, showing the relationships between different intensities of EA (1, 2, 4, 6, and 8 mA) and the rate of change change rate in jejunal pressure. **g** The integrate fitting curve showed the enhanced effect of EA with different intensities on jejunal motility in three groups. Data are expressed as mean ± SEM (n = 8 mice). $^*P < 0.05$ vs WT mice, $^{\#}P < 0.05$ vs $\beta_1\beta_2^{-/-}$ mice, independent t-test. WT, wild-type

inhibits gastrointestinal motility via the sympathetic pathway; in contrast, acupuncture at heterotopic points enhances gastrointestinal motility via the parasympathetic pathway. Our previous study has shown that EA at ST25 inhibits gastric and jejunal motility via the sympathetic pathway; however, EA at ST37 excites gastric and jejunal motility via the parasympathetic pathway [13, 40]. These results support the "homotopic and heterotopic acupoints" theory. We then turned our focus to the gastrointestinal effect of acupuncture at forelimb points such as LI11 (Quchi) and its underlying mechanism, because LI11 is an effective acupoint in regulating gastrointestinal motility. In fact, many acupuncturists select this point for treating gastrointestinal motility disorders in clinical practice [17–22]. The experimental exploration of the effect of acupuncture at LI11 in regulating gastrointestinal motility has not received much attention in the past. Qin [14], however, has reported that acupuncture at LI11 (containing afferents from the C5 spinal dorsal horn) is a heterotopic acupoint to the jejunum (T9–12); this treatment increases the amplitude of peristalsis waves and enhances jejunal motility in normal rats as well as constipated and diarrheic rats. In our study, we used an antagonist and agonist for both adrenoceptors and muscarinic receptors to identify the roles of the sympathetic and parasympathetic pathways in normal rats. In addition, we used gene knock-out mice ($\beta_1\beta_2^{-/-}$ mice and $M_2M_3^{-/-}$ mice) for further verification. As shown in Fig. 2, we found a clear promotion effect of EA at LI11 on jejunal motility, in experiments using both rats and mice. Further explorations of the underlying neural mechanisms are shown in Figs. 3 and 4. There were three notable results of this study: 1) EA stimulation did not enhance jejunal motility in the presence of atropine in rats (Fig. 4a); 2) after vagotomy, the effect of EA on jejunal motility disappeared in rats (Fig. 4b); and 3) EA stimulation at LI11 was less effective in $M_2M_3^{-/-}$ mice than in WT and $\beta_1\beta_2^{-/-}$ mice (Fig. 4c).

To clarify the effect and mechanism of EA at LI11 on jejunal motility, we used both an antagonist and agonist of adrenoceptors and muscarinic receptors to determine the roles of the sympathetic and parasympathetic pathways in normal rats. We used intravenous administration, and thus, the drugs acted systemically on the entire body rather than on only the target nerves. Therefore, the roles of the target nerves could not be specifically verified [41–46]. Because of this limitation, gene knockout animals were used in our study. These mice have frequently been used in studies of neurobiological mechanisms of acupuncture, and their reliability has been demonstrated in previous related studies [47]. The results of the gene knockout study also fully supported our scientific hypothesis. Notably, in the experiments with different EA intensities (Fig. 5), the rate of change of jejunal motility in the $\beta_1\beta_2^{-/-}$ mice greatly exceeded that of the WT mice. The former group of mice showed a large amplitude change, from 4 mA to 6 mA stimulation intensity, and the maximum stimulation after entering the plateau region was 2 mA higher than that of the WT animals. We propose that the effect of

stimulation at LI11 is primarily due to parasympathetic-M receptors. The mutual antagonistic effects between sympathetic and parasympathetic nerves may explain why the rate of change in beta receptor knockout animals subjected to acupuncture is stronger than that of WT mice.

In this study, we observed that the parasympathetic pathway is involved in EA at LI11, but we did not perform further studies of the sympathetic pathway. No sufficient evidence was found to demonstrate that LI11 stimulation inhibits sympathetic nerve activity, thus representing a limitation of our study that should be addressed in further research. However, our previous work has shown that stimulating ST37 (Shangjuxu) excites parasympathetic nerves, and stimulating ST25 (Tianshu) excites sympathetic nerves [40, 48]. All these results together support the "homotopic and heterotopic acupoints" theory proposed by Zhu Bing et al.

To address the mechanism of the effects of EA stimulation at LI11, we sought to characterize the somatic afferents of EA stimulation by using different stimulation intensities. Somatic afferent nerve fibres are composed of Aα- (group I), Aβ- (group II), Aδ- (group III) and C-fibres (group IV) [37, 49]. The mean stimulation thresholds for inducing firing in mouse Aδ- and C-fibres have been reported to be approximately 2 mA and 3 mA, respectively [37]. Thus, we chose different EA stimulation intensities (1, 2, 4, 6, and 8 mA) to test the responses in three types of mice ($\beta_1\beta_2^{-/-}$, $M_2M_3^{-/-}$ and WT mice). In normal mice (the WT mice group), EA at LI11 significantly increased jejunal motility at all intensities except 1 mA, and when the intensity exceeded 4 mA, the effect plateaued. These results verify that Aδ-fibres are activated by the stimulation when the intensity is maintained at 2 mA and that 4 mA can active C-fibres. The $M_2M_3^{-/-}$ group differed from the WT and $\beta_1\beta_2^{-/-}$ groups in that the rate of change remained under 105% for all stimulation intensities. This result suggests that activation of muscarinic receptors plays a key role in the effect of EA at LI11, thus further supporting further our hypothesis.

Conclusion

In summary, we clearly demonstrated the important role of the parasympathetic pathway in the promotion effect of EA stimulation at LI11 on jejunal motility. The intensity-dependent manner of EA stimuli indicates that Aδ-fibres and C-fibres may participate in the response to EA stimulation from 2 mA to 4 mA. LI11, a heterotopic point, also promotes jejunal motility under EA stimulation, similarly to the points on the hind paw. This study provides further evidence that acupuncture regulates gastrointestinal function via the somatic-autonomic reflex.

Acknowledgments
The authors thank Na Zhang, Yuqin Li and Yidan Wang for their assistance.

Funding
This work was supported by the National Key Basic Research Program (973 Program) [grant number 2011CB505206], the National Natural Science Foundation of China [grant numbers 81,202,744, 81,373,749, 81,574,071, 81,673,883], the Graduate Student Research Innovation Project of University in Jiangsu Province of China [grant number KYLX15_0995], and the People Programme (Marie Curie Actions) of the European Union's Seventh Framework Programme under REA grant agreement number PIRSES-GA-2013-612,589.

Authors' contributions
BX conceived and designed the experiments; YW, YL, NZ performed the experiments; XH and XS wrote the paper; ZY supervised the study. All authors have read and approved the final version of manuscript.

Authors' information
Xuanming Hu, Ph.D candidate, Major Research Direction: basic research of acupuncture treatment.

Competing interests
The authors declare that they have no competing interests.

References
1. Lauro A, Zanfi C, Dazzi A, di Gioia P, Stanghellini V, Pironi L, et al. Disease-related intestinal transplant in adults: results from a single center. Transplant Proc. 2014;46:245–8.
2. Chey WD, Kurlander J, Eswaran S. Irritable bowel syndrome: a clinical review. JAMA. 2015;313:949–58.
3. Törnblom H, Simrén M, Abrahamsson H. Gastrointestinal motility and neurogastroenterology. Scandinavian J Gastroenterology. 2015;50:685–97.
4. Kametani H, Sato A, Sato Y, Simpson A. Neural mechanisms of reflex facilitation and inhibition of gastric motility to stimulation of various skin areas in rats. J Physiol. 1979;294:407–18.
5. Sato A, Schmidt RF. Muscle and cutaneous afferents evoking sympathetic reflexes. Brain Res. 1966;2:399–401.
6. Sato A, Kaufman A, Koizumi K, Brooks CM. Afferent nerve groups and sympathetic reflex pathways. Brain Res. 1969;14:575–87.
7. Caulfield MP. Muscarinic receptors–characterization, coupling and function. Pharmacol Ther. 1993;58:319–79.
8. Noguchi E. Acupuncture regulates gut motility and secretion via nerve reflexes. Auton Neurosci. 2010;156:15–8.
9. Bayliss WM, Starling EH. The movements and innervation of the small intestine. J Physiol. 1899;24:99–143.
10. Kock NG. An experimental analysis of mechanisms engaged in reflex inhibition of intestinal motility. Acta Physiol Scand Suppl. 1959;47:1–54.
11. Jiang J, Yi Y, Zhan L. Acupuncture: a good choice to patients with intractable slow-transit constipation. Int J Color Dis. 2015;30:721–2.
12. Han G, Leem J, Lee H, Lee J. Electroacupuncture to treat gastroesophageal reflux disease: study protocol for a randomized controlled trial. Trials. 2016;17:246.
13. Yu Z, Zhang N, Lu CX, Pang TT, Wang KY, Jiang JF, et al. Electroacupuncture at ST25 inhibits jejunal motility: role of sympathetic pathways and TRPV1. World J Gastroenterol. 2016;22:1834–43.
14. Qin QG, Gao XY, Liu K, Yu XC, Li L, Wang HP, et al. Acupuncture at heterotopic acupoints enhances jejunal motility in constipated and diarrheic rats. World J Gastroenterol. 2014;20:18271–83.
15. Gao X, Qin Q, Yu X, Liu K, Li L, Qiao H, et al. Acupuncture at heterotopic acupoints facilitates distal colonic motility via activating M3 receptors and somatic afferent C-fibers in normal, constipated, or diarrhoeic rats. Neurogastroenterol Motil. 2015;27:1817–30.
16. Shen EY, Lai YJ. The efficacy of frequency-specific acupuncture stimulation on extracellular dopamine concentration in striatum—a rat model study. Neurosci Lett. 2007;415:179–84.
17. Xiong F, Wang Y, Li SQ, Tian M, Zheng CH, Huang GY. Electroacupuncture decreases the urinary bladder pressure in patients with acute gastrointestinal injury. J Huazhong Univ Sci Technol[Med Sci]. 2015;34(5):775–81.
18. Wu JN, Zhang BY, Zhu WZ, Du RS, Liu ZS. Ministered acupressure for treating adult psychiatric patients with constipation: a randomized controlled trial. Zhongguo Zhen Jiu. 2014;34(6):521–8.
19. Xu X. Zheng C1, Zhang M, Wang W, Huang GA. randomized controlled trial of acupuncture to treat functional constipation: design and protocol. BMC Complement Altern Med. 2014;29;14:423.
20. Chang XR, Yan J, Shen J, Liu M, Wang XJ. Observation on the therapeutic effect of needling method for harmonizing spleen-stomach on diabetic gastroparesis. Zhongguo Zhen Jiu. 2007;27(4):258–60.
21. Wang YL, Cao X, Liu ZC, Xu B. Observation on the therapeutic effect of electroacupuncture on simple obesity of gastrointestinal heat pattern/syndrome. World J Acupuncture-Moxibustion (WJAM). 2013;23:1–5.
22. Qin QG, Wang HP, Liu K, Zhao YX, Ben H, Gao XY, et al. Effects of acupuncture on intestinal motility: Agonism and antagonism. World Chin Med. 2013;8(3):262–6.
23. Jang JH, Lee DJ, Bae CH, Ha KT, Kwon S, Park HJ, et al. Changes in small intestinal motility and related hormones by acupuncture stimulation at Zusanli (ST 36) in mice. Chin J Integr Med. 2017;23(2):215–20.
24. Feng H, Yu Z, Xu B. Roles of TRPV1 receptor in electroacupuncture regulating the jejunal motility of mice: an experimental study. Zhongguo Zhong Xi Yi Jie He Za Zhi. 2014;34(7):859–63.
25. Yu Z, Xia YB, Lu MX, Lin J, Yu WJ, Xu B. Influence of electroacupuncture stimulation of "tianshu" (ST 25), "quchi" (LI 11) and "shangjuxu" (ST 37) and their pairs on gastric motility in the rat. Zhen Ci Yan Jiu. 2013;38(1):40–7.
26. Fang JQ, Zhang LL, Shao XM, Lian LL, Yu XJ, Dong ZH, et al. Effects of transcutaneous electrical acupoint stimulation combined with general anesthesia on changes of gastric dynamics in controlled hypotension dogs. Zhen Ci Yan Jiu. 2011;36(6):397–402.
27. Pang T, Lu C, Wang K, Liang C, Yu Z, Zhu B, et al. Electroacupuncture at ST25 inhibits Cisapride-induced gastric motility in an intensity-dependent manner. Evid Based Complement Alternat Med. 2016;2016:3457025.
28. Koloski NA, Talley NJ, Boyce PM. The impact of functional gastrointestinal disorders on quality of life. Am J Gastroenterol. 2000;95:67–71.
29. Quigley, Eamonn MM. Probiotics in functional gastrointestinal disorders: what are the facts? Curr Opin Pharmacol. 2008;8:704–8.
30. Schmulsom M, Corazziari E, Ghoshal UC, Myung SJ, Gerson CD, Quigley EM, et al. A four-country comparison of healthcare systems, implementation of diagnostic criteria, and treatment availability for functional gastrointestinal disorders a report of the Rome foundation working team on cross-cultural, multinational research. Neurogastroenterol Motil. 2014;26:1368–85.
31. Kaminski A, Kamper A, Thaler K. Antidepressants for the treatment of abdominal pain-related functional gastrointestinal disorders inchildren and adolescents. Cochrane Database Syst Rev. 2011;(7).
32. Lima FA, Ferreira LE, Pace FH. Acupuncture effectiveness as a complementary therapy in functional dyspepsia patients. Arq Gastroenterol. 2013;50:202–7.
33. Zhang X, Jin HF, Fan YH, Lu B, Meng LN, Chen JD. Effects and mechanisms of transcutaneous electroacupuncture on chemotherapy-induced nausea and vomiting. Evid Based Complement Alternat Med. 2014;2014:860631.
34. Ouyang H, Xing J, Chen J. Electroacupuncture restores impaired gastric accommodation in vagotomized dogs. Dig Dis Sci. 2004;49:1418–24.
35. Glickman-Simon R, Tessier J. Guided imagery for postoperative pain, energy healing for quality of life, probiotics for acute diarrhea in children, acupuncture for postoperative nausea and vomiting, and animal-assisted therapy for mental disorders. Explore (NY). 2014;10:326–9.
36. Pahlin PE, Kewenter J. Sympathetic nervous control of cat ileocecal sphincter. Am J Phys. 1976;231:296–305.
37. Li YQ, Zhu B, Rong PJ, Ben H, Li YH. Neural mechanism of acupuncture-modulated gastric motility. World J Gastroenterol. 2007;13:709–16.
38. Zhao YX, Cui CX, Qin QG, Gao JH, Yu XC, Zhu B. Effect of manual acupuncture on bowel motility in normal kunming mouse. J Tradit Chin Med. 2015;35:227–33.
39. Zhu B, Xu WD, Rong PJ, Ben H, Gao XY. By C-fiber reflex inhibition by electroacupuncture with different intensities applied at homotopic and heterotopic acupoints in rats selectively destructive effects on myelinated and unmyelinated afferent fibers. Brain Res. 2004;1011:228–37.
40. Yu Z, Cao X, Xia Y, Ren B, Feng H, Wang Y, et al. Electroacupuncture stimulation at CV12 inhibits gastric motility via TRPV1 receptor. Evid Based Complement Alternat Med. 2013;2013:294789.
41. Mason RP, Giles TD, Sowers JR. Evolving mechanisms of action of beta blockers: focus on nebivolol. J Cardiovasc Pharmacol. 2009;54(2):123–8.
42. Pertwee RG. Cannabinoids and the gastrointestinal tract. Gut. 2001;48:859–67.
43. Bertaccini G, Coruzzi G. Receptors in the gastrointestinal tract. Pharmacol Res Commun. 1987;19:87–118.

44. Allescher HD. Medicamentous modification of gastrointestinal motility and secretion. Z Gastroenterol. 1991;29:27–30.

45. Michel MC. Therapeutic modulation of urinary bladder function: multiple targets at multiple levels. Annu Rev Pharmacol Toxicol. 2015;55:269–87.

46. Nunes EJ1, Randall PA, Podurgiel S, Correa M, Salamone JD. Nucleus accumbens neurotransmission and effort-related choice behavior in food motivation: effects of drugs acting on dopamine, adenosine, and muscarinic acetylcholine receptors. Neurosci Biobehav Rev. 2013;37:2015–25.

47. Gao X, Zhao Y, Su Y, Liu K, Yu X, Cui C, et al. β1/2or M2/3Receptors Are Required for Different Gastrointestinal Motility Responses Induced by Acupuncture at Heterotopic or Homotopic Acupoints. PLoS One. 2016; 11(12):e0168200c.

48. Yuan M, Li Y, Wang Y, Zhang N, Hu X, Yin Y, et al. Electroacupuncture at ST37 enhances Jejunal motility via excitation of the parasympathetic system in rats and mice. Evid Based Complement Alternat Med. 2016;2016:3840230.

49. Ohsawa H, Yamaguchi S, Ishimaru H, Shimura M, Sato Y. Neural mechanism of pupillary dilation elicited by electro-acupuncture stimulation in anesthetized rats. J Auton Nerv Syst. 1997;64:101–6.

10

A survey of evidence users about the information need of acupuncture clinical evidence

Xiue Shi[1,2,3,4†], Xiaoqin Wang[1,2,3†], Yali Liu[1,2], Xiuxia Li[1,2], Dang Wei[1,2], Xu Zhao[1,5], Jing Gu[6] and Kehu Yang[1,2,3*]

Abstract

Background: The PRISMA statement was rarely used in the field of acupuncture, possibly because of knowledge gaps and the lack of items tailored for characteristics of acupuncture. And with an increasing number of systematic reviews in acupuncture, it is necessary to develop an extension of PRISMA for acupuncture. And this study was the first step of our project, of which the aim was to investigate the need for information of clinical evidence on acupuncture from the perspectives of evidence users.

Methods: We designed a questionnaire based on a pilot survey and a literature review of acupuncture systematic review or meta-analysis(SR/MA). Participants from five cities (Lanzhou, Chengdu, Shanghai, Nanjing and Beijing) representing the different regions of China, including clinicians, researchers and postgraduates in their second year of Master studies or higher level, were surveyed.

Results: A total of 269 questionnaires were collected in 18 hospitals, medical universities and research agencies, and 251 (93 %) with complete data were used for analysis. The average age of respondents was 33 years (SD 8.959, range 25–58) with male 43 % and female 57 %. Most respondents had less than 5 years of working experience on acupuncture, and read only one to five articles per month. Electronic databases, search engines and academic conferences were the most common sources for obtaining information. Fifty-six percent of the respondents expressed low satisfaction of the completeness of information from the literature. The eight items proposed for acupuncture SR/MAs received all high scores, and five of the items scored higher than eight on a scale zero to ten. The differences for the scores of most items between postgraduates and non-postgraduates were not statistically significant.

Conclusions: The majority of the respondents were not very satisfied with the information provided in acupuncture SRs. Most of the items proposed in this questionnaire received high scores, and opinions from postgraduates and non-postgraduates tended to agree on most items. Comments from the respondents can promote future work.

Keywords: Acupuncture SR/MAs, Information need, Questionnaire, Evidence users

Background

Reporting guidelines promote transparent and rigorous reporting. In 1996, several experts from the United States, United Kingdom and Canada worked together and published the Consolidated Standards of Reporting Trials (CONSORT) statement in Journal of the American Medical Association (JAMA), which started the rapid development of reporting guidelines in medical research [1]. With the evolving methodology of randomized controlled trials (RCT) and evidence-based medicine (EBM), CONSORT has been updated in 2001 and 2010 [2, 3], CONSORT 2010 being the latest version. CONSORT has been endorsed and uptaken after its release by several medical journals [4], and reporting guidelines have improved the quality of both the reporting and the methodology [5, 6]. Because different fields of medicine and different types of research data differ in characteristics, several extensions have been developed. The *STandards for Reporting*

* Correspondence: kehuyangebm2006@126.com
†Equal contributors
[1]Evidence-Based Medicine Center, School of Basic Medical Sciences, Lanzhou University, Lanzhou 730000, China
[2]Key Laboratory of Evidence Based Medicine and Knowledge Translation of Gansu Province, Lanzhou 730000, China
Full list of author information is available at the end of the article

Interventions in Clinical Trials of Acupuncture (STRICTA) was officially published in 2001, and was updated along with CONSORT in 2010 [7, 8]. Authors of acupuncture trials and systematic reviews have expressed their belief that STRICTA substantially contributes to the reporting of acupuncture interventions [9] and has significantly improved the reporting quality [10].

High-quality systematic reviews (SRs) of acupuncture form the best evidence to inform guidelines and clinical practice. Accurate and complete reporting enables readers to determine the internal and external validity of the research result, and editors and reviewers to make comprehensive and objective judgement effectively. The Preferred Reporting Items for Systematic reviews and Meta-Analyses (PRISMA) statement was developed for systematic reviews and meta-analyses (SR/MAs) [11]. Although PRISMA promotes the quality of the reporting and methodology of SR/MAs, in some specific areas, it cannot meet all the needs. The extensions PRISMA-Equity [12], PRISMA-Abstract [13], PRISMA-Protocol [14] and PRISMA-Network Meta-Analysis [15] were developed in 2012, 2013, 2015 and 2015, respectively. In 2012, the assessment of the published 476 acupuncture SRs/MAs with PRISMA and their included RCTs showed low quality in general. Information from those studies could not meet the needs of acupuncture practitioners, and therefore was not usable for implementation [16]. Furthermore, the results from a survey of the application status of the PRISMA statement indicated that it was rarely used in the field of acupuncture, possibly because of knowledge gaps among researchers. Another probable reason was lack of items tailored for the characteristics of acupuncture [17]. On the other hand, research in acupuncture develops rapidly with an increasing number of studies published every year [18]. Thus, it is necessary to develop an extension of PRISMA for acupuncture, and implement it along with PRISMA.

Our project aims to develop a reporting guideline for acupuncture SR/MAs. This project consists of three phases: the investigation about the requirements of evidence users for the information needs of reporting of acupuncture SR/MAs; three rounds of Delphi process; and a face-to-face meeting for reaching consensus. This paper described the first phrase, where we aimed to conduct a survey among the evidence users about their information needs, to directly capture their opinions about the current reporting of evidence and the further needs on information reported in acupuncture SR/MAs. Before this survey, we conducted a pilot study in Lanzhou on the questionnaire, and found that most of the questions and items were highly valued by the participants. We also investigated the reporting rates of the items in acupuncture SR/MAs, and found a range of 6.3 to 73.7 % [19]. In this survey, with comments from users and evidence from the literature review, we aimed to design a rigorous and valid questionnaire, and to conduct a survey among acupuncture clinicians, researchers, teachers, and postgraduates across the whole country. Based on this survey, we will draft the items for acupuncture SR/MAs reporting for the Delphi process in next period.

Methods

Design of the questionnaire

We designed a questionnaire containing three main parts: 1) demographic information of the respondent, including sex, age, occupation, education, and professional title; 2) the experience, awareness and knowledge on the clinical evidence of acupuncture, including the duration of career, working fields, and reading behavior, 3) the importance of the proposed items from the perspectives of evidence users, including background information about acupuncture, diagnostic criteria of Chinese medicine, types and details of acupuncture, outcome measures of the effects, experience of the operators, and the rationale of the follow-up time. Furthermore, respondents were invited to provide any item they thought important but were missing in our list. The initial items in part three were based on the analysis of existing reporting guidelines, such as STRICTA and PRISMA, and a systematic review of 476 SR/MAs on acupuncture [16] (see Additional file 1 for a copy of the questionnaire).

The questions were designed to be easy to complete, with several pre-defined options from which the respondents could simply choose their answer. An open-ended response marked "other" was added into some questions if necessary. Respondents were asked to score the reporting items for the necessity and feasibility of inclusion in SR/MAs of acupuncture using the Likert scale [20] ranging from zero (not necessary) to ten (essential). For the eight items need to be rated, each question included a space for "explanation" in the end for respondents who were willing to provide more details.

Method to conduct survey

We conducted a pilot survey by two trained investigators (XQW, DW) in Lanzhou to find out necessary adjustment and to evaluate the feasibility in an attempt to predict an appropriate sample size and improve the study design prior to performing the formal one. Then, the two trained investigators completed the formal survey between April and June, 2014 by distributing and collecting the questionnaires in person, which could prevent the low response rate of electronic questionnaire. Our investigators were responsible only for distributing the material, interpreting the background, and checking with the respondents to ensure the completeness of the questionnaires. For subjective questions, the respondents were asked to fill it themselves without our investigators' interfering.

In the formal survey, we visited Traditional Chinese Medicine agencies, hospitals and colleges in five cities (Lanzhou, Chengdu, Shanghai, Nanjing and Beijing).

With the inclusion criterion that respondents must have acupuncture clinical experience more than 1 year, we surveyed clinicians, researchers, postgraduates in their second year or higher, and doctors majoring in acupuncture. We surveyed at least 50 individuals in each city, with about 40 % of respondents being students. Acupuncture students, practitioners and researchers have a critical role in bridging evidence and practice, and their opinions are mainly based on practical work which can provide valuable experience on what is the most urgently needed information in acupuncture SR/MAs. Before we distributed the questionnaire, we identified a liaison person in every city, and collected information about the respondents in advance. Then, the investigator visited the respondents one by one. This investigation was approved by the Research Ethics Committee of the First Hospital of Lanzhou University, Lanzhou, China (approval number: LDYYL2013-0007). All the participants were required to sign informed consent. We marked student or non-student on the left top of each questionnaire to avoid errors.

Data analysis

Data were processed using Epidata 3.1 and analyzed with software Excel 2013. For the close-ended question with given options, we used frequencies and percentages to summarize the results. For evaluating the importance of the proposed items, we used mean value of the score, and analyzed the difference between postgraduates and non-postgraduates (including clinicians and researchers) with independent-Sample T-test with the SPSS Statistics 19 software. Additional items provided by respondents beyond this questionnaire were listed in a table. We abstracted all the questionnaire independently and grouped them according to the type of suggestion or opinion on reporting. All discrepancies were discussed and agreed on for final interpretation.

Results

A total of 269 questionnaires were collected, of which 251 (93 %) were used for analysis and 18 (7 %) were excluded because of missing data (Fig. 1). Of the included questionnaires, 52 (21 %) were from Lanzhou, 50 (20 %) from Chengdu, 48 (19 %) from Nanjing, 55 (22 %) from Shanghai, and 46 (18 %) from Beijing. The demographic and socioeconomic characteristics of the respondents are shown in Table 1. The average age was 33 years (SD = 9.0, range 25–58).

Table 2 showed the findings on the respondents' experience and knowledge on clinical evidence of acupuncture. More than half of the respondents had work experience of less than 5 years. The main work of most respondents was clinical treatment with acupuncture. On the other hand, a notable percentage of the participants were involved in more than three types of work. Most of the respondents read one to five articles each month. According to the response, electronic databases, printed professional journal, academic conferences, search engines, and ancient literature were all commonly used to obtain information. Forty-three of the respondents chose at least three or more approaches. The most popular type of literature read by the respondents was RCT, and for the satisfaction of the completeness of information in acupuncture literature, only 2 % were very satisfied.

For the reporting items in our questionnaire, mean scores were all above five. Table 3 presents the respondents' ranking of each item. The additional suggestions proposed by the respondents about what should be presented in acupuncture SR/MAs were shown in Table 4.

Discussion

Our survey and questions were designed for acupuncture evidence users with the hope of collecting reporting items for acupuncture SR/MAs, which was different from STRICA for reporting interventions in clinical trials of acupuncture. To ensure the representativeness, we discussed how to select the participants considering various aspects, including geographic location, gender, and work experience. We visited participants from five cities located in south, north, north-west and south-west China, and included about 40 % students. We surveyed students who

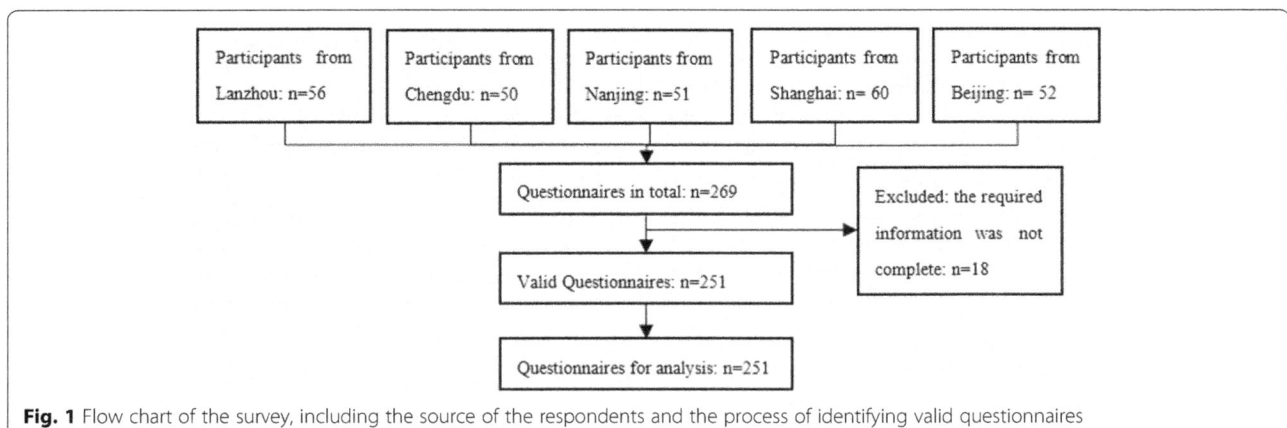

Fig. 1 Flow chart of the survey, including the source of the respondents and the process of identifying valid questionnaires

Table 1 Characteristics of the respondents

Variable	Categories	Respondents: n (%)
Total		251
Age	20 ~ 30	130 (52 %)
	30 ~ 40	75 (30 %)
	40 ~ 50	32 (13 %)
	≥50	14 (6 %)
Sex	Male	142 (57 %)
	Female	109 (43 %)
Education	Medical Doctor	42 (17 %)
	Master	161 (64 %)
	Bachelor	46 (18 %)
	Beneath Bachelor	2 (1 %)
Occupation	Postgraduate student specializing in acupuncture	95 (38 %)
	Clinician practicing acupuncture	126 (50 %)
	Others (including teachers and researchers)	30 (12 %)
Health worker grade[a]	Senior	39 (16 %)
	Vice-senior	30 (12 %)
	Middle	43 (17 %)
	Primary or below	51 (20 %)
	No title	88 (35 %)
Specialty	Western Medicine	3 (1 %)
	Traditional Chinese Medicine (TCM)	236 (94 %)
	Integrative Medicine	12 (5 %)

[a]This refers to the category of title obtained after passing a qualifying test

were at least in the second year of their Master studies, and having completed an internship on acupuncture for at least one year, to avoid surveying participants whose knowledge of acupuncture is too limited to provide practical response. We recruited the participants from universities conducting research and teaching in TCM and their affiliated hospitals, research institutes for acupuncture, and TCM hospitals, to be able to fully reflect the need of scientific research among the various groups of evidence users.

Our findings were not optimistic in terms of the reading behavior of the respondents. Most of the respondents read one to five relevant articles per month, and surprisingly, we found also respondents who never read the literature. Yet most of the participants could give advice about the information they need in an article, based on their clinical experience of acupuncture. Forty-three percent of the respondents were not satisfied with the adequacy of information reported in SR/MAs, which corresponds to the poor reporting quality of acupuncture SR/MAs [16].

Acupuncture is used for various kinds of diseases [21] which differ from each other in terms of theoretical and

evidence basis. The authors should clearly describe the theoretical knowledge on the use of acupuncture for this disease to promote the rapid understanding for readers. Acupuncture is characterized by a broad diversity of styles and approaches in both East Asia and Western countries [22], and the ways of conducting acupuncture and the theories behind these different styles also differ [23]. Therefore the appropriate background information on the style, and theoretical basis of acupuncture for the specific disease should be reported.

In general, there are two different sets of diagnostic criteria: syndrome differentiation used in Traditional Chinese Medicine, and diagnostic criteria of diseases used in Western medicine [24]. These criteria should be interpreted in completely different ways, and it is important to indicate which set of criteria, or both, should be used. There are diverse types of needles, and nine classical acupuncture needles are always mentioned, which include filiform needle, shear needle, round-pointed needle, spoon needle, lance needle, round-sharp needle, stiletto needle, long needle and big needle [25]. With different functions [26], it is necessary to state which type of needles the study can be applied to. At the same time, the details of the acupuncture intervention including numbers of needles, names of acupoints, depths of puncture, de-qi or not, and times for needle retention, will all influence the treatment effect. As for judgement on effect, there are many indicators used only in acupuncture, such as acupuncture-tailored symptomatic relief and adverse effects like bleeding. Between 2000 and 2009, 95 cases of serious adverse events were reported [27]. However, many such events have not been reported among adequately-trained acupuncturists, and they should therefore not be considered inherent to acupuncture, but instead being due to malpractice of acupuncturists [28]. Therefore, a qualified acupuncturist is needed to ensure the effectiveness and safety of the treatment. The necessary follow-up time differs greatly between different conditions, and the patients treated with acupuncture also need to be followed up for possible side effects.

Our results showed a high acceptability and recognition for most items among the respondents (Table 3). The mean scores of the third, fourth, fifth, sixth and eighth item were higher than eight, the first item was 7.2, while items two and seven were lower than six. But we did not exclude or include any items in this period. Instead, we would like to integrate these items with additional comments from the respondents in order to form the checklist of items for the following Delphi process. We also compared the mean scores between postgraduates and NPs (including methodologists, acupuncture clinicians, researchers and teachers), using the independent-sample T-test. The results of the T-test showed that the difference of the mean scores between postgraduates and NPs were

Table 2 Findings on respondents' experience and knowledge on clinical evidence of acupuncture

Subjects	Options	Respondent: n (%)		
		Postgraduates (95)	Non-postgraduates[b] (156)	Total
Years of experience in acupuncture	<5 years	79 (83 %)	49 (31 %)	128 (51 %)
	5-10 years	14 (15 %)	46 (29 %)	60 (24 %)
	10-20 years	1 (1 %)	25 (16 %)	26 (10 %)
	>20 years	1 (1 %)	36 (24 %)	37 (15 %)
Main work related to acupuncture (multiple answers allowed)	Clinical treatment	87 (92 %)	141 (90 %)	228 (91 %)
	Rehabilitation care	26 (27 %)	45 (29 %)	71 (28 %)
	Clinical research	49 (52 %)	85 (54 %)	134 (53 %)
	Basic research	17 (18 %)	37 (24 %)	54 (22 %)
	Review	12 (13 %)	16 (10 %)	28 (11 %)
	Writing SR/MA	9 (9 %)	10 (6 %)	19 (8 %)
	Writing clinical guidelines	2 (2 %)	6 (4 %)	8 (3 %)
	Acting as a reviewer	0 (0 %)	8 (5 %)	8 (3 %)
	Editor	0 (0 %)	1 (0.4 %)	1 (0.4 %)
	Others	0 (0 %)	3 (2 %)	3 (1 %)
Papers on acupuncture read per month	>10	17 (18 %)	35 (22 %)	52 (21 %)
	5–10	25 (26 %)	42 (27 %)	67 (27 %)
	1–5	48 (51 %)	76 (49 %)	124 (49 %)
	0	5 (5 %)	3 (2 %)	8 (3 %)
Ways of obtaining information on acupuncture (multiple answers allowed)	Medical databases	83 (87 %)	130 (83 %)	213 (85 %)
	Printed professional journals	21 (22 %)	65 (42 %)	86 (34 %)
	Academic meetings	30 (32 %)	82 (53 %)	112 (45 %)
	Search engines	40 (42 %)	79 (51 %)	119 (47 %)
	Ancient literature bibliographies	38 (40 %)	61 (40 %)	99 (39 %)
	Others	1 (1 %)	3 (2 %)	4 (16 %)
Types of studies most commonly read (multiple answers allowed)	RCTs	68 (72 %)	104 (67 %)	172 (69 %)
	Observational studies	52 (55 %)	75 (48 %)	127 (51 %)
	Basic research	37 (39 %)	78 (50 %)	115 (46 %)
	Reviews	32 (34 %)	48 (31 %)	80 (32 %)
	SRs/MAs	29 (31 %)	63 (0 %)	92 (37 %)
	Clinical practice guidelines	25 (26 %)	65 (42 %)	90 (36 %)
	Ancient literature	27 (28 %)	61 (39 %)	88 (35 %)
	Others	1 (1 %)	3 (2 %)	4 (2 %)
Satisfaction of the information acquired from the literature	Very satisfied	1 (1 %)	1 (1 %)	2 (2 %)
	Satisfied	56 (59 %)	85 (54 %)	141 (56 %)
	Sometimes satisfied	28 (29 %)	54 (35 %)	82 (33 %)
	Not satisfied	10 (11 %)	16 (10 %)	26 (10 %)

[b]Non-postgraduates include clinicians and researchers

non-significant (p value ≥ 0.05) for six of the eight items, and the p-value was close to 0.05 also for the two remaining ones where the difference was found significant (7.5 and 7.7). This indicated that the experienced acupuncture workers and the less experienced postgraduates tend to put similar attention on the most items, that is, both groups demanded more complete information in acupuncture SR/MAs. For details of acupuncture interventions and qualification of acupuncture clinicians in methods, postgraduates gave higher scores compared with non-postgraduates, which might be related with their experience.

Table 3 Scores of the candidate items

Score		1	2	3	4	5	6	7	8	9	10	Mean	p (independent-sample T-test)
7.1	Total	6	9	14	17	24	18	18	48	25	72	7.2	
	P[c]	2	5	1	5	9	7	7	15	11	33	7.6	0.109
	NP[d]	4	4	13	12	15	11	11	33	14	39	7.0	
7.2	Total	19	11	14	15	33	18	23	37	21	60	6.6	
	P	9	3	4	5	12	8	8	13	13	20	6.6	0.895
	NP	10	8	10	10	21	10	15	24	8	40	6.6	
7.3	Total	3	2	0	4	18	15	9	40	33	127	8.6	
	P	1	1	0	0	7	6	5	16	13	46	8.5	0.954
	NP	2	1	0	4	11	9	4	24	20	81	8.6	
7.4	Total	2	0	2	4	15	9	12	46	45	116	8.6	
	P	1	0	1	1	9	2	1	19	18	43	8.6	0.700
	NP	1	0	1	3	6	7	11	27	27	73	8.7	
7.5	Total	1	0	3	9	12	8	14	37	42	125	8.7	
	P	1	0	2	2	7	4	8	15	15	41	8.4	0.044
	NP	0	0	1	7	5	4	6	22	27	84	8.8	
7.6	Total	1	2	3	6	8	13	16	42	42	118	8.6	
	P	1	2	0	2	2	6	5	19	16	42	8.5	0.560
	NP	0	0	3	4	6	7	11	23	26	76	8.7	
7.7	Total	17	11	25	17	38	36	20	45	16	26	5.9	
	P	11	3	9	7	18	12	7	17	4	7	5.5	0.047
	NP	6	8	16	10	20	24	13	28	12	19	6.2	
7.8	Total	3	2	5	8	14	24	21	55	34	85	8.0	
	P	2	1	2	3	5	13	6	20	13	30	7.8	0.286
	NP	1	1	3	5	9	11	15	35	21	55	8.1	

[c]P: Postgraduates; [d]NP: Non-postgraduates, including clinicians and researchers of acupuncture
7.1 Provide the theoretical basis of acupuncture used for the target disease in background/introduction
7.2 Provide the style of acupuncture treatment (e.g. traditional Chinese acupuncture, South Korean acupuncture) in background/introduction
7.3 Provide the diagnostic criteria in methods (TCM syndrome and/or diagnostic criteria of diseases according to Western medicine)
7.4 Provide types of acupuncture interventions in methods (e.g. type of acupunctures like percussopunctator and needles, and any other intervention like sham acupuncture)
7.5 Provide details of acupuncture interventions in methods (e.g. number of needles, names of acupoint, depth of puncture, relevant body response, needling manipulation, time for needle retention, types of needles)
7.6 Provide indicators of effect judgement in methods (e.g. Visual Analogue Scale (VAS))
7.7 Provide the qualification (e.g. career and other experience) of acupuncture clinicians in methods
7.8 Provide the follow-up time along with rationality in results

For additional comments in Table 4, the top five mentioned items (mentioned by seven or more respondents) were carefully analyzed. The 7.9.1 and 7.9.2 were not tailored for acupuncture, and they have already been mentioned in PRISMA. As for the 7.9.3 and 7.9.5, they were similar or close to 7.1 and 7.4 respectively. And 7.9.4 will be integrated in the item checklist in the future period.

Our study has both strengths and limitations. We designed the questionnaire based on a pilot study and a literature review, combining the two key factors in evidence based medicine—— evidence and practitioners' experience [29]. We designated two researchers to distribute and collect printed questionnaires and some explanatory materials without interfering the answer process, which helped us improve the response rate [30, 31]. We proposed eight items collected from current literature in our questionnaire, which probably does not cover all relevant issues for reporting SR/MAs of acupuncture. However, the open ended comments from the respondents gave us useful suggestions for further improvement. We limited our survey to five cities, but these cities represent in the different regions of China. We also considered the representative from the aspects of gender, geography, clinical experience, and experience in literature. The participants are representative of typical users of systematic reviews on acupuncture. Acupuncture is mainly practiced in specialized and general hospitals,

Table 4 Additional items proposed by respondents

Items	Content	Respondents (n)
7.9.1	Specify whether the included studies were RCTs and describe the method of randomization.	10
7.9.2	Specify the statistical and data processing methods, and estimate the statistical power of the data analysis.	8
7.9.3	Discuss the rationale and mechanism of action for acupuncture in modern medicine.	7
7.9.4	Describe the safety and adverse effects (both long term and short term) of acupuncture, such as epilepsy.	7
7.9.5	Provide the effect and reproducibility of acupuncture, including the description of effect evaluation time and indicators and patient outcomes.	7
7.9.6	Describe the demographic information (e.g. age, sex), physical status, medical history and conditions.	5
7.9.7	Describe the method, including study design, quality assessment, and bias control.	4
7.9.8	Describe whether the preferences and values of the patients were considered or not.	3
7.9.9	Describe the follow-up time, result, and the loss to follow-up and corresponding solutions.	3
7.9.10	Describe the origin and development of acupuncture.	3
7.9.11	Describe the status quo of research on diseases and acupuncture both at home and abroad.	3
7.9.12	Analyzing the results and presenting the discussion.	3
7.9.13	Description of the blinding method of the included studies.	2
7.9.14	Providing the references of the study.	2
7.9.15	Description of the limitations and implications of the study.	2
7.9.16	Description of the sample method and size.	1
7.9.17	Description of the innovations and strengths of the study.	1
7.9.18	Description of which type of clinical research is suitable for acupuncture.	1
7.9.19	Description of the Ethics Committee review and registration status.	1
7.9.20	Description of the conclusion of the study and the clinical evidence on acupuncture.	1
7.9.21	Declaration of the funding of the study.	1
7.9.22	Description of the environment of study implementation (such as primary health setting or one of the top three hospitals).	1
7.9.23	Description of the standard of syndrome differentiation and treatment.	1

In addition to the eight items proposed in our questionnaire, some respondents also gave suggestions on other information

where the health care workers are in general well educated and involved in research. In China, acupuncture is not commonly practiced in local health centers or private clinics, where the health care workers tend to be less well educated [32, 33]. In the next period, relevant experts will be identified and surveyed with an online questionnaire, and the results of this survey, including the comments and additional items suggested by the respondents, will be properly considered and integrated.

Conclusions

Most clinicians, researchers and students involved in acupuncture were not satisfied with the information provided in acupuncture SRs. This indicates the need for promoting the more complete and critical information reporting of acupuncture SR/MAs. Most of the items proposed in the questionnaire scored highly, and there were only small, mostly non-significant, differences between the opinions from postgraduates and more experienced NPs. The open-ended questions for respondents for collecting comments and additional items provided us with a lot information, which would promote our work in next step.

Abbreviations
CONSORT: Consolidated Standards of Reporting Trials; EBM: Evidence-based medicine; JAMA: Journal of the American Medical Association; PRISMA: Preferred Reporting Items for Systematic reviews and Meta-Analyses; RCT: Randomized controlled trial; SR/MA: Systematic review or meta-analysis; STRICTA: STandards for Reporting Interventions in Clinical Trials of Acupuncture; TCM: Traditional Chinese medicine

Acknowledgments
The authors wish to thank Yajun Wang, Huijuan Tan, Guanghui An and Hao Chen with their help with the planning of survey, and Janne Estill for polishing the paper.

Funding
This study is supported by the National Natural Science Foundation of China (General Program, ID: 81373882), and the funding had no role in study design, collection, analysis and interpretation of data, writing of the report, and decision to submit the article for publication.

Authors' contributions

XES, XQW and KHY contributed to the conception and design, as well as acquisition of data of this study. XQW and DW performed the statistical analysis and drafted the manuscript. XZ and JG participated in the whole survey and helped to revise the manuscript. All authors read and approved the final manuscript.

Competing interests

The authors declare that there is no conflict of interest regarding the publication of this paper.

Author details

[1]Evidence-Based Medicine Center, School of Basic Medical Sciences, Lanzhou University, Lanzhou 730000, China. [2]Key Laboratory of Evidence Based Medicine and Knowledge Translation of Gansu Province, Lanzhou 730000, China. [3]Chinese GRADE Center, Lanzhou 730000, China. [4]Gansu Rehabilitation Center Hospital, Lanzhou 730000, China. [5]Department of Hypertension, Lanzhou University Second Hospital, Lanzhou 730000, China. [6]Gansu University of Chinese Medicine, Lanzhou 730000, China.

References

1. Centre for Reviews and Dissemination. Systematic reviews: CRD's guidance for undertaking reviews in health care. York: CRD; 2009. Available at http://www.york.ac.uk/inst/crd/pdf/Systematic_Reviews.pdf. Accessed 16 Oct 2014.
2. Moher D, Schulz KF, Altman DG. The CONSORT statement: revised recommendations for improving the quality of reports of parallel-group randomised trials. Lancet. 2001;357(9263):1191–4.
3. Schulz KF, Altman DG, Moher D. CONSORT 2010 statement: updated guidelines for reporting parallel group randomised trials. BMC Med. 2010;8(1):18.
4. Endorsers. http://www.consort-statement.org/about-consort/endorsers. Accessed 21 Jan 2015.
5. Mannocci A, Saulle R, Colamesta V, D'Aguanno S, Giraldi G, Maffongelli E, et al. What is the impact of reporting guidelines on Public Health journals in Europe? The case of STROBE, CONSORT and PRISMA. J Public Health (Oxf). 2014;37(4):737–40.
6. Panic N, Leoncini E, de Belvis G, Ricciardi W, Boccia S. Evaluation of the endorsement of the preferred reporting items for systematic reviews and meta-analysis (PRISMA) statement on the quality of published systematic review and meta-analyses. PLoS ONE. 2013;8(12):e83138.
7. Wu TX, representative. Revised STandards for Reporting Interventions in Clinical Trials of Acupuncture (STRICTA): extending the CONSORT statement. Chin J Evid-based Med. 2010;10(10):1228–39.
8. Extensions. http://www.consort-statement.org/extensions? ContentWidgetId = 559. Accessed 21 Jan 2015.
9. Prady SL, MacPHERSON H. Assessing the utility of the standards for reporting trials of acupuncture (STRICTA): a survey of authors. J Altern Complement Med. 2007;13(9):939–43.
10. Hammerschlag R, Milley R, Colbert A, Weih J, Yohalem-Ilsley B, Mist S, Aickin M. Randomized controlled trials of acupuncture (1997–2007): an assessment of reporting quality with a CONSORT-and STRICTA-based instrument. Evid Based Complement Alternat Med. 2011;2011:25. Article ID 183910. doi:10.1155/2011/183910.
11. Moher D, Liberati A, Tetzlaff J, Altman DG, PRISMA Group. Preferred reporting items for systematic reviews and meta-analyses: the PRISMA statement. Ann Intern Med. 2009;151(4):264–9.
12. Welch V, Petticrew M, Tugwell P, Moher D, O'Neill J, Waters E, et al. PRISMA-Equity 2012 extension: reporting guidelines for systematic reviews with a focus on health equity. PLoS Med. 2012;9(10):e1001333.
13. Beller EM, Glasziou PP, Altman DG, Hopewell S, Bastian H, Chalmers I, et al. PRISMA for Abstracts: reporting systematic reviews in journal and conference abstracts. PLoS Med. 2013;10(4):e1001419.
14. Moher D, Shamseer L, Clarke M, Ghersi D, Liberati A, Petticrew M, et al. Preferred reporting items for systematic review and meta-analysis protocols (PRISMA-P) 2015 statement. Syst Rev. 2015;4:1.
15. Hutton B, Salanti G, Caldwell DM, Chaimani A, Schmid CH, Cameron C, et al. The PRISMA extension statement for reporting of systematic reviews incorporating network meta-analyses of health care interventions: checklist and explanations. Ann Intern Med. 2015;162(11):777–84.
16. Liu Y, Zhang R, Huang J, Zhao X, Liu D, Sun W, et al. Reporting Quality of Systematic Reviews/Meta-Analyses of Acupuncture. PLoS ONE. 2014;9(11): e113172.
17. Wang XQ, Wei D, Liu YL, Wu CL, Ji K, Wei JQ, et al. A survey of application status of the PRISMA statement. Chin J Evid-based Med. 2014;14(9):1160–4 [Article in Chinese].
18. Wang C, He WJ, Guo Y. Analysis on acupuncture related articles published in periodicals in Science Citation Index(SCI)in 2008. Zhongguo Zhen Jiu. 2010;30(9):755–8.
19. Liu YL. Research on the Quality of Systematic Reviews and Randomized Controlled Trials of Acupuncture and Cognition of Reporting Guideline. Lanzhou University, 2012. [Article in Chinese]
20. Dawes JG. Do data characteristics change according to the number of scale points used? An experiment using 5 point, 7 point and 10 point scales. Int J Mark Res. 2008;51(1).
21. Acupuncture. Available at: https://en.wikipedia.org/wiki/Acupuncture. Accessed 6 Jan 2016.
22. Birch S, Felt R. Understanding acupuncture. Edinburgh: Churchill Livingstone; 1999.
23. Western medical acupuncture: a definition. Available at: http://your-gp.com/western-acupuncture-vs-traditional-acupuncture/. Accessed 6 Jan 2016.
24. Jiang M, Lu C, Zhang C, Yang J, Tan Y, Lu A, et al. Syndrome differentiation in modern research of traditional Chinese medicine. J Ethnopharmacol. 2012;140(3):634–42.
25. http://www.acupuncturemoxibustion.com/acupuncture/nine-classical-needles/. Accessed 6 Jan 2016.
26. Zhang TS, Jin CN, Guan F, et al. The history and development of new nine-needle. Chin Acupunct Moxibustion. 2009;07:591–4 [Article in Chinese].
27. Ernst E, Lee MS, Choi TY. Acupuncture: does it alleviate pain and are there serious risks? A review of reviews. PAIN®. 2011;152(4):755–64.
28. Xu S, Wang L, Cooper E, Zhang M, Manheimer E, Berman B, et al. Adverse events of acupuncture: a systematic review of case reports. Evid Based Complement Alternat Med. 2013;2013.
29. Sackett DL, Rosenberg WM, Gray JA, Haynes RB, Richardson WS. Evidence based medicine: what it is and what it isn't. BMJ. 1996;312(7023):71.
30. Nulty DD. The adequacy of response rates to online and paper surveys: what can be done? Assess Eval High Educ. 2008;33(3):301–14.
31. Asch DA, Jedrziewski MK, Christakis NA. Response rates to mail surveys published in medical journals. J Clin Epidemiol. 1997;50(10):1129–36.
32. Lin ML. Comparison of the Present Situations of Acupuncture and Moxibustion among China Mainland and Taiwan Region. Nanjing University of Chinese Medicine. 2007. [Article in Chinese]
33. Li ZC. Analysis on Resource Allocation and Utilization in Township Hospitals Under Health Reform in China. Chinese Health Econ. 2009;28(5):31–3 [Article in Chinese].

11

Evaluating validity of various acupuncture device types: a random sequence clinical trial

Jungtae Leem[1,2†], Jimin Park[3†], Gajin Han[1,4], Seulgi Eun[5], Meena M. Makary[5,6], Kyungmo Park[5], Junhee Lee[1,7*] and Sanghoon Lee[1,3] [iD]

Abstract

Background: Although various placebo acupuncture devices have been developed and used in acupuncture research, there is controversy concerning whether these devices really serve as appropriate placebos for control groups.

Methods/Design: The proposed study is a single-center prospective random sequence participant- and assessor-blinded trial with two parallel arms. A total of 76 participants will be randomly assigned to Group 1 or Group 2 in a 1:1 ratio. Group 1 will consist of Sham Streitberger's needle, Real Streitberger's needle, and Phantom acupuncture session. Group 2 will consist of Park Sham device with real needle, Park Sham device with sham needle, and no treatment session. Participants will have a total of three acupuncture sessions in a day. The primary endpoint is blinding test questionnaire 1. Secondary endpoints are the Bang's blinding index, the Massachusetts General Hospital Acupuncture Sensation Scale index, and physiological data including heart rate, heart rate variability, and skin conductance response.

Discussion: This trial will evaluate the relevance of using placebo acupuncture devices as controls using a validation test procedure.

Trial registration: Clinical Research Information Service: KCT0001347.

Keywords: Placebo acupuncture, Blinding, Validation, Park sham device, Streitberger's needle, Phantom acupuncture

Background

Acupuncture is a treatment modality that has been used in Eastern Asia for more than 2000 years. An increased interest in the clinical effects of acupuncture has also been expressed in the West in recent years. In a 1997 report on the effects of acupuncture, the National Institutes of Health (NIH) stressed the need for evidence of efficacy [1]. Subsequently, the number of randomized controlled clinical trials (RCTs) using acupuncture to treat various conditions has rapidly increased; however, many acupuncture clinical trials have methodological limitations. Establishing appropriate placebo control groups is one of several issues. Ideally, placebo acupuncture should satisfy two conditions: (1) it should be indistinguishable from real acupuncture to blinded participants, and (2) it should be physiologically inert. Various placebo acupuncture devices that satisfy these conditions have been developed and used in acupuncture clinical trials.

Currently, there are two types of acupuncture controls: (1) sham acupuncture, in which real acupuncture needles are inserted into the skin either fully at non-acupuncture points or superficially at acupuncture points, non-acupuncture points, or non-relevant acupuncture points with certain conditions, and (2)

* Correspondence: ssljh@hanmail.net
†Equal contributors
[1]Korean Medicine Clinical Trial Center, College of Korean Medicine, Kyung Hee University, Seoul, South Korea
[7]Department of Sasang Constitutional Medicine, College of Korean Medicine, Kyung Hee University, Seoul, South Korea
Full list of author information is available at the end of the article

placebo acupuncture, which uses non-penetrating acupuncture devices (i.e., blunt tip needles or non-needle devices) [2].

Various non-penetrating placebo acupuncture devices such as Streitberger's needle, the Park sham device (PSD), and the Takakura needle have been developed. The first device, Streitberger's needle, was developed in 1998 and used a plastic ring covered with a plastic sheet to place the needle [3]. When the practitioner taps the needle, it moves inside the handle and appears as if the acupuncture needle punctures the skin. However, it does not puncture the skin, but only a pricking sensation is felt by the patient because the tip is blunt.

In 1999, Park et al. developed the PSD which was similar to Streitberger's needle [4]. The PSD included a flange with adhesive tape and a guide tube to place the placebo needle on the acupuncture point, while Streitberger's needle used a plastic ring and sheet. Although these two placebo acupuncture devices were successfully applied to blinded participants and their use validated, there still remains the limitation that they induce physiological activity by touching the skin.

In 2014, Lee et al. developed a novel form of placebo acupuncture, phantom acupuncture, which induces participant expectation without any tactile stimulation such as palpation, needle insertion, or manipulation and which was also validated using blinded participants [5]. However, complex equipment is needed to perform phantom acupuncture. Therefore, it may be difficult to apply phantom acupuncture in clinical acupuncture trials.

Although various placebo acupuncture devices have been developed and used in acupuncture research, there is controversy concerning whether these devices are really appropriate for placebo control groups.

This trial will evaluate various placebo acupuncture devices that have been used in acupuncture clinical trials using a validation test to determine if they are suitable to be used in control groups.

Methods/Design
Objectives
The objectives of this trial are to evaluate the validity of different types of placebo acupuncture devices and determine their suitability for use as placebos in clinical trials.

Trial design and study setting
This study will be a single center, prospective, randomized, random sequence, participant and assessor blinded trial with two parallel arms.

We will conduct the study in the Kyung Hee University Medical Center.

There are arm1 (Group1) and arm2 (Group2) in our trial that is separated. Each group has three different intervention sessions in random sequence. The order of intervention will be randomized.

Inclusion and exclusion criteria
Participants who meet the following criteria will be included irrespective of previous acupuncture experience: (1) healthy participants 20–50 years old, and (2) participants who can communicate and complete the questionnaire.

Participants will be excluded if they meet any of the following criteria: (1) individuals who have taken medications during the prior month that could influence trial results (e.g. medications for epilepsy, depression, panic disorders, schizophrenia, etc.), (2) pregnant or breastfeeding women, (3) Korean Medicine Doctors (KMD) or Korean Medicine University students (because we think that they can distinguish between placebo and real acupuncture better than the general population), (4) individuals who drank alcohol or coffee, or overworked the day before or the day of the experiment, and (5) individuals who are determined to be unsuitable for following the study protocol by the researcher.

Recruitment
We will upload an advertisement to the hospital and university homepages, and place a poster advertisement on the bulletin boards of the hospital and university. Potential participants will call the clinical research coordinator (CRC) and will be pre-screened for eligibility. Eligible participants will make an appointment. When potential participants visit the hospital, the investigator will provide information about volunteering and explain the risks and benefits of the research. When the individuals agree to enroll in the research, they will sign an informed consent form.

Randomization and allocation concealment
After signing the informed consent form, the participants will be randomized to Group 1 or Group 2. Group 1 will receive the Real Streitberger's needle (Real ST), Sham Streitberger's needle (Sham ST), and Phantom acupuncture (PHNT); Group 2 will receive the PSD with a real needle (Real Park), the PSD with a sham needle (Sham Park), and no treatment (No treat). The treatment orders in both groups will be randomized. A computerized balanced block randomization will be performed by an independent clinical research coordinator (CRC) using R version 3.1.2 with 'block random' function. The CRC will send an e-mail regarding the name, random number, and treatment order of enrolled participants to the practitioners and operators. This e-mail will be documented in the trial master file (TMF).

Blinding

Participants will be blinded in this trial. However, it is almost impossible to blind practitioners and operators because they need to know which acupuncture devices to use. They will not be allowed to communicate with the participants concerning the type of acupuncture devices and the purpose of the study. Outcome assessors and statisticians will also be blinded to treatment allocation.

Intervention

Study flow

The study flow will be as follows. Group 1 will consist of Sham ST, Real ST, and PHNT. Group 2 will consist of Real Park, Sham Park, and No treatment. Groups 1 and 2 are separate groups; participants allocated to Group 1 will not receive Real Park, Sham Park, and No treatment and vice versa. Participants will have a total of three sessions (acupuncture or no treatment) in a day (Fig. 1). Before acupuncture treatment, the investigator will explain to participants that they will receive three different types of acupuncture except for the no treatment session. Participants will not know that placebo acupuncture occurred until all sessions are completed. To avoid order effect, the order of the three treatment sessions in each group will be randomly assigned by the CRC. Before the first session, the CRC will collect demographic information (e.g., age, sex) and baseline data (e.g., vital signs, acupuncture expectation questionnaire (AEQ) [6], and bodily sensation questionnaire (BSQ)). After each treatment session, participants will complete the blinding test questionnaire 1 (BTQ 1) and acupuncture sensation questionnaire (ASQ) and will be asked about adverse events (AEs). After completion of the third BTQ 1 and ASQ, an independent assessor will inform the participants of the use of placebo acupuncture and instruct them to complete the blinding test questionnaire 2 (BTQ 2).

Procedures of each session

Physiological data including heart rate (HR) and skin conductance response (SCR) will be measured by an operator during each session to quantify the autonomic nervous system (ANS) response (Fig. 2). We will record three tonic responses (before, during, and after acupuncture treatment) and one phasic response (during stimulation).

1. Stabilization: After all preparations (e.g., attaching electrodes, checking the ECG and SCR wave patterns) are complete, participants will lie on the bed for 5 to10 min to stabilize.
2. Tonic response before acupuncture: We will measure the tonic ANS response before acupuncture treatment during 5 min of resting.
3. Needle insertion and rest: We will insert the acupuncture needle and induce the de-qi sensation for 1 min and explain to participants that the response induced by needle insertion will be measured. To minimize the influence of the acupuncture insertion, participants will be rested for 1 min.
4. Phasic response during stimulation: The practitioner will approach her hand to the left ST 36 acupuncture point and rotate the needle eight times within 3 min according to an audio signal relayed via a headphone. The stimulation timing will be pseudo-randomly set by computer (Psychtoolbox and Matlab, The MathWorks Inc., MA, USA).
5. Rest: To minimize the influence of the acupuncture stimulation, participants will be rested for 1 min.
6. Tonic response during acupuncture: We will measure the tonic ANS response for 5 min during acupuncture treatment.
7. Needle removal and rest: We will remove the acupuncture needle for 1 min. To minimize the

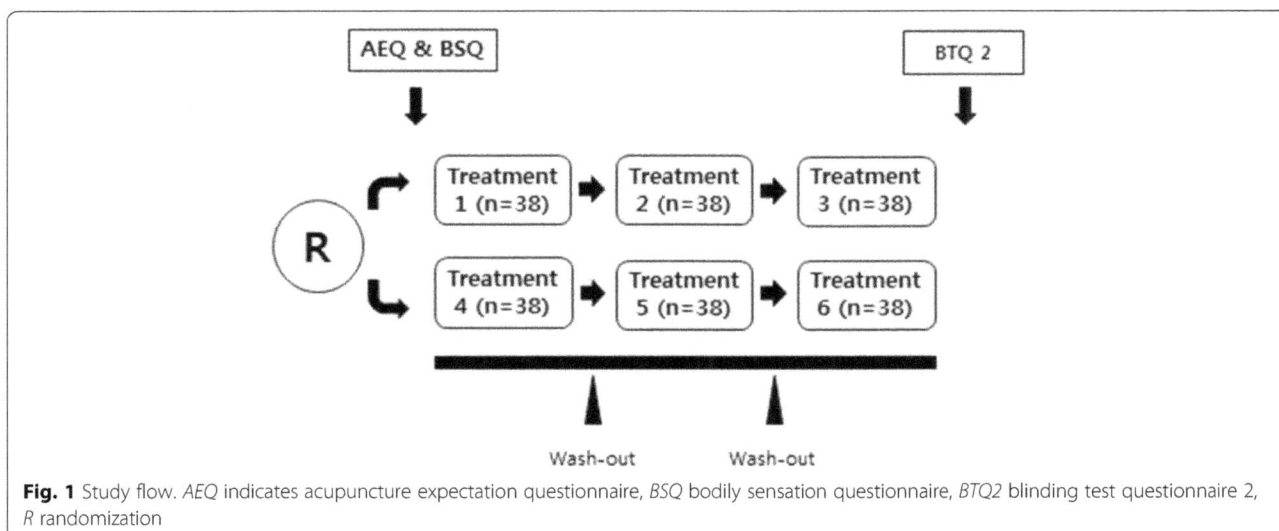

Fig. 1 Study flow. *AEQ* indicates acupuncture expectation questionnaire, *BSQ* bodily sensation questionnaire, *BTQ2* blinding test questionnaire 2, *R* randomization

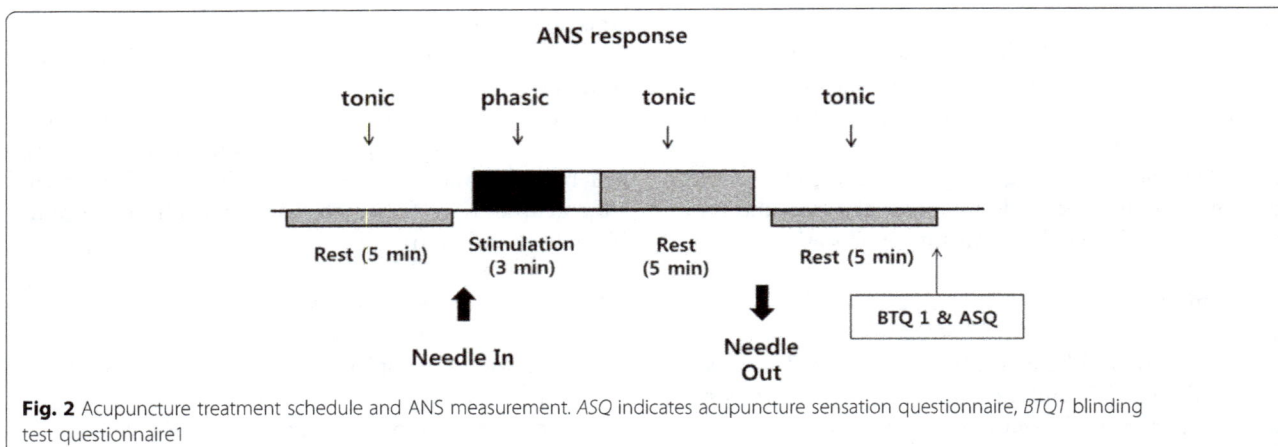

Fig. 2 Acupuncture treatment schedule and ANS measurement. *ASQ* indicates acupuncture sensation questionnaire, *BTQ1* blinding test questionnaire1

influence of the acupuncture needle removal, participants will be rested for 1 min.

8. Tonic response after acupuncture: We will measure the tonic ANS response for 5 min after the acupuncture needle is removed.

Acupuncture treatment setting and equipment

The acupuncture treatment room setting will be modified from a previous study by Lee et al. [5] and is shown in Fig. 3. Participants will lie on the bed in a supine position. A visual barrier will prevent participants from viewing their leg and the acupuncture treatment procedure directly.

Acupuncture stimulation will be recorded simultaneously and will be shown to the participants through a ceiling monitor in real time for 3 min. Before the stabilization phase, the operator will show the acupuncture point and movement of their legs through the ceiling monitor so that participants will have body ownership via the image.

Details of the acupuncture treatment plans are shown in Table 1.

Phantom acupuncture and no treatment session

In PHNT, practitioners will not provide any tactile stimulation and will only approach their hand to the left ST 36 acupuncture point without touching. A recorded video clip of the participant's Real ST session will be played during the PHNT session. If the PHNT session is scheduled as the first session, we will play a video from another participant with similar skin color and leg hair.

In the No treatment session, practitioners will inform participants that they will not receive any treatment. A blinding questionnaire will not be completed; recorded physiological data will be used as a baseline. In order to ensure comparability, participants will undergo the same procedure except they will be shown a 3 min video clip that is not related to acupuncture but has a similar background color and shows some type of artificial movement

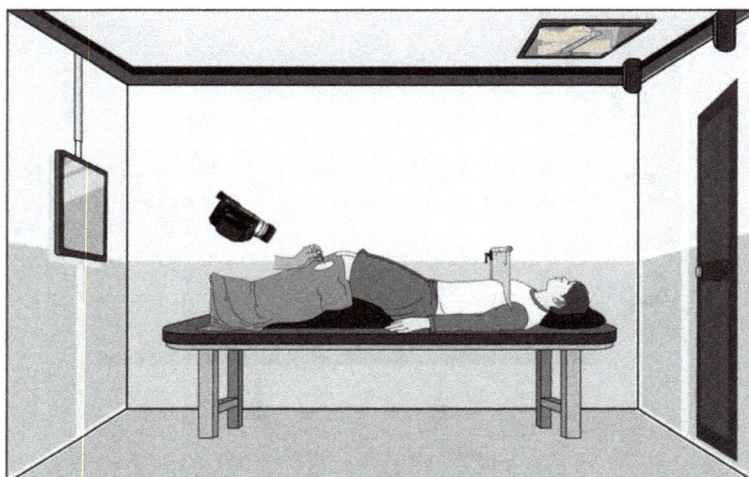

Fig. 3 Acupuncture treatment setting

Table 1 Details of acupuncture treatments (STRICTA 2010 checklist)

Item		Detail
1. Acupuncture rationale	1a) Style of acupuncture	Manual acupuncture based on traditional Korean medicine theory
	1b)Reasoning for treatment provided, based on historical context, literature sources, and/or consensus methods, with references where appropriate	Consensus of the KMD
	1c)Extent to which treatment was varied	All participants will receive standardized treatment
2. Details of needling	2a) Number of needle insertions per subject per session	1
	2b) Names of points used	Left ST36
	2c) Depth of insertion, based on a specified unit of measurement	15 mm
	2d) Response sought	De-qi
	2e) Needle stimulation :	During 3 min of phasic session, manual stimulation will be conducted eight times based on an audio signal received via a headphone. Interval between each manual stimulation is from 10 to 14 s. For each manual stimulation, the acupuncture needle will be rotated five times during 3 s.
	2f) Needle retention time	11 min
	2g) Needle type	[Group 1] Real Streitberger's needle; 0.25 × 40 mm sterilized stainless steel needle (Asia-med GmbH & Co. KG, Kirchplatz 1, Germany).
		[Group 2] PSD; 0.25 × 40 mm sterilized stainless steel needle (Park sham Device, Acuprime, Exter, UK).
3. Treatment regimen	3a) Number of treatment sessions	3 sessions
	3b) Frequency and duration of treatment sessions	3 sessions for 1 day
		(30 min washout period between each session)
4. Other components of treatment	4a) Details of other interventions administered to the acupuncture group	None
	4b) Setting and context of treatment, including instructions to practitioners, and information and explanations to patients	The study will be conducted in the Kyung Hee University Medical Center. All information except the objective of trial and acupuncture types will be provided to the participants.
5. Practitioner background	5) Description of participating acupuncturists	Licensed KMD with at least 5 years of clinical practice experience
6. Control interventions	6a) Rationale for the control or comparator in the context of the research question, with sources that justify this choice	Validated placebo acupuncture devices will be used in control sessions.
	6b) Precise description of the control or comparator. If sham acupuncture or any other type of acupuncture-like control is used, provide details as for Items 1 to 3 above.	The order of three treatments in each group will be randomized.
		[GROUP 1]1) Sham Streitberger' needle: 0.25 × 40 mm sterilized stainless steel needle (Special No. 16 of Asia-med GmbH & Co. KG, Kirchplatz 1,Germany) will be used.The appearance, acupuncture point, stimulation method, and duration will be the same with the real Streitberger's needle.
		2) Phantom acupuncture: There is no tactile stimulation to ST 36. To induce credibility that participants are treated with acupuncture, the video clip of the previously recorded Streitberger's needle session will be shown.

	[GROUP 2]1) PSD with sham needle: 0.25×40 mm sterilized stainless steel needle (Park sham Device, Acuprime, Exter, UK) will be used. The appearance, acupuncture point, stimulation method, and depth will be the same with the PSD as with the real needle. 2) No treatment: There is no acupuncture treatment. To induce the attention effect as in the other sessions, a neutral image will be provided instead of an acupuncture treatment image.

KMD Korean Medicine Doctor; *PSD* park sham device

that would occur with same stimulation time point during an acupuncture session.

Outcome measurement
Primary endpoint
BTQ 1 : After each acupuncture session, participants will complete the BTQ 1. BTQ1 consists of five questions. If a participant completes all five questions without any doubt or asking, we will conclude blinding is succeeded. If participants mention strange aspect of the questionnaire or reply they did not receive acupuncture treatment, conclude that blinding is failed. Otherwise, we will conclude that blinding is succeeded.

Secondary endpoints

Bang's blinding index (BI) After all the sessions are finished, participants will complete the BTQ 2. At this time, participants will be told that a placebo acupuncture session occurred. We will calculate the BI from the BTQ 2 [7]. The range of BI is -100 to 100 %; 0 % means random guessing (e.g., 50 % correct and 50 % incorrect) and 100 % means complete unblinding (i.e., all responses are correct), -100 % means opposite of guessing (e.g., all responses are incorrect) [8]. Thus, the BI is the proportion of participants who guessed their treatment arm correctly beyond chance [9, 10].

Massachusetts General Hospital (MGH) Acupuncture Sensation Scale (MASS) Index by de-qi sensation questionnaire (DSQ) The MASS measures the sensation caused by acupuncture stimulation. It consists of 12 descriptions: soreness, aching, deep pressure, heaviness, fullness/distention, tingling, numbness, sharp pain, dull pain, warmth, cold, and throbbing. The MASS index is a weighted average based on a formula [11]. We will determine the MASS using the DSQ.

Heart rate, heart rate variability, and skin conductance response Participants will rest for 5 to10 min before we measure their tonic response to stabilize the electrocardiogram and SCR wave pattern. We will record the HR and SCR throughout the study using a PowerLab Data acquisition system/800, Bio amplifier/ML132, GSR

Amplifier/ML116 (AD instruments, Australia) with a 400 Hz sampling rate. To measure HR, participants will be placed on the bed and three electrodes (3M disposable PAD 2223) will be attached beneath the clavicles and the left rib. Then, we will remove power noise frequency at 60 Hz and detect the R peak to measure the HR. To measure the SCR, we will apply a gel to the index and third fingers and attach electrodes [5, 12].

The HR and SCR will be measured during the tonic and phasic responses. For the tonic responses, the mean HR and SCR will be measured before, during, and after the acupuncture treatment session for 5 min.

The HRV will be calculated by evaluating the R peak. In the time domain analysis, we will calculate the standard deviation of all R-R intervals (SDNN) and the root-mean-square of the successive difference (RMS-SD). For the frequency domain analysis, we will calculate the high frequency value (HF), low frequency value (LF), total power, and the LF/HF ratio [13, 14].

In the phasic event related SCR responses, the average of the maximum score change and the area under the curve (AUC) will be estimated. We will also calculate the stimulation/baseline SCR ratio of the score change and the AUC.

Sample size calculation
This will be a kind of mechanism study, so we did not follow the general method to calculate sample size. It is known that a sample size of 12 or more is adequate for a pilot study [15, 16]. We concluded that we will have sufficient analytical power if our sample size is greater than 12. We decided that we need to enroll at least 30 participants in our pilot study for each session assuming a drop-out rate of approximately 20 %. We calculated a sample size of 37.5 and rounded to this to 38 resulting in a total sample size of 76 participants.

Statistical analysis
As our design has two independent groups that acquire comparability by randomization, we can compare variables not only within each group, but also between groups.

The primary outcome of our research will be to compare the blinding rates of the placebo acupuncture devices studied within and between groups. We will also conduct several exploratory secondary outcome analyses. Expectation for acupuncture (measured by AEQ) [6], previous acupuncture experiences, and age will be considered as covariates. We will analyze physiological data in three tonic responses (before, during, and after acupuncture) and during phasic responses. We will not statistically compare the Bang's BI [9]. Instead, we will calculate the point estimate and 95 % confidence interval of Bang's BI.

For dichotomous variables (i.e., blinding rate), within group comparison will be performed using Cochran's Q test for Group 1 (Sham ST, Real ST, and PHNT) and McNemar's test for Group 2 (Sham, Real Park). We will not check the blinding of the No treatment session. Comparisons of blinding rates between group devices (Sham ST vs Sham Park or PHNT vs Sham Park) will be performed using the chi-square test, and comparisons within group devices (PHNT vs Sham ST) will be performed using McNemar's test. For continuous variables (i.e., the MASS index, De-qi sensation, physiological data such as HR, HRV, and SCR), within group comparisons will be performed using repeated measured ANOVA for Group 1 and paired t-test for Group 2. We will use the independent t test for comparisons between group.

When we analyze physiological data, we will use the both change ratio contrast to baseline and absolute value. Change ratio and absolute value of HR and SCR will be compared for three separate windows during the tonic responses (before vs during vs after acupuncture session). As absolute change value is very dependent on baseline value, it will be used as covariates.

Quality control

Before the study begins, we will conduct several simulations using our colleagues and volunteers to identify any problems with our study protocol. Practitioners will conduct acupuncture sessions according to the standard operating procedure (SOP) of our study. We will have researcher meetings regularly to discuss issues that may be raised by investigators and participants such as protocol revisions, serious adverse events, and participant recruitment.

Safety and adverse event outcomes

When each session is completed, the assessor will ask if any AE occurred and it will be documented in the CRF. If any AEs occur, the type of AE, start/end date, severity, manner of report, course, outcome, causality with acupuncture treatment, and actions taken will be documented and appropriate treatment will be provided to the participants.

Ethics approval and registration

This study has been approved by the Institutional Review Board of Kyung Hee University Korean Medicine Hospital (KOMCIRB-140923-HR-008). Written informed consent will be obtained from all participants. This study has been registered with the Clinical Research Information Service (CRIS), Republic of Korea, KCT0001347 (registered: January 15th, 2015).

Discussion

This trial was designed to investigate if various placebo acupuncture devices are appropriate for control groups in acupuncture research. We will evaluate the blinding of participants and also measure physiological parameters such as HR, HRV, and SCR. In addition, we will investigate the effects of various factors on blinding and physiological parameters. We will examine the effects of the bodily sensation, de-qi sensation (i.e., acupuncture-evoked sensations including numbness, heaviness, soreness, or distention), or patient expectation for acupuncture on blinding and physiological parameters.

Acupuncture treatment is composed of a variety of components such as acupuncture point selection, skin penetration, stimulation dose (diameter, length, and number of needles, needling depth, and stimulation method), patient expectation, and practitioner-patient relationship [2]. However, studies on how each factor affects the total therapeutic effect are lacking. In this study, we are going to dis-associate a range of acupuncture treatment factors using a validation test of three types of placebo acupuncture techniques that have different components.

Other researchers have developed placebo acupuncture devices and evaluated their relevance using validation tests.

Streitberger et al. performed a validation study that investigated if acupuncture- naïve healthy participants ($n = 60$) could feel the difference between a real acupuncture needle and a placebo acupuncture device [3]. They showed that the participants could not distinguish between the two needles and suggested Streitberger's needle as a credible placebo treatment. Also White et al. conducted a validation test of Streitberger's needle in participants waiting for orthopedic hip and knee joint replacement [17]. Most participants could not distinguish penetration with a real acupuncture needle from that with a placebo needle. However, in two similar treatments, almost 40 % were able to discern a difference between real and placebo acupuncture treatment administered by the male practitioner only. This shows that it is important how two interventions are delivered and that standardization of treatment technique is strictly required.

The PSD developed by Park et al. was validated in two randomized controlled trials (RCTs) in acute stroke patients and acupuncture-naïve, healthy volunteers [18]. The study was designed to evaluate if PSD was indistinguishable from a real acupuncture needle and if PSD induced de-qi. They found that PSD was indistinguishable and inactive (in terms of de-qi), thus it is a valid placebo control for acupuncture research.

However, these previous two devices touch the skin and thus induce a physiological effect. To overcome this limitation, Lee et al. developed a phantom acupuncture technique that imitates the acupuncture treatment ritual without any tactile stimulation [5]. They showed the credibility of phantom acupuncture without somatosensory components of real acupuncture in healthy participants.

In summary, three types of placebo acupunctures were all evaluated to blinded participants using validation tests. In this study, by measuring blinding, de-qi sensation, and various physiological parameters such as HR, HRV, and SCR, we will investigate if placebo acupuncture techniques are indistinguishable from real acupuncture and physiologically inert.

This trial will evaluate the relevance of using placebo acupuncture devices in control groups using a validation test of various placebo acupuncture devices that have been used in acupuncture research.

Trial status
This trial is currently recruiting participants.

Abbreviations
AEQ: acupuncture expectation questionnaire; ANS: quantify autonomic nervous system; ASQ: acupuncture sensation questionnaire; BTQ: blinding test questionnaire; BSQ: bodily sensation questionnaire; BI: blinding index; CRC: clinical research coordinator; CRF: case report form; DSQ: de-qi sensation questionnaire; HRV: heart rate variability; IRB: Institutional Review Board; KMD: Korean Medicine Doctor; MASS Index: Massachusetts General Hospital Acupuncture Sensation Scale index; No treat: no treatment session; PHNT: phantom acupuncture; PSD: park sham device; Real Park: park sham device with real needle; Real ST: Real Streitberger's needle treatment; Sham Park: park sham device with sham needle; Sham ST: Sham Streitberger's needle treatment; SCR: skin conductance response; SOP: standard operation procedures; TMF: trial master file.

Competing interests
The authors declare they have no conflicts of interest.

Authors' contributions
SHL is as a principal investigator. KMP, SGE, MM, and JTL settled research environment and manage devices. JMP and GJH will conduct acupuncture procedure simulation and complete case report form. KMP, JMP, GJH, JTL, and SGE revised study protocol. JMP drafted the protocol and communicated with IRB. GJH prepared trial master file and concerned ethical issues. JTL coordinated practical feedback. SGE and MM undertake electronic equipment and program code. JTL and JMP wrote the final manuscript. JHL contributed in obtaining research fund for the trial and settled study design and statistical analysis.. All authors read and approved the final manuscript.

Acknowledgements
This study was supported by the Traditional Korean Medicine R&D program funded by the Ministry of Health and Welfare through the Korean Health Industry Development Institute (KHIDI) (No. HI13C0700), And it was also supported by a grant of the Traditional Korean Medicine R&D Project, Ministry of Health & Welfare, Republic of Korea. (HI13C0580)
We thank Prof. Nobuari Takakura for his advice on the research.

Author details
[1]Korean Medicine Clinical Trial Center, College of Korean Medicine, Kyung Hee University, Seoul, South Korea. [2]Department of Clinical Research of Korean Medicine, College of Korean Medicine, Kyung Hee University, Seoul, South Korea. [3]Department of Acupuncture and Moxibustion, College of Korean Medicine, Kyung Hee University, Hoegi-dong 1, Dongdaemun-gu, Seoul 130-701, Republic of Korea. [4]Department of Gastroenterology, College of Korean Medicine, Kyung Hee University, Seoul, South Korea. [5]Department of Biomedical Engineering, Kyung Hee University, Yongin, Gyeonggi, South Korea. [6]Systems and Biomedical Engineering Department, Faculty of Engineering, Cairo University, Giza, Egypt. [7]Department of Sasang Constitutional Medicine, College of Korean Medicine, Kyung Hee University, Seoul, South Korea.

References
1.   NIH Consensus Conference. Acupuncture. JAMA. 1998;280:1518–24.
2.   Zhu D, Gao Y, Chang J, Kong J. Placebo acupuncture devices: considerations for acupuncture research. Evid-Based Complement Altern Med ECAM. 2013;2013:628907.
3.   Streitberger K, Kleinhenz J. Introducing a placebo needle into acupuncture research. Lancet. 1998;352:364–5.
4.   Park J, White A, Lee H, Ernst E. Development of a new sham needle. Acupunct Med. 1999;17:110–2.
5.   Lee J, Napadow V, Kim J, Lee S, Choi W, Kaptchuk TJ, et al. Phantom acupuncture: dissociating somatosensory and cognitive/affective components of acupuncture stimulation with a novel form of placebo acupuncture. PLoS One. 2014;9, e104582.
6.   Dennehy EB, Webb A, Suppes T. Assessment of beliefs in the effectiveness of acupuncture for treatment of psychiatric symptoms. J Altern Complement Med N Y N. 2002;8:421–5.
7.   Bang H, Ni L, Davis CE. Assessment of blinding in clinical trials. Control Clin Trials. 2004;25:143–56.
8.   Bang H, Flaherty SP, Kolahi J, Park J. Blinding assessment in clinical trials: a review of statistical methods and a proposal of blinding assessment protocol. Clin Res Regul Aff. 2010;27:42–51.
9.   Lee H, Bang H, Kim Y, Park J, Lee S, Lee H, et al. Non-penetrating sham needle, is it an adequate sham control in acupuncture research? Complement Ther Med. 2011;19 Suppl 1:S41–8.
10. Kolahi J, Bang H, Park J. Towards a proposal for assessment of blinding success in clinical trials: up-to-date review. Community Dent Oral Epidemiol. 2009;37:477–84.
11. Kong J, Gollub R, Huang T, Polich G, Napadow V, Hui K, et al. Acupuncture de qi, from qualitative history to quantitative measurement. J Altern Complement Med N Y N. 2007;13:1059–70.
12. Chang D-S, Kim Y-J, Lee S-H, Lee H, Lee I-S, Park H-J, et al. Modifying bodily self-awareness during acupuncture needle stimulation using the rubber hand illusion. Evid-Based Complement Altern Med ECAM. 2013;2013:849602.
13. Chung JWY, Yan VCM, Zhang H. Effect of acupuncture on heart rate variability: a systematic review. Evid Based Complement Alternat Med. 2014;2014, e819871.
14. Evrengül H, Tanriverdi H, Dursunoglu D, Kaftan A, Kuru O, Unlu U, et al. Time and frequency domain analyses of heart rate variability in patients with epilepsy. Epilepsy Res. 2005;63:131–9.
15. Hertzog MA. Considerations in determining sample size for pilot studies. Res Nurs Health. 2008;31:180–91.
16. Julious SA. Sample size of 12 per group rule of thumb for a pilot study. Pharm Stat. 2005;4:287–91.
17. White P, Lewith G, Hopwood V, Prescott P. The placebo needle, is it a valid and convincing placebo for use in acupuncture trials? A randomised, single-blind, cross-over pilot trial. Pain. 2003;106:401–9.
18. Park J, White A, Stevinson C, Ernst E, James M. Validating a new non-penetrating sham acupuncture device: two randomised controlled trials. Acupunct Med J Br Med Acupunct Soc. 2002;20:168–74.

12

Implementation of tobacco cessation brief intervention in complementary and alternative medicine practice

Emery R. Eaves[1*], Amy Howerter[2], Mark Nichter[3], Lysbeth Floden[4], Judith S. Gordon[2], Cheryl Ritenbaugh[2] and Myra L. Muramoto[2]

Abstract

Background: This article presents findings from qualitative interviews conducted as part of a research study that trained Acupuncture, Massage, and Chiropractic practitioners' in Arizona, US, to implement evidence-based tobacco cessation brief interventions (BI) in their routine practice. The qualitative phase of the overall study aimed to assess: the impact of tailored training in evidence-based tobacco cessation BI on complementary and alternative medicine (CAM) practitioners' knowledge and willingness to implement BIs in their routine practice; and their patients' responses to cessation intervention in CAM context.

Methods: To evaluate the implementation of skills learned from a tailored training program, we conducted semi-structured qualitative interviews with 54 CAM practitioners in Southern Arizona and 38 of their patients. Interview questions focused on reactions to the implementation of tobacco cessation BIs in CAM practice.

Results: After participating in a tailored BI training, CAM practitioners reported increased confidence, knowledge, and motivation to address tobacco in their routine practice. Patients were open to being approached by CAM practitioners about tobacco use and viewed BIs as an expected part of wellness care.

Conclusions: Tailored training motivated CAM practitioners in this study to implement evidence-based tobacco cessation BIs in their routine practice. Results suggest that CAM practitioners can be a valuable point of contact and should be included in tobacco cessation efforts.

Keywords: Tobacco cessation, Behavioral intervention, Complementary and alternative medicine, CAM

Background

Tobacco use is the leading cause of preventable death in the United States [1–4]. Research has shown that receiving cessation advice from any health care professional increases quit rates [5–7] and that advice and support from more than one type of health professional can substantially increase readiness to quit [8–10]. The present study aimed to assess the feasibility and impact of training complementary and alternative medicine (CAM) practitioners' (Chiropractors, Licensed/Certified Massage Therapists, and Acupuncturists) to become part of such a network of health professionals providing cessation intervention. CAM practitioners were provided with a tailored training in implementing a tobacco cessation brief intervention (BI) in their routine practice that included guiding patients towards evidence-based cessation tools like quitlines or nicotine-replacement options. This article reports the results of qualitative evaluation of the implementation of tobacco cessation BI in CAM practice following tailored training. Results included the perspectives of practitioners that participated in the study and their patients.[1]

* Correspondence: emery.eaves@nau.edu
[1]Department of Anthropology, Northern Arizona University, 5 E. McConnell Drive, PO Box: 15200, Flagstaff, AZ 86011-5200, USA
Full list of author information is available at the end of the article

Increases in tobacco screening initiatives have improved practitioner screening for tobacco use [11, 12] and there has been some movement in overall quit rates in the US [13], however, a substantial number of adult smokers continue to struggle to remain tobacco free. Health care practitioners are unlikely to assist with tobacco cessation if they are not confident in their ability and knowledge to assist [14–16] and many report time constraints as the biggest barrier to effectively assisting a patient with tobacco cessation [11]. Although tobacco cessation BI training for both health care practitioners and laypersons can effectively extend the reach of tobacco intervention [17, 18], training initiatives are almost exclusively focused on conventional medical professionals in clinical settings [19, 20]. Our training was designed in accordance with the 2008 Clinical Practice Guideline for Tobacco Use [21] to increase the number of contacts with health professionals screening for tobacco use, assessing for readiness to quit, and utilizing motivational interviewing techniques to encourage patients who are resistant to cessation attempts. Compared to biomedical practitioners, interactions with CAM practitioners are typically longer, more frequent, and more focused on wellness care [22]. Further, a considerable proportion of US adults (33.2% in 2012), [23] including approximately 1.5 million smokers, seek care from CAM practitioners annually [24, 25]. The potential reach of CAM practitioners in promoting tobacco cessation has unfortunately been largely overlooked by cessation initiatives [15, 26]. Following the successful implementation of the CAMR training intervention, this paper presents the results of qualitative interviews assessing the implementation of tobacco BIs in CAM practice from the perspectives of both practitioners and patients.

Methods

Qualitative results presented in this article were collected as part of a larger study, CAM Reach (CAMR) (NCI RO1 CA137375) [26, 27], that trained Acupuncture, Chiropractic, and Massage Therapy practitioners to implement tobacco cessation brief intervention (BI) in their practice. The training was specifically tailored and adapted for use in CAM practice settings.

Prior to CAMR intervention development, investigators conducted semi-structured, open-ended qualitative key informant interviews with local CAM practitioners chosen for expertise in their discipline and connectedness with professional peers (see Muramoto et al. [26] for a description of these interviews as part of the intervention development process, including themes covered, participant quotations, and in-depth interviewing methods).

Key informants in those interviews raised three primary concerns [26] that would be addressed in the CAMR study:

- First, that regularly raising the issue of tobacco cessation might compromise their relationship with patients, particularly those whose key complaints may not be seen by the patient as tobacco-related.
- Second, given that most patients pay for CAM services out-of-pocket, practitioners were concerned that promoting cessation might cause patients to leave their practice.
- Third, practitioners were concerned that introducing cessation materials, such as pamphlets or posters, to new patients might be perceived as a "sales pitch" aimed at promoting additional, fee-based products or services [26].

Four months after CAMR training, a second phase of qualitative interviews assessed practitioners' experiences after participating in the training. The purpose of these qualitative interviews was to determine whether tailoring BI training to address key informants' concerns was effective in making the BI a routine and accepted part of CAM practice. This article is focused on analysis of data from the second phase of qualitative inquiry, conducted with the CAMR study practitioners and their patients after participation in tailored training.

The CAMR training and practice system intervention (CAMR Study intervention, Table 1) tailored BI training to the everyday reality of CAM practice settings with specific emphasis on addressing potential concerns. The goal of the training was to increase practitioners' sense of self-efficacy and comfort in initiating BIs by teaching practitioners to deliver tobacco cessation advice to patients in non-intrusive ways that could be easily incorporated in their practice.

Qualitative methods

The qualitative component of the CAMR study was designed and conducted by an interdisciplinary team of public health and medical researchers and medical anthropologists. It consisted of telephone interviews with practitioners and patients ranging from 10 to 55 min in length. Semi-structured interview guides allowed interviewers to explore the concerns raised during key informant interviews [26] and to cover other aspects of their training and experience, but included some set questions that all participants were asked to respond to (See Additional file 1).

Practitioner interviews

Practitioners from all three cohorts (chiropractic, acupuncture, massage therapy) who participated in CAMR

Table 1 Summary of CAMR study

Overall objective	• Train chiropractors, acupuncturists and massage therapists to perform tobacco BIs with their patients
Aims	• Evaluate the effectiveness of the CAMR training by studying practitioner BI behavior and patient tobacco cessation activity. • Conduct a qualitative study with a sub-sample of enrolled practitioners and patients to examine factors associated with implementing tobacco cessation BIs
Design and methods	• Single group, Pre/post post design; assessments measured knowledge, attitudes, beliefs and confidence about tobacco BIs (assessed at baseline, and 3-, 6-, 9- and 12-months post-training). • Training was a one-day, in-person workshop and included a one-hour in-situ "practice patient" learning activity 1–2 weeks later. • Practitioners were provided tobacco cessation materials (pamphlets and posters) to display in their practices and distribute to their patients. • After the CAMR training, research staff visited practices every 2–4 weeks for 3 months, to encourage practitioners to incorporate study patient materials and implement tobacco cessation activities into routine practice. • N = 99 practitioners (30 chiropractors, 27 acupuncturists and 42 massage therapists) enrolled in the study. • N = 595 clients of enrolled practitioners participated in the study. • Of these participants, 54 practitioners and 38 patients were selected for qualitative interviews spread across all three cohorts.

training were eligible to participate in qualitative interviews based on self-reported tobacco cessation BI- related activity in the past 3 months. BI-related activity indicators were: (1) reports of BIs with patients who use tobacco; (2) distribution of tobacco cessation related materials; (3) referral of patients to Public Health Service guideline-based tobacco cessation treatment; and/or (4) conversations with non-tobacco users exposed to second-hand smoke. Interview questions asked about interactions with both established and new patients, the contexts in which conversations about tobacco were introduced, patients' reactions to the discussion, and the use of tobacco related educational materials.

Patient interviews

Patients were eligible to participate in qualitative interviews if they had visited their practitioner within the previous three months and reported conversations with their practitioner about tobacco use or second-hand smoke. Patient interviews focused on how appropriate or intrusive it was for CAM practitioners to ask about tobacco use; changes in patients' thinking about tobacco use following BIs; and how CAMR patient education materials were used or passed on.

Qualitative participants

Of 99 practitioners and 595 patients enrolled in the study, 54 practitioners and 38 patients participated in qualitative interviews (see Table 2 for number eligible based on meeting criteria of having conducted a BI in the past 3 months, and response rates). Optimally, practitioners were interviewed multiple times, at 3 months, 7 months, and 1 year post-training to assess implementation over time. Patients were interviewed once to assess perception of the brief intervention delivered by a CAM practitioner, and those who reported intention to quit or active quit attempts discussed with practitioners were interviewed again three months later. One hundred and one practitioner interviews and 50 patient interviews were included in this analysis.

Qualitative analysis

Semi-structured qualitative interviews were audio-recorded and transcribed verbatim. The research team analyzed qualitative data using constant comparative analysis [28, 29] and phenomenological analysis methodologies [30, 31]. The coding scheme used to code data was based on initial thematic analysis and additional codes were added when new themes became apparent. In-depth thematic coding was conducted using ATLASti qualitative data analysis software [32]. Thematic analysis of data included a "mechanical" stage (organizing and dividing the data into a useful scheme/codebook), and an "interpretive" stage (identifying criteria for organizing thematic codes) [33]. Phenomenological analysis is a method of contextualizing participants' experiences and gaining in-depth understanding of how their interpretation of the meaning in their experiences impacts behavior [30, 31].

Six coders were involved in coding the transcripts. Reliability among coders was established through a process of regular meetings of all coders during which they discussed differences in their coding of a single transcript until there was consensus among coders as to the

Table 2 Numbers of practitioners and patients eligible to participate in qualitative interviews and response rates among those eligible[a]

		Months 3–4	Months 7–9	Month 12	Total
Practitioners	# eligible	n = 45	n = 45	n = 43	n = 133
	# completed	n = 38	n = 32	n = 31	n = 101
	Response rate	84.4%	71.1%	72.1%	75.9%
Clients	# eligible	n = 13	n = 37	n = 21	n = 71
	# completed	n = 10	n = 26	n = 14	n = 50
	Response rate	76.9%	70.3%	66.7%	70.4%

[a]Practitioners were eligible to participate in qualitative interviews if they reported having discussed tobacco use or second-hand smoke with patients during their interactions in the past 3 months. Patients were eligible if they reported having seen tobacco-related materials or having discussed tobacco use or second-hand smoke with practitioners in the past 3 months

definition and scope of the themes. This reliability procedure was intended to critically reflect on disagreements and improve analytical consistency, not to measure percentage of agreement [34, 35]. Coded qualitative data were analyzed by a researcher not involved in the study design or coding process (EE) to reduce potential bias in results that can be produced when initial expectations of interviewers drive themes [35]. Using thematically grounded qualitative analysis, the research team was attentive to both emergent themes and topics of interest such as how practitioners and patients engaged with the topic of tobacco use and second hand smoke exposure.

Results

The CAMR training and practice system intervention (CAMR Study intervention, Table 1) tailored BI training to the everyday reality of CAM practice settings with specific emphasis on addressing potential concerns. The goal of the training was to increase practitioners' sense of self-efficacy and comfort in initiating BIs by teaching practitioners to deliver tobacco cessation advice to patients in non-intrusive ways that could be easily incorporated in their practice.

We first highlight findings from qualitative interviews specifically addressing the three concerns described by the initial key informants. Strategies found useful in implementing tobacco BIs in routine CAM practice are then briefly considered.

Concern 1: Potential harm to the patient-practitioner relationship

Practitioners' perspective

Prior to the training, even if questions about tobacco were included on patient intake forms, practitioners rarely followed up on reports of tobacco use. After the training, however, practitioners reported greater understanding of the connections between tobacco use and common patient complaints (e.g. pain, impaired healing). Feeling more able to describe the relevance of their cessation advice increased practitioners' confidence and motivation to discuss tobacco cessation. One practitioner, for example, explained that learning about how tobacco use impacts tissue healing motivated her to address tobacco with a patient.

> I was more comfortable with learning how to put together the detriments of smoking, linking it with something that would be occurring. For instance, a massage client who has a stiff shoulder and upper back issues. He's a smoker and through the training I learned that because smoking inhibits some of the circulation and it doesn't allow muscles and tissue to heal as readily as a nonsmoker, I was able to bring that up. (Massage Therapist, 4 months post-training)

Connections between tobacco and pain were described as a helpful way to begin a BI (i.e. introduce the topic of tobacco) and as a key motivation to address tobacco use with patients.

> I didn't realize that tobacco was tied to pain levels. I didn't realize that people would not heal as quickly if they smoked. It's good to be able to point that out to patients, that we've been working on this problem and some of the reason you still have pain could be because you're still smoking. (Acupuncturist, 4 months post-training)

Patients' perspective

CAMR BI training encouraged practitioners to assess patients' readiness to quit and to support patients accordingly. If a patient had not thought about quitting or was contemplating a possible quit, for example, information was offered about both the general harm of smoking and possible links between smoking and current health problems. If and when a patient was ready to take steps toward planning or executing a quit attempt, practitioners offered practical advice, including referral to an Arizona statewide quit line (ASHline) where patients could obtain behavioral support and information about medications that might help with the process of quitting. Practitioners were taught to offer advice in a motivational, supportive manner and to refrain from proscriptive advice. Patients corroborated this in descriptions of how practitioners approached them about tobacco use. Notably, this approach did not compromise, but rather strengthened practitioner-patient relationships and was viewed as an act of caring. Patients who were interested in quitting tobacco reported that their practitioners were a nonjudgmental source of information and support for achieving their goals. One patient, for example, identified this approach to behavior change as empowering.

> She made me feel empowered. She made me feel whole, that it was okay where I was right there, and that I could move forward to what I really truly wanted. It was just important that I really wanted it. It had to be a conscious choice of mine that I wanted it, not somebody else wanted it. ... I just felt empowered—empowered and accepted, and not judged at all. (Acupuncture patient, 12 months post-training)

Concern 2: Intrusiveness of BI in CAM practice

Practitioners' perspective

Several practitioners in this study reported that prior to the CAMR training they were apprehensive about approaching patients about tobacco use. After participating in the training, however, they described being far more comfortable approaching patients using the skills they had learned. Practitioners explained that learning to approach tobacco-users as a source of information and referral gave them the confidence to approach patients. Also notable, as illustrated in the following quote, practitioners reported surprise that tobacco users were less defensive about talking about tobacco than they had anticipated.

> It surprised me that it wasn't as difficult as you think. The resistance isn't there as much as you think it is. Because with the training, with the material, it's not as much as like a parent to a child lecture. It's more like, "Here, I want to help you," and we've got tools. (Chiropractor, 7 months post-training)

As one practitioner explained, the training helped practitioners put aside personal biases and approach tobacco-addicted patients with empathy and support.

> I'm definitely more willing to bring up tobacco outside of the initial intake form. I'm more willing to—more able to talk to people about it. Before, I had a hard time because I'm not a smoker, and I don't like smoking. I don't enjoy it in any sense, anywhere for anybody, and so I always felt like I maybe would come off as a little too biased and a little too headstrong, and so I was hesitant because I didn't want to offend anybody, but now I feel a lot better about it. (Chiropractor, 12 months post-training)

Patients' perspective

Contrary to Practitioners' concern that patients might resist tobacco intervention, patients noted that wellness and lifestyle recommendations from their CAM practitioners were an expected part of seeking these therapies. This discrepancy between practitioners' concerns and patients' expectations regarding tobacco intervention has also been reported in dental and primary care settings [36, 37]. As one patient reported, not only was a frank discussion about tobacco use seen as an acceptable part of a CAM practice, it was valued as an important part of a wellness consultation

> Yes, it's appropriate... It definitely adds value to going to the appointment; I'm having the therapy because it's more than just the massage. It's also how that affects your entire life and what things you can do to achieve more benefits from the massage. (Massage client, 4 months post-training)

Concern 3: The possibility of cessation support being perceived as a "sales-pitch"
Practitioners' perspective

As part of the training, practitioners were offered continuing education credits and training completion

certificates. Although some did not see value in a certificate that did not contribute to their licensing, most described the credential as increasing their legitimacy and patients' receptivity to the information they offered.

> It gives it a professional look rather than just me by myself saying, "Oh, you should think about quitting." It gives me the nice documentation and presentation look of it: that I did go through training, I did learn about this, I did take continuing education on it, and it is through a well-known university, University of Arizona... A lot of them say, "Oh, the University of Arizona does this. Oh, that's so neat." I guess it validates the information, and it gives it substance. (Licensed Massage Therapist (LMT), 7 months post-training)

Printed educational materials given to practitioners as part of the CAMR training figured prominently into practitioners' descriptions of implementing the BI. Instead of seeming like a sales-pitch for additional services, the materials, in combination with techniques for non-confrontational communication provided as part of the training, were a way to provide information about the benefits of quitting tobacco without being pushy or discouraging patients from returning.

> I've noticed that having the pamphlets available to the patient makes it a lot easier because it's a way of conversing about the different aspects of quitting and having medications available, having ASH Line available. Then being able to just—if they're not real open to it, just say, "Okay, well, here, take these. If you'd like to continue the conversation, we can. I'll follow up later." (Acupuncturist, 12 months post-training)

The CAMR training addressed a broad range of tobacco-related topics including availability of the state quit line (ASHline), how to refer patients for quit coaching, and basic information about cessation medications should they be asked direct questions by patients (e.g. most commonly used, which are available without prescription, referring patients to pharmacists or physicians for more information about cessation medications). This knowledge of quit-related resources further increased practitioners' credibility as sources of cessation advice for patients who were interested in their assistance.

Patients' perspective

When asked whether they felt the BI was an appropriate part of CAM therapeutic interaction, patients reported that rather than feeling pressured to accept—or pay for—additional forms of treatment, patients saw CAM practitioners as resources for wellness information and support. For example, a long time massage patient expressed initial concerns about her practitioner becoming involved in tobacco BI training. After seeing the materials offered in a supportive way, however, she revised her initial impression and described the information on quitting smoking as an additional form of wellness support.

> [The practitioner] has a little area where people sit when they first come in. I thought, "Oh, God, is she gonna start advertising with us, and hitting us with stuff?" ... At first it kind of put me off. Then I realized that it was yet another avenue of talking about a healthy body and keeping one's body healthy. Actually, I really sort of admired her for doing that. (Massage Client, 4 months post-training)

Strategies for implementing brief tobacco intervention in routine CAM practice

CAMR training was designed to complement the holistic approach common to all three types of CAM practice in the study. Practitioners were offered evidence-based techniques for effective communication and behavioral intervention. All three types of practitioners reported that as a result of the CAMR training, they were more likely to discuss tobacco use with patients. The training provided strategies for approaching patients in non-judgmental and supportive ways. Practitioners mentioned that the availability of pamphlets, posters, and certificates of training completion all enhanced their credibility as sources of tobacco cessation information. This identity contributed to their readiness to initiate discussions about tobacco use, pass on information, and make referrals to cessation services.

> I've always asked if they smoked before [CAM] Reach, but now I have the education and the resources to follow up and do something about it rather than it just being another question on the intake form. I believe that it will remain the same, and I believe I'll still be following up with clients and asking them because it seems to give my clients and I a closer relationship as far as their health is concerned. They share more when they realize I care about everything, not just coming in and giving a massage and leaving. (LMT, 12 months post-training)

As practitioners became aware of tobacco's centrality to treating common ailments, they described increased motivation to engage in cessation efforts as a core means to achieve wellness goals.

> I have to admit that I really did not pursue [tobacco] until I became a part of this [study]... I really did not

pursue it. Now it's just a regular part of my history taking... I love being a source of information for people that are interested in how we can live healthier lives, so that's perfect for me. (Chiropractor, 3 months post-training)

CAM practitioners were trained in how to answer basic questions about nicotine replacement and other tobacco cessation medications, but reported being asked infrequently about them. They were, however, grateful to have this information included as part of the training as it boosted their confidence to talk to patients and enabled them to be seen as credible sources of information and referral. CAM practitioners who had been asked about cessation medications generally referred patients to primary care physicians and provided other types of support during the quitting process.

Practitioners noted that referring patients for cessation services did not constitute a statement about the limitations of their discipline, but rather that CAM practice is a site for making contact with and advising patients. If other support is required, CAM providers who are trained in tobacco cessation can advise, and in some cases arrange, for additional support, information, and resources.

> Acupuncture is much better at treating other things than tobacco cessation. The way I would look at it is that at least if somebody were willing to come in for tobacco cessation, it means that they're thinking of quitting. That, whether it's acupuncture or anything else, is a good thing. (Acupuncturist, 4 months post-training)

Discussion & Conclusion

Despite interest in wellness promotion and contact with large numbers of people seeking wellness care in the U.S., CAM practitioners are rarely included in tobacco cessation initiatives [24]. CAM practitioners are well-positioned to encourage tobacco cessation [38] and contrary to popular misconceptions, see about the same proportion of smokers as do other types of health professionals [24]. When compared with typical biomedical consultations, consultations with CAM providers are longer, more frequent, and more wellness focused [39]. These qualitative data collected as part of the CAMR study found that when offered the opportunity to be trained in evidence-based tobacco cessation BIs, CAM practitioners were interested in learning BI skills and implementing them in tobacco-cessation [26, 27]. This analysis of the implementation of tobacco cessation BI in routine CAM practice after participation in the CAMR study training suggests that it is feasible and acceptable to Chiropractic, Massage, and Acupuncture practitioners as well as to their patients who use tobacco.

After participation in tailored tobacco cessation intervention training as part of the CAMR study, practitioners reported confidence, knowledge, and motivation to address tobacco use. Based on their experience, practitioners described positive responses from patients regardless of their readiness to quit. In study interviews, patients reported openness to being approached by CAM practitioners about tobacco use and saw such inquiry as part of highly-valued, patient-centered care and a holistic approach to wellness. Cessation materials and certificates of training from a respected university increased CAM practitioners' credibility as knowledgeable cessation resources. These qualitative findings suggest that with training tailored to their practice-related concerns, CAM practitioners can be valuable points of contact for reaching patients who desire help with tobacco cessation.

Endnote

[1]Note that chiropractors and acupuncturists typically refer to persons receiving their treatments as "patients", whereas massage therapists usually use "clients". For simplicity, in this paper we use "patients."

Acknowledgements

Funding for this study was provided by a grant from the National Institutes of Health National Cancer Institute (NIH-NCI) (R01-CA137375-01A1). The authors would like to thank the CAM practitioners who participated in training and interviews and in formative research, as well as the patients who were willing to participate in this research.

Funding

Funding for this study was provided by a grant from the National Institutes of Health National Cancer Institute (NCI RO1 CA137375). Data collection, analysis, and reporting was conducted solely by the authors with no input from the funding source.

Authors' contributions

EE performed qualitative analysis and interpretation of data and drafted and revised the manuscript. AH was involved with coding and helped draft and revise the manuscript. LF was involved with data collection and coding and helped draft the manuscript. MN was involved in study design and data collection and helped revise the manuscript. JG was involved with study design, revision, and approved the final the manuscript. CR was involved with study design, revision, and approved the final manuscript. MM was the study PI and was involved with study design, data collection, revision, and approved the final manuscript. All authors read and approved the final manuscript.

Competing interests

The authors declare that they have no competing interests.

Author details

[1]Department of Anthropology, Northern Arizona University, 5 E. McConnell Drive, PO Box: 15200, Flagstaff, AZ 86011-5200, USA. [2]Department of Family and Community Medicine, College of Medicine, University of Arizona, 1450 N Cherry Ave, Tucson, AZ 85719, USA. [3]School of Anthropology, College of Social and Behavioral Sciences, Department of Family and Community Medicine, College of Medicine, University of Arizona, P.O. Box 210030, Tucson, AZ 85721-0030, USA. [4]Department of Pharmacy Practice & Science, College of Pharmacy, University of Arizona, 1295 N. Martin, PO Box 210202, Tucson, AZ 85721, USA.

References

1. Campbell J, Mays MZ, Yuan NP, Muramoto ML. Who are health influencers? Characterizing a sample of tobacco cessation interveners. Am J Health Behav. 2007;31(2):181–92.
2. Cigarette smoking among adults–United States. MMWR. Morbidity and mortality weekly report 2002. 2000;51(29):642–5.
3. Shafey O, Dolwick S, Guindon GE. In: Tobacco control country profiles. vol. 356. Atlanta: American Cancer Society; World Health Organization, International Union Against Cancer; 2003: 28–31.
4. Nguyen KH. State-Specific Prevalence of Current Cigarette Smoking and Smokeless Tobacco Use Among Adults—United States, 2014. MMWR Morb Mortal Wkly Rep. 2016;65
5. Gorin SS, Heck JE. Meta-analysis of the efficacy of tobacco counseling by health care providers. Cancer Epidemiol Biomark Prev. 2004;13(12):2012–22.
6. Hollis JF, Bills R, Whitlock E, Stevens VJ, Mullooly J, Lichtenstein E. Implementing tobacco interventions in the real world of managed care. Tob Control. 2000;9(suppl 1):i18–24.
7. Rollnick S, Butler CC, Stott N. Helping smokers make decisions: the enhancement of brief intervention for general medical practice. Patient Educ Couns. 1997;31(3):191–203.
8. An LC, Foldes SS, Alesci NL, Bluhm JH, Bland PC, Davern ME, et al. The impact of smoking-cessation intervention by multiple health professionals. Am J Prev Med. 2008;34(1):54–60.
9. Flocke SA, Stange KC. Direct observation and patient recall of health behavior advice. Prev Med. 2004;38(3):343–9.
10. Vijayaraghavan M, Yuan P, Gregorich S, Lum P, Appelle N, Napoles AM, et al. Disparities in receipt of 5As for smoking cessation in diverse primary care and HIV clinics. Preventive Medicine Reports. 2017;6:80–7.
11. Treating tobacco use and dependence: 2008 Update U.S. Public Health Service clinical practice guideline executive summary. Respiratory care. 2008;53(9):1217–22.
12. Borland R, Partos TR, Yong HH, Cummings KM, Hyland A: How much unsuccessful quitting activity is going on among adult smokers? Data from the International Tobacco Control Four Country cohort survey. Addiction (Abingdon, England) 2012, 107(3):673–682.
13. U.S. Department of Health and Human Services. The Health Consequences of Smoking —50 Years of Progress: A Report of the Surgeon General. Atlanta, GA: U.S. Department of Health and Human Services, Centers for Disease Control and Prevention, National Center for Chronic Disease Prevention and Health Promotion, Office on Smoking and Health, 2014.
14. Schnoll RA, Rukstalis M, Wileyto EP, Shields AE. Smoking cessation treatment by primary care physicians: an update and call for training. Am J Prev Med. 2006;31(3):233–9.
15. Gordon JS, Istvan J, Haas M. Tobacco cessation via doctors of chiropractic: results of a feasibility study. Nicotine & tobacco research: official journal of the Society for Research on Nicotine and Tobacco. 2010;12(3):305–8.
16. Coan L, Windsor LJ, Romito LM. Increasing tobacco intervention strategies by oral health practitioners in Indiana. American Dental Hygienists Association. 2015;89(3):190–201.
17. Muramoto ML, Hall JR, Nichter M, Nichter M, Aickin M, Connolly T, et al. Activating lay health influencers to promote tobacco cessation. Am J Health Behav. 2014;38(3):392–403.
18. Muramoto ML, Wassum K, Connolly T, Matthews E, Floden L. Helpers program: a pilot test of brief tobacco intervention training in three corporations. Am J Prev Med. 2010;38(3 Suppl):S319–26.
19. Muramoto ML, Connolly T, Strayer LJ, Ranger-Moore J, Blatt W, Leischow R, et al. Tobacco cessation skills certification in Arizona: application of a state wide, community based model for diffusion of evidence based practice guidelines. Tob Control. 2000;9(4):408–14.
20. Zhu SH, Nguyen QB, Cummins S, Wong S, Wightman V. Non-smokers seeking help for smokers: a preliminary study. Tob Control. 2006;15(2):107–13.
21. Fiore M, Jaen CR, Baker T, Bailey W, Benowitz N, Curry S, Dorfman S, Froelicher E, Goldstein M, Healton C: Treating tobacco use and dependence: 2008 update. 2008.
22. Heiligers PJ, de Groot J, Koster D, van Dulmen S. Diagnoses and visit length in complementary and mainstream medicine. BMC Complement Altern Med. 2010;10:3.
23. Clarke TC, Black LI, Stussman BJ, Barnes PM, Nahin RL. Trends in the use of complementary health approaches among adults: United States. National health statistics reports. 2002–2012;2015(79):1–16.
24. Hamm E, Muramoto ML, Howerter A, Floden L, Govindarajan L. Use of provider-based complementary and alternative medicine by adult smokers

in the United States: comparison from the 2002 and 2007 NHIS survey. American journal of health promotion: AJHP. 2014;29(2):127 31.

25. Barnes PM, Bloom B, Nahin RL. Complementary and alternative medicine use among adults and children: United States. National health statistics reports. 2007;2008(12):1–23.

26. Muramoto ML, Matthews E, Ritenbaugh CK, Nichter MA. Intervention development for integration of conventional tobacco cessation interventions into routine CAM practice. BMC Complement Altern Med. 2015;15(1):96.

27. Muramoto ML, Howerter A, Matthews E, Floden L, Gordon JS, Nichter M, et al. Tobacco brief intervention training for chiropractic, acupuncture, and massage practitioners: protocol for the CAM reach study. BMC Complement Altern Med. 2014;14(1):510.

28. Bernard HR: Research methods in anthropology: qualitative and quantitative approaches: Rowman Altamira; 2011.

29. Trotter Ii RT. Qualitative research sample design and sample size: resolving and unresolved issues and inferential imperatives. Prev Med. 2012;55(5):398–400.

30. Larkin M, Watts S, Clifton E. Giving voice and making sense in interpretative phenomenological analysis. Qual Res Psychol. 2006;3(2):102–20.

31. Pietkiewicz I, Smith JA. A practical guide to using interpretative phenomenological analysis in qualitative research psychology. Psychological Journal. 2014;20(1):7–14.

32. NVivo qualitative data analysis Software; QSR International Pty Ltd. Version 10. In.; 2014.

33. Guest G, MacQueen KM, Namey EE: Applied thematic analysis: sage; 2011.

34. Armstrong D, Gosling A, Weinman J, Marteau T. The place of inter-rater reliability in qualitative research: an empirical study. Sociology. 1997;31(3):597–606.

35. Pope C, Ziebland S, Mays N. Analysing qualitative data. BMJ. 2000;320(7227):114–6.

36. Campbell HS, Sletten M, Petty T. Patient perceptions of tobacco cessation services in dental offices. J Am Dent Assoc. 1999;130(2):219–26.

37. Gordon JS, Andrews JA, Albert DA, Crews KM, Payne TJ, Severson HH. Tobacco cessation via public dental clinics: results of a randomized trial. Am J Public Health. 2010;100(7):1307–12.

38. Bodeker G, Kronenberg F. A public health agenda for traditional, complementary, and alternative medicine. Am J Public Health. 2002;92(10):1582–91.

39. Nahin RL, Barnes PM, Stussman BJ, Bloom B. Costs of complementary and alternative medicine (CAM) and frequency of visits to CAM practitioners: United States. National health statistics reports. 2007;2009(18):1–14.

13

Early electroacupuncture treatment ameliorates neuroinflammation in rats with traumatic brain injury

Wei-Chen Tang[1], Yao-Chin Hsu[2], Che-Chuan Wang[3,4,5], Chiao-Ya Hu[4], Chung-Ching Chio[4] and Jinn-Rung Kuo[4,6,7*]

Abstract

Background: Neuroinflammation is the leading cause of neurological sequelae after traumatic brain injury (TBI). The aim of the present study was to investigate whether the neuroprotective effects of electroacupuncture (EA) are mediated by anti-neuroinflammatory effects in a rat model of TBI.

Methods: Male Sprague-Dawley rats were randomly divided into three groups: sham-operated, TBI control, and EA-treated. The animals in the sham-operated group underwent a sham operation, those in the TBI control group were subjected to TBI, but not EA, and those in the EA group were treated with EA for 60 min immediately after TBI, daily for 3 consecutive days. EA was applied at the acupuncture points GV20, GV26, LI4, and KI1, using a dense-dispersed wave, at frequencies of 0.2 and 1 Hz, and an amplitude of 1 mA. Cell infarction volume (TTC stain), neuronal apoptosis (markers: TUNEL and Caspase-3), activation of microglia (marker: Iba1) and astrocytes (marker: GFAP), and tumor necrosis factor (TNF)-α expression in the microglia and astrocytes were evaluated by immunofluorescence. Functional outcomes were assessed using the inclined plane test. All tests were performed 72 h after TBI.

Results: We found that TBI-induced loss of grasp strength, infarction volume, neuronal apoptosis, microglial and astrocyte activation, and TNF-α expression in activated microglia and astrocytes were significantly attenuated by EA treatment.

Conclusions: Treatment of TBI in the acute stage with EA for 60 min daily for 3 days could ameliorate neuroinflammation. This may thus represent a mechanism by which functional recovery can occur after TBI.

Keywords: Astrocyte, Electroacupuncture, Microglia, Neuronal apoptosis, Traumatic brain injury, Tumor Necrosis factor-α

Background

Neuroinflammation is the major cause of disability and death after traumatic brain injury (TBI). Activated astrocytes and microglia are markers of neuroinflammation after TBI [1, 2]. These activated cells can release tumor necrosis factor-alpha (TNF-α) and can signal neuronal apoptosis and impair brain function [3, 4]. Therefore, attenuating reactive microgliosis and astrogliosis may be a promising strategy for the treatment of the neurological sequelae of TBI.

Electroacupuncture (EA), a highly popular traditional Chinese therapy, is also widely used in the USA, with 2.1 million adults undergoing EA per year [5]. Previous studies have demonstrated the beneficial effects of EA on stroke [6–8], spinal cord injury [9], arthritis [10], and sciatica [11]. Recently, we have demonstrated that application of EA 60 min post-TBI has neuroprotective effects on neuronal cells. These effects might be attributable to the anti-apoptotic effects of EA, as demonstrated in the injured cortex in a fluid-percussion model of TBI [12]. However, the effects of EA on neuroinflammation after TBI still require clarification.

In this study, we tested the hypothesis that EA therapy attenuates TBI-induced cerebral injury and improves

* Correspondence: kuojinnrung@gmail.com
[4]Department of Medical research, Chi-Mei Medical Center, Tainan, Taiwan
[6]Department of Biotechnology, Southern Taiwan University of Science and Technology, Tainan, Taiwan
Full list of author information is available at the end of the article

neurological outcomes by inhibiting activation of microglia and astrocytes, as well as TNF-α expression in activated microglia and astrocytes, after TBI. To this end, we assessed neuronal apoptosis and TNF-α expression in activated microglia and astrocytes in the ischemic cortex at 72 h after TBI. We also compared motor deficits and cerebral infarction volume after TBI in rats that did or did not receive EA therapy for 60 min per day for 3 days.

Methods

Animals

Adult male Sprague-Dawley (SD) rats, weighing 360 ± 20 g, were used in these experiments. All experimental procedures conformed to the NIH guidelines and were approved by the Institutional Animal Care and Use Committee (IACUC) of Chi Mei Medical Center (IACUC Approval NO 10012722). Care was taken to minimize discomfort of the animals during surgery and the recovery period. At the end of the experiments, the rats were sacrificed with an overdose of urethane.

Traumatic brain injury

Animals were anesthetized by intramuscular administration of a mixture of ketamine (44 mg/Kg, Nankuang Pharmaceutical, Tainan, Taiwan), atropine (0.02633 mg/kg, Sintong Chemical Ind. Co., Taoyuan, Taiwan), and xylazine (6.77 mg/kg, Bayer, Berlin, Germany). Using a stereotaxic frame, a craniectomy defect with a 2-mm radius was created in the right parietal cortex. Then, a fluid percussion device (VCU Biomedical Engineering, Richmond, VA, USA) was connected, and the brain was injured with a 2.0–2.2 atm, 25-ms percussion. This method produces moderately severe brain trauma, as described by McIntosh et al. [13]. Detailed procedures are previously described [12].

Treatment intervention

The rats were randomly divided into three groups: Sham operation, TBI control, and EA treatment immediately after TBI. EA was applied at the acupuncture points Baihui (GV20), Shuigou (GV26), Hegu (LI4), and Yongquan (KI1) (WHO standard names), using a dense-dispersed wave at frequencies of 0.2 and 1 Hz, and an amplitude of 1 mA (low frequency 5-channel TENS Unit and Electrical Needle Stimulator, model 05B, Ching Ming Medical Device Co., Ltd., Taipei, Taiwan) for 60 min per day, for 3 days. For each group of measurement parameters, we used six rats. The experimental endpoint was measured 3 days after TBI as lateral fluid percussion causes motor dysfunction from 3 days to 1 year after TBI [14].

Cerebral infarction assay

The infarction volume was measured using triphenyltetrazolium chloride (TTC) staining at 72 h after TBI. TTC staining was performed as described previously [15]. Under deep anesthesia (sodium pentobarbital, 100 mg/kg, i.p.), the animals were administered an intracardiac perfusion of saline. The brain tissue was then removed, immersed in cold saline for 5 min, and sliced into 2.0-mm-thick sections. The brain slices were incubated in 2% TTC dissolved in phosphate-buffered saline (PBS) for 30 min at 37 °C, and then fixed in 5% formaldehyde solution. The infarction volume, as revealed by negative TTC stains, indicating dehydrogenase-deficient tissue, was measured in each slice and summed using computerized planimetry (Media Cybernetics, Inc. Washington Street, Rockville, USA). The infarction volume was calculated as 2 mm (thickness of the slice) × [the sum of the infarction areas in all brain slices (mm^2)].

Motor function evaluation

An inclined plane was used to measure limb strength. The animals were placed facing right and then facing left, perpendicular to the slope of a plane inclined at 55° (20 cm × 20 cm buffer-ribbed surface) [16]. To determine the maximum angle at which an animal could remain on the inclined plane, the angle was increased or decreased in increments of 5°. Motor deficits were measured at the left- and right-side maximal angles, at 72 h after TBI.

Immunofluorescence assays

At 72 h after TBI, consecutive 6-μm thick sections, corresponding to coronal coordinates 2.0–7.0 mm posterior to the bregma, were obtained as described previously [17]. Activated microglia and astrocytes were evaluated by detecting Iba1- and GFAP-positive cells, respectively, using an immunofluorescence assay [18]. TNF-α expression in the activated microglia and astrocytes was investigated by detecting Iba1/GFAP plus TNF-α-positive cells using an immunofluorescence assay. Apoptotic neuronal cells were identified by double-staining with terminal deoxynucleotidyltransferase-mediated dUTP-biotin nick-end labeling (TUNEL) or Caspase-3 and Neu-N staining [19]. The following antibodies were used: a monoclonal mouse anti-Iba1 antibody (ab1211, Abcam, Boston, MA, USA) at a 1:400 dilution, detected with a DyLight® 594 anti-mouse (IgG) antibody (ab96873, Abcam) at a 1:400 dilution; a polyclonal rabbit anti-TNF-α antibody (ab6671, Abcam) at a 1:200 dilution, detected with an Alexa-Fluor® 488 anti-rabbit (IgG) antibody (ab150063, Abcam) at a 1:1000 dilution; a monoclonal mouse anti-NeuN antibody (ab104224, Abcam) at a 1:1000 dilution, detected with a DyLight® 594 anti-mouse (IgG) antibody (ab96873, Abcam) at a 1:400 dilution; a monoclonal mouse anti-GFAP antibody (ab10062, Abcam) at a 1:1000 dilution, detected with a DyLight® 594 anti-mouse (IgG) antibody (ab96873, Abcam) at a 1:400 dilution; a monoclonal rabbit anti-Caspase-3 antibody (#9664, Cell Signaling Technology, Beverly, MA, USA) at a 1:400 dilution, detected with an Alexa Fluor® 488 anti-rabbit (IgG) antibody (ab150073, Abcam) at a 1:1000 dilution. The number of positively stained cells was calculated in five coronal sections corresponding to peri-lesional of ipsilateral cortex (original magnification, 400 × (10 × 40)) and expressed as the mean number of positive cells in all five sections from each rat using computerized planimetry (Image-Pro Plus Media Cybernetics, Inc., Rockville, MS, USA).

Statistical analysis

The results are expressed as the means ± standard deviation. A two-way analysis of variance for repeated measurements was used for factorial experiments, and Dunnett's test was used for post hoc multiple comparisons among means. Differences were considered significant at $p < 0.05$. All data were analyzed with Sigma Plot version 11.0 for Windows (Systat Software, San Jose, CA, USA).

Results

Effects of EA on functional outcome measures assessed on the inclined plane

The maximal grip angle of rats at 72 h after TBI was significantly lower than that of the sham controls (51.1° ± 0.43° versus 57.2° ± 0.66°, respectively, $p < 0.001$). The TBI-induced motor dysfunction was significantly improved by EA treatment (TBI group versus EA group, 51.1° ± 0.43° versus 56.1° ± 1.33°, $p < 0.01$; Fig. 1).

EA significantly decreases TBI-induced cerebral infarction volume

At 72 h following TBI, the TTC-stained volume was significantly higher in the infracted area of TBI controls than in the corresponding area of the sham controls (139.4 ± 13.8 mm^3 versus 0, $p < 0.001$; $n = 6$ per group). The TBI-induced infarction volume was significantly decreased by EA treatment (TBI group versus EA group, 139.4 ± 13.8 mm^3 versus 101.8 ± 14.2 mm^3, $p < 0.05$; $n = 6$ per group; Fig. 2).

EA decreases neuronal apoptosis in the peri-lesional cortex after TBI

First, using the Caspase-3 assay, we found that the number of Caspase-3 expressing neurons (i.e., double-positive for Neu-N and Caspase-3) in the peri-lesion cortex was significantly higher in the TBI group at 72 h after TBI than in the sham controls (12.0 ± 2.02 and 0 ± 0, respectively; $p < 0.001$; $n = 6$ both groups). However, this number was significantly reduced after EA treatment (TBI group versus EA group, 12.0 ± 2.02 versus 5.4 ± 1.99; $p < 0.05$; $n = 6$ both groups; Fig. 3).

Then, using the TUNEL assay, we found that the number of apoptotic neuronal cells (positive for Neu-N plus TUNEL staining) in the peri-lesional cortex was significantly higher in the TBI group at 72 h after TBI than in the sham controls (37.0 ± 3.08 and 0 ± 0, respectively; $p < 0.001$; $n = 6$ both groups). Moreover, this number was

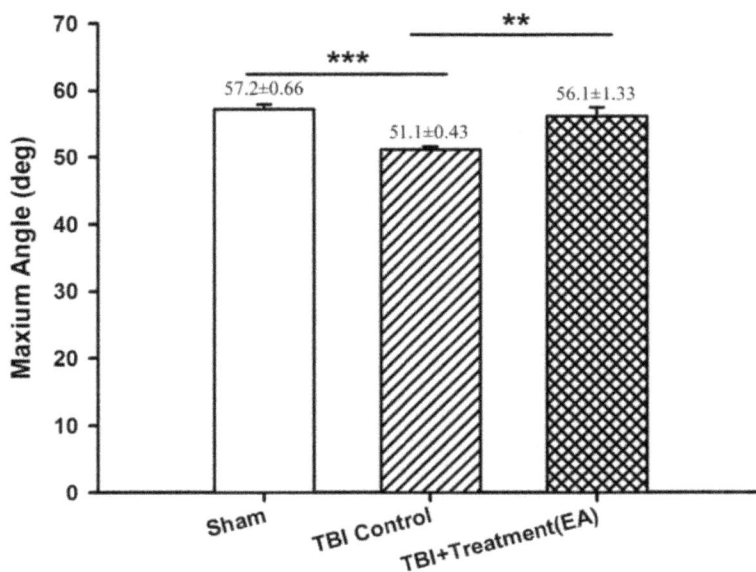

Fig. 1 The effects of electroacupuncture (EA) treatment on traumatic brain injury (TBI)-induced motor deficits, as investigated using the inclined plane test to determine the maximum grasp angle at 72 h after TBI. ***$p < 0.001$ compared with the sham group; **$p < 0.01$ compared with EA treatment in the TBI group, $n = 6$ in each group

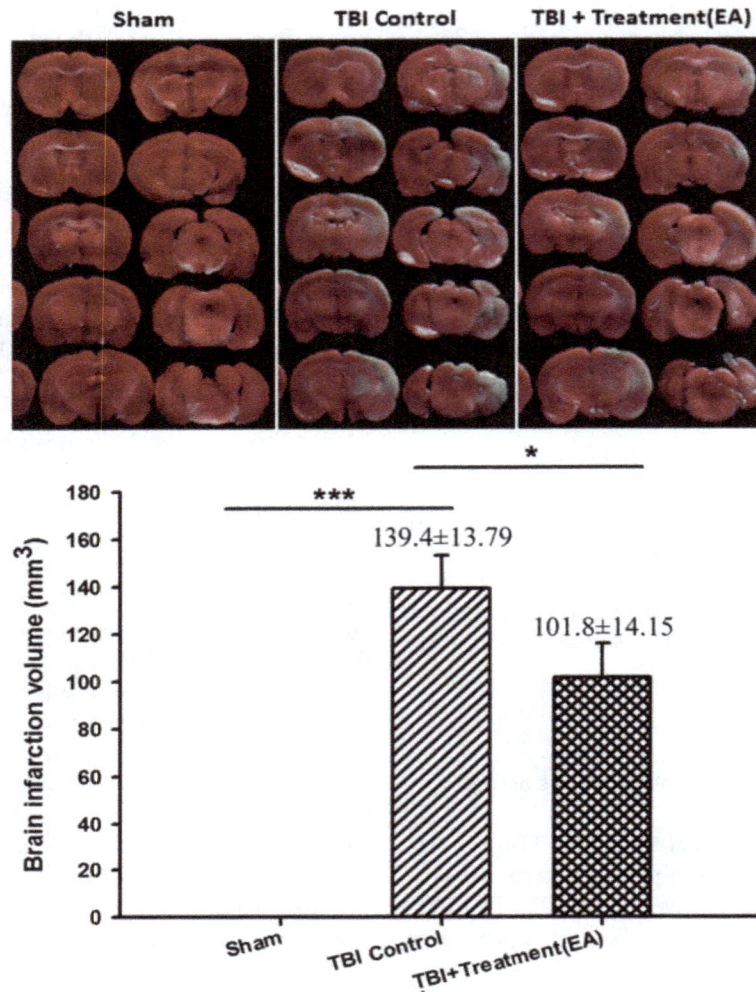

Fig. 2 The effects of electroacupuncture (EA) on traumatic brain injury (TBI)-induced infarction volume in the ischemic cortex at 72 h after TBI, ***p < 0.001 compared with the sham group; *p < 0.05 compared with EA treatment in the TBI group, n = 6 in each group

significantly reduced after EA treatment (TBI group versus EA group, 37.0 ± 3.08 versus 23.4 ± 1.73; p < 0.01; n = 6 both groups; Fig. 4).

EA attenuates activation of microglia and astrocytes in the peri-lesional cortex

We evaluated microglial and astroglial activation and tested the possibility that EA might suppress TBI-induced brain microgliosis and astrogliosis. Microgliosis was represented by microglia with an amoeboid morphology, with retracted, thickened processes and an enlarged soma. Iba1-DAPI and GFAP-DAPI double-staining showed that the number of microglia was significantly increased in the peri-lesional cortex of the TBI rats than in the sham rats. EA significantly attenuated this TBI-induced activation of microglia (p < 0.01, Fig. 5) and astrocytes (p < 0.01, Fig. 6).

EA attenuates TNF-α expression in activated microglia and astrocytes in the peri-lesional cortex

We evaluated TNF-α expression in activated microglia and tested the possibility that EA might attenuate TBI-induced neuroinflammation. As predicted, the expression of Iba1 plus TNF-α and GFAP plus TNF-α in the peri-lesioned cortex was significantly higher in the TBI rats than in the sham rats. However, EA significantly reduced the TBI-induced TNF-α expression in activated microglia (p < 0.01, Fig. 7) and astrocytes (p < 0.01, Fig. 8).

Discussion

In the current study, treatment of TBI with EA for 60 min per day for 3 days, using low frequencies of 0.2 and 1 Hz and an intensity of 1 mA, during the acute injury phase, was shown to decrease neuroinflammation and the expression of factors associated with neuronal apoptosis. This may represent a

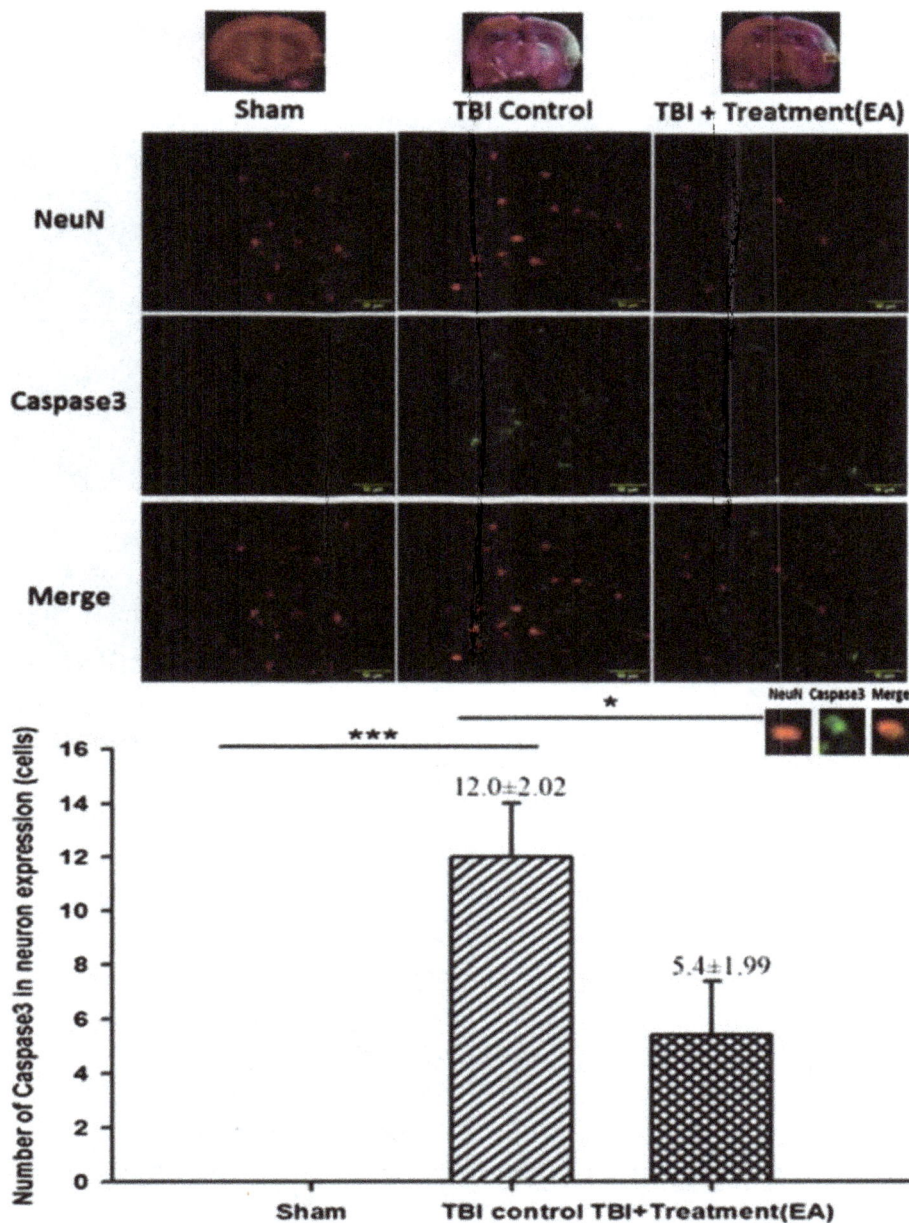

Fig. 3 The effects of electroacupuncture (EA) treatment on Caspase-3 expression in cortical neurons (markers: Caspase-3 plus Neu-N) at 72 h after traumatic brain injury (TBI), ***$p < 0.001$, compared with the sham group; *$p < 0.05$ compared with EA treatment in the TBI group, $n = 6$ in each group. The areas measured for TTC staining are marked with squares in the top panel

mechanism by which functional recovery may occur after TBI.

Most acupuncture-related research in Chinese medicine employs "acupoint groups", which comprise two or more acupoints. Therefore, the therapeutic roles and mechanisms of single, specific acupoints are difficult to discern in these studies. Rather, the majority of acupuncture experimental research describes the synergistic effects of "acupoints groups". Xu et al. investigated the effects of acupuncture at

the acupoints Baihui (GV 20) and Zusanli (ST36) in an ischemia – reperfusion injury model after middle cerebral artery occlusion. They found that TNF-α expression was lower in the EA group than in the model and sham-operated groups [7]. In a study by Cheng et al., acupuncture at the Baihui (GV 20) and Dazhui (GV14) acupoints significantly downregulated the expression of TNF-α, GFAP, S100B, and nuclear factor-kB in the ischemic cortical penumbra [8]. Jiang et al. selected Shuigou (GV 26) and Fengfu

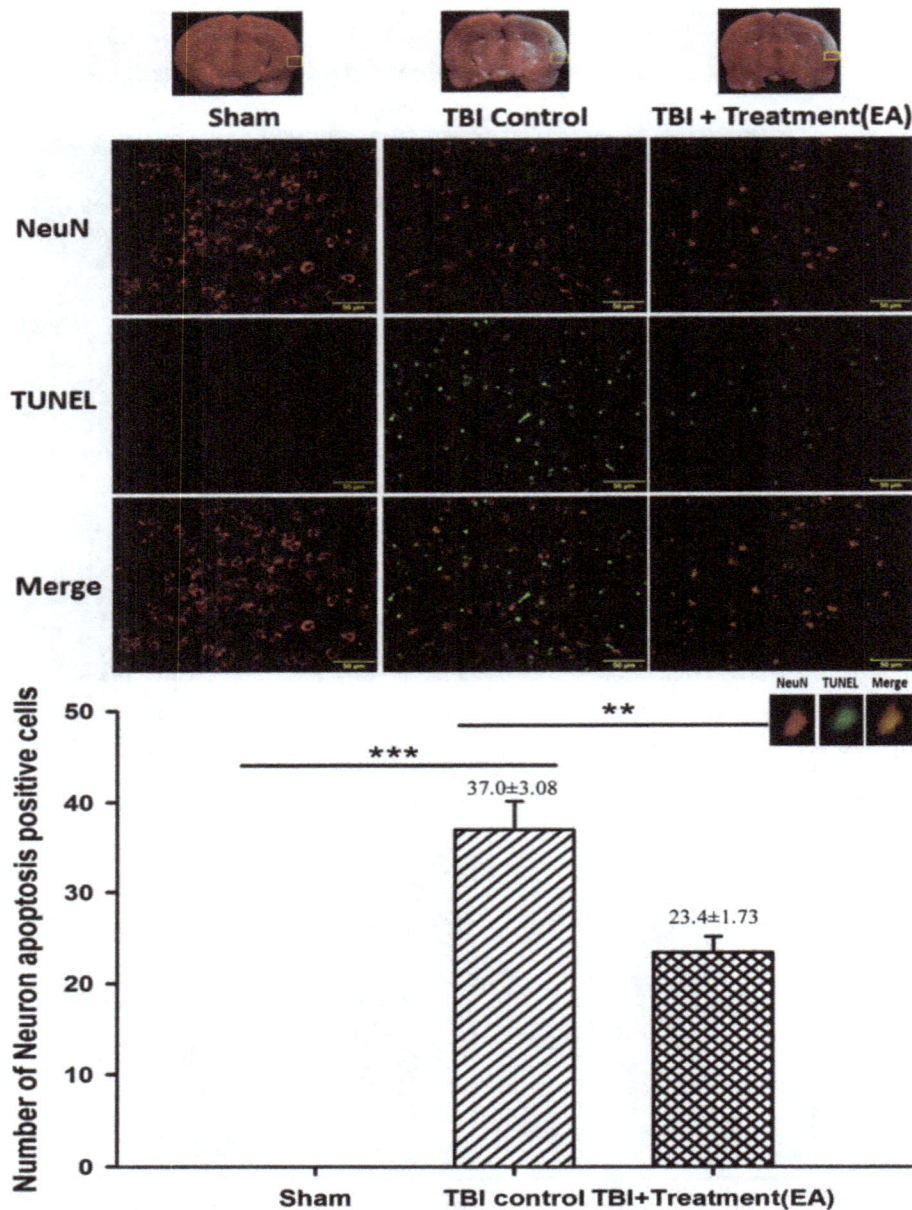

Fig. 4 The effects of electroacupuncture (EA) treatment on traumatic brain injury (TBI)-induced neuronal apoptosis (markers: Neu-N plus TUNEL) at 72 h after TBI, ***$p < 0.001$ compared with the sham group; **$p < 0.01$ compared with EA treatment in the TBI group, $n = 6$ in each group. The areas measured for TTC staining are marked with squares in the top panel

(DU16) for acupuncture treatment of traumatic spinal cord injury and found that EA had anti-oxidative, anti-inflammatory, and anti-apoptotic effects as indicated by reduced expression of inflammatory cytokines, including TNF-α [9]. Gu et al. treated patients that had undergone laparoscopic cholecystectomy (LC) at Hegu (LI 4), Neiguan (PC6), Zusanli (ST 36), and Yanglingquan (GB 34), and found that the TNF-α levels decreased significantly at 3 days after LC [20]. In the current study, EA was applied at the acupuncture points GV20, GV26, LI4, and KI1; we found that this significantly attenuated neuroinflammation in a TBI model.

Related studies on EA therapy have employed different EA parameters, including EA frequency, waveform, and intensity. Liu et al. have reported that EA at a frequency of 2 and 5 Hz, 0.4–10 mA, with an intermittent waveform, was more effective for treatment of sciatica [11]. Chan et al. previously reported that EA at 2 Hz (low frequency) can provide neuroprotection by preserving retinal function in glaucomatous rats [21]. Kuai

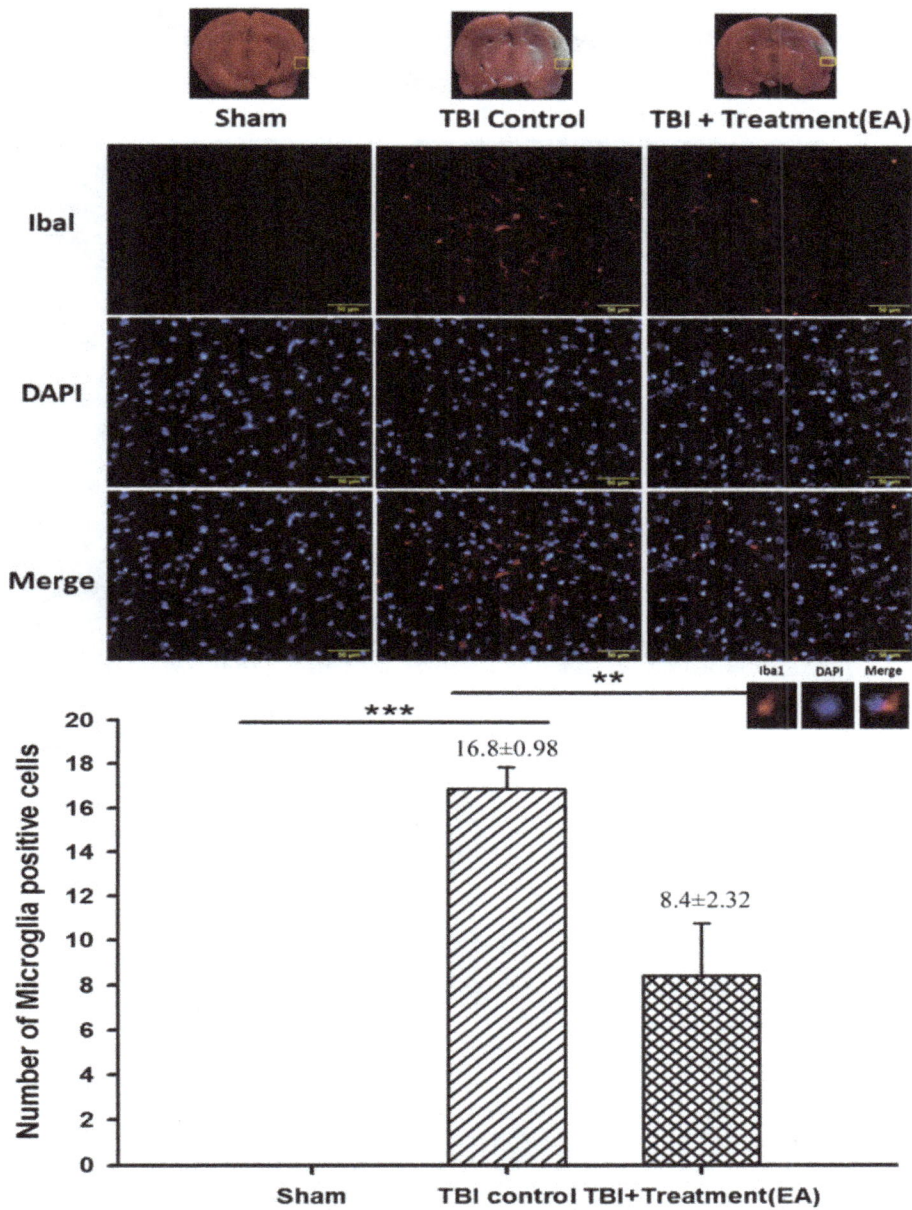

Fig. 5 The effects of electroacupuncture (EA) treatment on the activation of microglia in the ischemic cortex (markers: Iba1 plus DAPI) at 72 h after traumatic brain injury (TBI). ***$p < 0.001$ compared with the sham group; **$p < 0.01$ compared with EA treatment in the TBI group, $n = 6$ in each group. The areas measured for TTC staining are marked with squares in the top panel

et al. compared the effects of EA between different waveforms (continuous, intermittent, and sound-electric waves); EA treatment of arthritis with intermittent waves increased the β-endorphin content in tissues with local inflammation [10]. Chuang et al. demonstrated that 60 min of EA treatment in the acute stage of TBI could show a better outcome than a 30-min treatment, as determine from an increase in the regional blood flow and attenuation of neuroinflammation-associated parameters [12].

In the current study, EA with sparse-dense wave of low frequency (0.2 Hz/1 Hz) and intensity of 1 mA was applied for 60 min daily for 3 days. Therefore, the therapeutic time used was 2–3 times that used in previous studies. This design was consistent with that used by Gu et al. [20], who used the same sparse-dispersed wave. Results of both studies showed that TNF-α levels were decreased in the injured tissues after EA treatment. In future, the efficacy of intermittent and sparse-dense waveforms should be compared, and the correlation

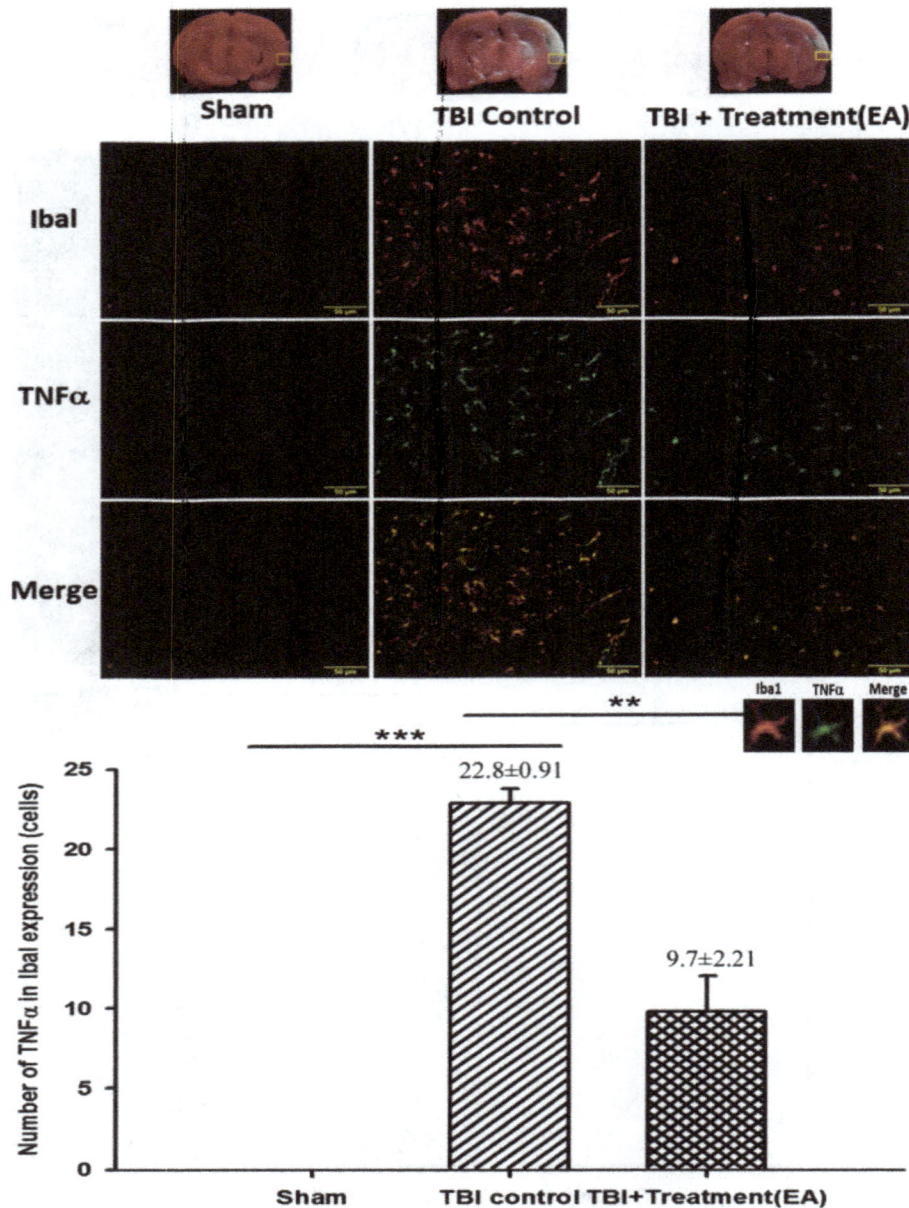

Fig. 6 The effects of electroacupuncture (EA) treatment on activation of cortical astrocytes (markers: GFAP plus DAPI) at 72 h after traumatic brain injury (TBI), ***$p < 0.001$ compared with the sham group; **$p < 0.05$ compared with EA treatment in the TBI group, $n = 6$ in each group. The areas measured for TTC staining are marked with squares in the top panel

between TNF-α levels and different EA waveforms should be investigated.

The timeline of TNF-α release varies, ranging from 1 h to months after TBI [22, 23]. Our findings on TNF-α expression and neuroinflammation at 72 h after TBI are in line with many previous results. TNF-α expression was significantly higher in the lesion boundary zone in TBI-control rats at 72 h post-TBI than in rats with TBI who were treated with simvastatin [24], etanercept [2, 25], hyperbaric oxygen therapy [26], or EA [12]. Similarly, in the current study, we found numerous Caspase-3- and TUNEL-positive neurons in the ischemic cortex of TBI animals; these were significantly reduced in the EA treatment group, suggesting that EA treatment alleviates neuronal apoptosis. Based on these results, we propose that TNF-α is produced by activated microglia and astrocytes after TBI, thus activating the neuronal apoptosis pathway, and that these adverse effects could be attenuated by EA treatment [27].

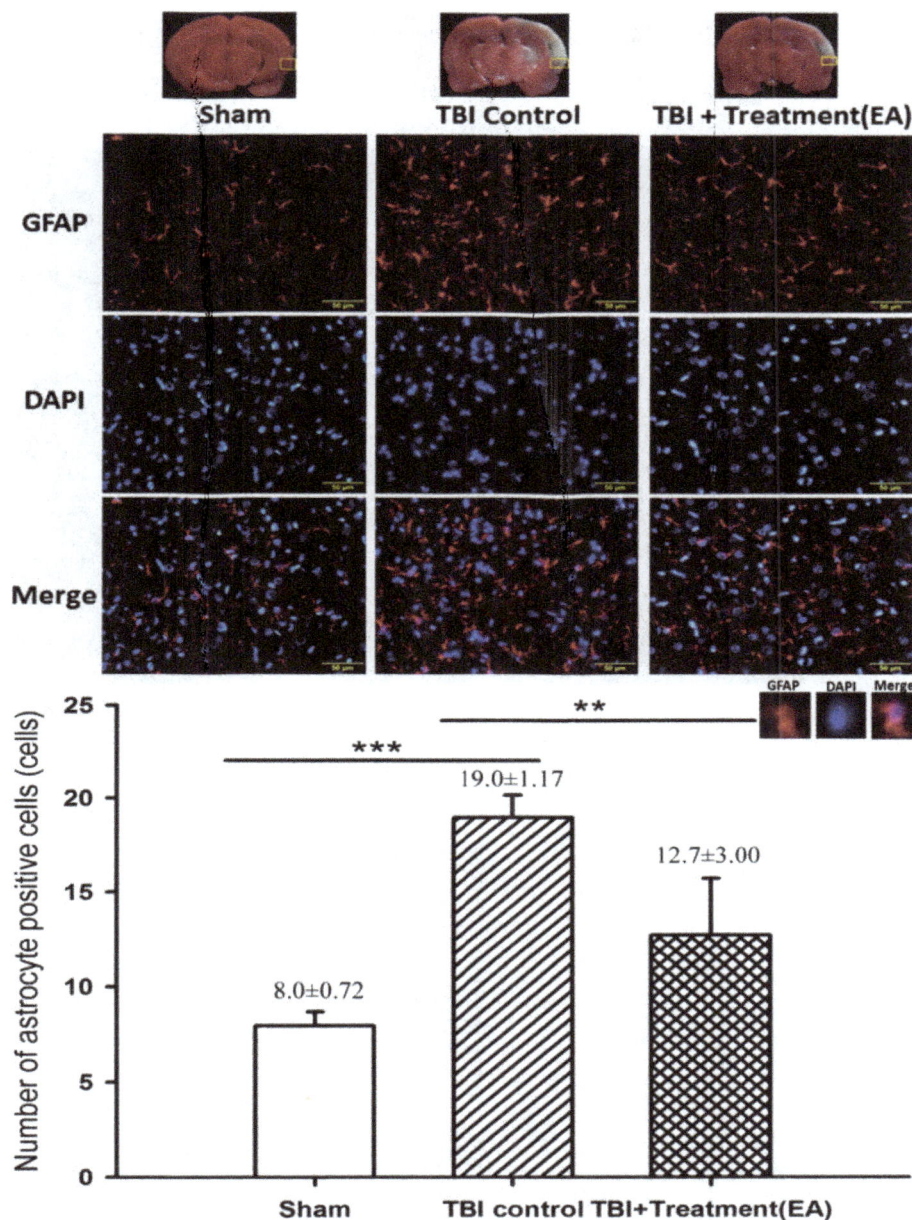

Fig. 7 The effects of electroacupuncture (EA) treatment on tumor necrosis factor (TNF)-α expression in activated microglia in the ischemic cortex (markers: Iba1 plus TNF-α) at 72 h after traumatic brain injury (TBI), ***p < 0.001 compared with the sham group; **p < 0.01 compared with EA treatment in the TBI group, n = 6 in each group. The areas measured for TTC staining are marked with squares in the top panel

Besides affecting glial TNF-α expression, as shown in this study, EA has multiple other effects in several animal models. For example, EA activates the α7 nicotinic acetylcholine receptors to attenuate inflammatory processes, thereby providing protection against cerebral ischemic injury [6]. EA also increases brain-derived neurotrophic factor expression in heat stroke [28], modulates the NF-E2 related factor 2/antioxidant response element pathway to provide protection against endotoxic shock-induced acute lung injury [29], and inhibits the ERK1/2-Egr-1 signaling pathway, thereby protecting cardiomyocytes in a mouse model of myocardial ischemia – reperfusion [30]. Thus, we believe that EA therapy may be useful for patients with TBI because of these effects. We suggest that application of EA in the acute stage of TBI may have clinical benefits.

Silver [31] demonstrated that, after TBI, glial scar formation, particularly those involving astrocytes, interfered with functional neuronal regeneration. In the present study, the TBI-induced astrogliosis was significantly attenuated by EA therapy at 72 h after TBI. Therefore, we

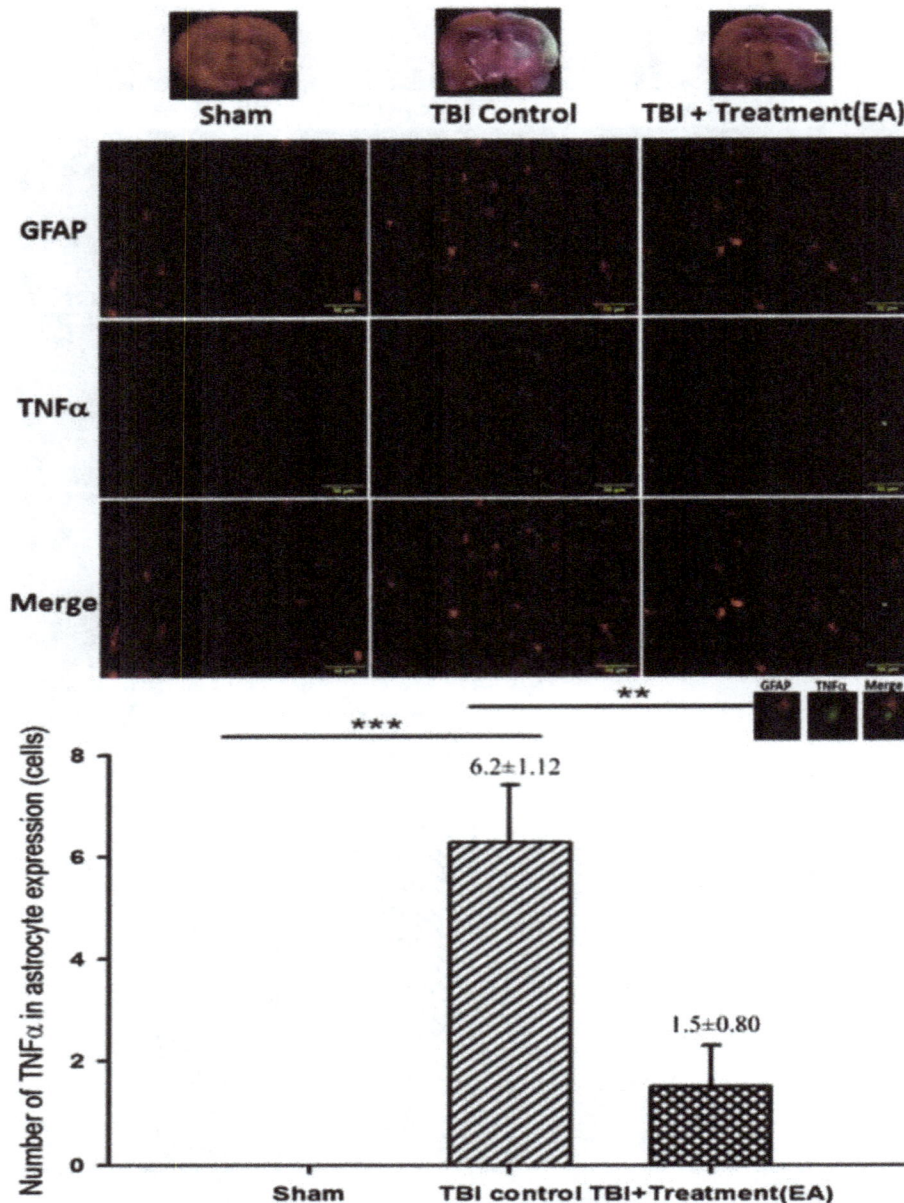

Fig. 8 The effects of electroacupuncture (EA) treatment on tumor necrosis factor (TNF)-α expression in cortical astrocytes (markers: GFAP plus TNF-α) at 72 h after traumatic brain injury (TBI), ***$p < 0.001$ compared with the sham group; **$p < 0.01$ compared with EA treatment in the TBI group, $n = 6$ in each group. The areas measured for TTC staining are marked with squares in the top panel

propose that EA may have beneficial effects on neuronal regeneration.

In order to avoid interference of the effects of different treatments, recent acupuncture studies have used a sham acupuncture group as the control against which to compare the results of the experimental group. The non-acupoints are usually situated adjacent to actual acupoints, and in several experimental animal models, they have been separated by a distance of <5 mm [29, 32, 33] or have been far away from the actual acupoints [34]. For example,

Zhang et al. showed that the therapeutic effects of EA applied to actual acupoints on TNF-α expression were better than the effects of EA administered at non-acupoints in a Wistar rat abdominal adhesion model [32], and Yu et al. reported the same effects in an endotoxic shock-related lung injury model in rabbits [29]. Furthermore, in SD rat models equivalent to those used in our study, Du et al. demonstrated the same results in an abdominal adhesion model even though the rats' weights were less than those in our study [33]. Finally, Eshkevari et al. described the same results in a cold stress model in rats with weights similar to those in our study [34]. Therefore, our study did not include a non-acupoint group, but focused on comparing whether EA delivered at acupoints could notably improve the injured cortex after TBI.

Some limitations of the current study should be considered. First, only male rats were investigated. Future studies should evaluate whether EA protects female rats from TBI-induced neurobehavioral and pathological changes. Second, only one method (the inclined plane test) was used to evaluate functional outcomes, due to limited equipment availability. Third, we were unable to characterize changes in the injured brain that occurred on each day within the 3-day EA treatment window after TBI. Therefore, a time-series imaging study using this experimental TBI model/EA treatment paradigm should be conducted in future. Fourth, we did not perform EA at non-acupoints. Results from an appropriate control groups are required to clarify the specific effects of EA stimulation of acupoints and other influences.

Conclusions

Electroacupuncture delivered for 60 min daily for 3 consecutive days ameliorates TBI in the acute stage in a rat model, by attenuating TNF-α expression in activated microglia and astrocytes and reducing neuronal apoptosis, thus contributing to improved functional outcomes. Therefore, EA may be a promising treatment strategy for TBI.

Acknowledgements
The authors thank Chi-Mei Medical Center, Tainan, Taiwan, for instrument support.

Funding
This work was supported by Chi-Mei Medical Center, grant number CMFHR10315.

Authors' contributions
Author contributions to the study and manuscript preparation are as follows. Contributors WCT and JRK both contributed to the writing of this manuscript; CYH, YCH and CCC were the main researcher who provided the innovative idea that was the focus of this study; CYH and CCW revised the manuscript and coordinated the study of related research; JRK was responsible for the final submission after full revision, acceptance of the manuscript and for organizing the research group.

Competing interests
The authors declare that they have no competing interests.

Ethics approval and consent to participate
Affidavit of Approval of Animal Use Protocol, Chi-Mei Medical Center. Statement: The animal use protocol listed below has been reviewed and approved by the Institutional Animal Care and Use Committee (IACUC). Protocol Title: Anti-inflammation effects and mechanism of electroacupuncture after traumatic brain injury in a rat model.
IACUC Approval No.: 102122306.
Valid Period of Protocol: 01/01/2014 ~ 31/12/2014
Principal Investigator (PI): Yao-Chin Hsu.

Author details
[1]Department of Chinese Medicine, Tainan Municipal An-Nan Hospital, Tainan, Taiwan. [2]Department of Chinese Medicine, Chi-Mei Medical Center, Tainan, Taiwan. [3]Department of Neurosurgery, Chi-Mei Medical Center, Tainan, Taiwan. [4]Department of Medical research, Chi-Mei Medical Center, Tainan, Taiwan. [5]Department of Child Care, Southern Taiwan University of Science and Technology, Tainan, Taiwan. [6]Department of Biotechnology, Southern Taiwan University of Science and Technology, Tainan, Taiwan. [7]Traumatic Brain Injury Center, Chi Mei Hospital, No. 901, Zhonghua Rd., Yongkang Dist., Tainan City 710, Taiwan, ROC.

References
1. Block ML, Hong JS. Microglia and inflammation mediated neurodegeneration: multiple triggers with a common mechanism. Prog Neurobiol. 2005;76(2):77–98.
2. Chio CC, Lin JW, Chang MW, Wang CC, Kuo JR, Yang CZ, Chang CP. Therapeutic evaluation of etanercept in a model of traumatic brain injury. J Neurochem. 2010;115(4):921–9.
3. Zhang D, Hu X, Qian L, O'Callaghan JP, Hong JS. Astrogliosis in CNS pathologies: is there a role for microglia? Mol Neurobiol. 2010;41(2–3):232–41.
4. Cheong CU, Chang CP, Chao CM, Cheng BC, Yang CZ, Chio CC. Etanercept attenuates traumatic brain injury in rats by reducing brain TNF- alpha contents and by stimulating newly formed neurogenesis. Mediators Inflamm. 2013;2013:620837.
5. Mayer DJ. Acupuncture: an evidence-based review of the clinical literature. Annu Rev Med. 2000;51:49–63.
6. Wang Q, Wang F, Li X, Yang Q, Li X, Xu N, Huang Y, Zhang Q, Gou X, Chen S, et al. Electroacupuncture pretreatment attenuates cerebral ischemic injury through alpha7 nicotinic acetylcholine receptor-mediated inhibition of high-mobility group box 1 release in rats. J Neuroinflammation. 2012;9:24.
7. Xu H, Sun H, Chen SH, Zhang YM, Piao YL, Gao Y. Effects of acupuncture at Baihui (DU20) and Zusanli (ST36) on the expression of heat shock protein 70 and tumor necrosis factor α in the peripheral serum of cerebral ischemia-reperfusion-injured rats. Chin J Integr Med. 2014;20(5):369–74.
8. Cheng CY, Lin JG, Tang NY, Kao ST, Hsieh CL. Electroacupuncture-like stimulation at the Baihui (GV20) and Dazhui (GV14) acupoints protects rats against subacute-phase cerebral ischemia-reperfusion injuries by reducing S100B-mediated neurotoxicity. PLoS One. 2014;9(3):e91426.
9. Jiang SH, Tu WZ, Zou EM, Hu J, Wang S, Li JR, Wang WS, He R, Cheng RD, Liao WJ. Neuroprotective effects of different modalities of acupuncture on traumatic spinal cord injury in rats. Evid Based Complement Alternat Med. 2014;2014:431580.
10. Kuai L, Yang H-Y, Liu T-Y, Gao M. Analgesic effects of electroacupuncture of different pulse waveforms in the rat of adjuvant arthritis. Chin Acupunct Moxibustion. 2005;25(1):68–71.
11. Liu X, Liu Z-S, Shi-xi H. Literature analysis of electroacupuncture stimulation index on the treatment of sciatica. Chin Acupunct Moxibustion. 2009;29(12):1026–8.
12. Chuang CH, Hsu YC, Wang CC, Hu C, Kuo JR. Cerebral blood flow and apoptosis-associated factor with electroacupuncture in a traumatic brain injury rat model. Acupunct Med. 2013;31(4):395–403.
13. McIntosh TK, Vink R, Noble L, Yamakami I, Fernyak S, Soares H, Faden AL. Traumatic brain injury in the rat: characterization of a lateral fluid-percussion model. Neuroscience. 1989;28(1):233–44.
14. Pierce JE, Smith DH, Trojanowski JQ, McIntosh TK. Enduring cognitive, neurobehavioral and histopathological changes persist for up to one year following severe experimental brain injury in rats. Neuroscience. 1998;87(2):359–69.

15. Wang Y, Lin SZ, Chiou AL, Williams LR, Hoffer BJ. Glial cell line-derived neurotrophic factor protects against ischemia-induced injury in the cerebral cortex. J Neurosci. 1997;17(11):4341–8.

16. Hallam TM, Floyd CL, Folkerts MM, Lee LL, Gong QZ, Lyeth BG, Muizelaar JP, Berman RF. Comparison of behavioral deficits and acute neuronal degeneration in rat lateral fluid percussion and weight-drop brain injury models. J Neurotrauma. 2004;21(5):521–39.

17. Kuo JR, Lo CJ, Chang CP, Lin KC, Lin MT, Chio CC. Agmatine-promoted angiogenesis, neurogenesis, and inhibition of gliosis-reduced traumatic brain injury in rats. J Trauma. 2011;71(4):E87–93.

18. Koshinaga M, Katayama Y, Fukushima M, Oshima H, Suma T, Takahata T. Rapid and widespread microglial activation induced by traumatic brain injury in rat brain slices. J Neurotrauma. 2000;17(3):185–92.

19. Mullen RJ, Buck CR, Smith AM. NeuN, a neuronal specific nuclear protein in vertebrates. Development. 1992;116(1):201–11.

20. Gu CY, Shen LR, Ding YH, Lou Y, Wu HG, Shi Z, Ma XP. Effect of different anesthesia methods on immune function in patients of laparoscopic cholecystectomy in peri-operational period. Zhongguo Zhen Jiu. 2011;31(3):236–40.

21. Chan HHL, Leung MCP, So K-F. Electroacupuncture provides a new approach to neuroprotection in rats with induced glaucoma. J Altern Complement Med. 2005;11(2):315–22.

22. Ross SA, Halliday MI, Campbell GC, Byrnes DP, Rowlands BJ. The presence of tumour necrosis factor in CSF and plasma after severe head injury. Br J Neurosurg. 1994;8(4):419–25.

23. Holmin S, Mathiesen T. Long-term intracerebral inflammatory response after experimental focal brain injury in rat. Neuroreport. 1999;10(9):1889–91.

24. Li B, Mahmood A, Lu D, Wu H, Xiong Y, Qu C, Chopp M. Simvastatin attenuates microglial cells and astrocyte activation and decreases interleukin-1beta level after traumatic brain injury. Neurosurgery. 2009;65(1):179–85. discussion 185–176.

25. Chio CC, Chang CH, Wang CC, Cheong CU, Chao CM, Cheng BC, Yang CZ, Chang CP. Etanercept attenuates traumatic brain injury in rats by reducing early microglial expression of tumor necrosis factor-alpha. BMC Neurosci. 2013;14:33.

26. Lim SW, Wang CC, Wang YH, Chio CC, Niu KC, Kuo JR. Microglial activation induced by traumatic brain injury is suppressed by postinjury treatment with hyperbaric oxygen therapy. J Surg Res. 2013;184(2):1076–84.

27. Elmore S. Apoptosis: a review of programmed cell death. Toxicol Pathol. 2007;35(4):495–516.

28. Kim MW, Chung YC, Jung HC, Park MS, Han YM, Chung YA, Maeng LS, Park SI, Lim J, Im WS, et al. Electroacupuncture enhances motor recovery performance with brain-derived neurotrophic factor expression in rats with cerebral infarction. Acupunct Med. 2012;30(3):222–6.

29. Yu JB, Shi J, Gong LR, Dong SA, Xu Y, Zhang Y, Cao XS, Wu LL. Role of Nrf2/ARE pathway in protective effect of electroacupuncture against endotoxic shock-induced acute lung injury in rabbits. PLoS One. 2014;9(8), e104924.

30. Zhang J, Song J, Xu J, Chen X, Yin P, Lv X, Wang X. ERK1/2-Egr-1 signaling pathway-mediated protective effects of electroacupuncture in a mouse model of myocardial ischemia-reperfusion. Evid Based Complement Alternat Med. 2014;2014:253075.

31. Silver J, Miller JH. Regeneration beyond the glial scar. Nat Rev Neurosci. 2004;5(2):146–56.

32. Zhang L, Wang H, Huang Z, Shi X, Hu S, Gaischek I, Litscher D, Wang L, Litscher G. Inhibiting effect of electroacupuncture at zusanli on early inflammatory factor levels formed by postoperative abdominal adhesions. Evid Based Complement Alternat Med. 2014;2014:950326.

33. Du MH, Luo HM, Tian YJ, Zhang LJ, Zhao ZK, Lv Y, Xu RJ, Hu S. Electroacupuncture ST36 prevents postoperative intra-abdominal adhesions formation. J Surg Res. 2015;195(1):89–98.

34. Eshkevari L, Permaul E, Mulroney SE. Acupuncture blocks cold stress-induced increases in the hypothalamus-pituitary-adrenal axis in the rat. J Endocrinol. 2013;217(1):95–104.

14

Electroacupuncture at acupoint ST 37(Shangjuxu) improves function of the enteric nervous system in a novel mouse constipation model

Chao Liang[1†], Kaiyue Wang[2†], Bin Xu[1] and Zhi Yu[1*]

Abstract

Background: Electroacupuncture (EA) at acupoint ST 37 (Shangjuxu) has been used to alleviate gastrointestinal symptoms and improve gastrointestinal motility. However, the mechanisms by which EA affects the enteric nervous system (ENS) have scarcely been investigated. In this study, we investigated whether EA could improve ENS function.

Methods: A constipation model was established by gastric instillation of ice-cold saline daily for 14 days. The constipated mice were divided into two groups: the model group, which was not treated, and the EA group, which received EA at ST 37 at a frequency of 2–15 HZ and an amplitude of 1 mA for 15 min a day for 3 days. A further six mice were included as a non-constipated control group. After EA treatment, intestinal propulsion and defecation time were measured. Additionally, in jejunum, ileum and proximal colon myenteric plexus, the expressions of PGP9.5 and nNOS were measured by immunohistochemistry.

Results: The EA group demonstrated significant improvements in carbon propulsion rates and defecation time compared to model group ($P < 0.05$). In addition, after EA, the PGP9.5 and nNOS expression in jejunum, ileum and proximal colonic myenteric plexus was back to normal levels.

Conclusion: This study suggests that EA stimulation at ST 37 is capable of ameliorating intestinal motility dysfunction, and can partly restore enteric neuron function. The ENS can participate in changes in intestinal motility by affecting inhibitory neurons.

Keywords: Electroacupuncture(EA), Enteric nervous system(ENS), Gastrointestinal (GI), Neuronal nitric oxide synthase (nNOS)

Background

Constipation is a symptom of underlying defects in transit of fecal mass through the gut or in defecation, and is a commonly diagnosed functional gastrointestinal (GI) disorder. Constipation is usually associated with a number of diseases, and is characterized by a series of complex GI symptoms in the absence of mechanical obstruction of the GI tract [1, 2]. Diet, side effects of medication, and hormonal disorders may induce constipation [3–5]. Therapy for

constipation is largely directed towards treating the symptoms, and most of the treatment methods are uniformly effective [6]. However, these treatments do not address the underlying dysfunction in the GI tract that results in constipation.

Acupuncture as one of the most frequently applied methods in Traditional Chinese Medicine, which has a history of more than 3000 years, has gained increased popularity. In recent years, electroacupuncture (EA) at different acupoints has come to be recognized as a potential effective therapy to treat GI disorder. Preclinical researches have shown that ST 37 could increase GI transit, relieve defecation difficulty and improve life quality [7–9], and indicated that it is effective for constipation. Previous

* Correspondence: mickey28282@sina.com
†Equal contributors
[1]Nanjing University of Chinese Medicine, Nanjing 210046, Jiangsu Province, China
Full list of author information is available at the end of the article

experiments have shown chronic and recurrent cold water irritation to stomach might cause long-term effects on bowel movements, which resulted in the GI motility, such as inhibited jejunal and colonic motility [10, 11]. In a cold water-induced rat model of constipation, EA stimulation at ST 37 increases faecal water content, defaecation frequency and GI transit [12, 13]. ST37 has a positive effect on objective markers of constipation. It is believed that acupuncture at different acupoints exerts different effects on internal organs to restore the homeostatic balance [14–16]. Most previous research has focused on the effects on central and peripheral neural pathways in EA's ameliorating effects on intestinal motility [17]. However, the effects and mechanisms of EA on the enteric nervous system (ENS) have not been widely investigated. The purpose of this study was to investigate whether EA affects the ENS, and to explore local neural mechanism of EA in the gut.

Methods

Animals

C57BL/6 J mice (SPF-grade, 3-week-old males, 20–25 g) were purchased from the Model Animal Research Center of Nanjing University (Nanjing, China, license number: SCXK 2013–0005). Animals were housed in a room with 12 h light–dark cycle (turn on at 8:00 a.m.) maintained at 22 ± 2 °C with 60 % humidity and ad libitum access to food and water. All experimental manipulations were undertaken in accordance with the Principles of Laboratory Animal Care and the Guide for the Care and Use of Laboratory Animals, published by the National Science Council, China.

Experimental model of constipation

The mice were randomly divided into two groups: a 0–4 °C saline-treated group ($n = 40$), and a normal feeding group ($n = 10$), randomly numbered, and raised in single cages that allowed normal access to food and water. Wire netting was used to facilitate the separation and collection of stools. The constipation model was established by gastric instillation of ice-cold (0–4 °C) saline daily for 14 days [18]. To eliminate the influence of biological rhythms, intragastric administrations were conducted at 8:00 am daily for 14 d. Animals were initially administered ice-cold (0–4 °C) saline at a dose of 0.2 mL/mouse, and then the dose was increased by 0.05 mL/mouse every 5 d. Control mice were raised normally without intragastric administration of ice-cold saline.

Materials

Materials used in this study include wire netting (to facilitate the separation and collection of stools); a precision electronic balance (Sartorius Co, Beijing, China); ceramic cups (high temperature-resistant, radius: 2 cm, high: 3.5 cm).

Drugs included saline (Sodium chloride injection; Nanjing Chemical Reagent Co, Jiangsu, China), acacia gum (Gum Arabic powder; BASF Chemical Co, Tianjin, China), and black or red carbon powder (Color toner; Sanheng Information Technology Co). Primary antibodies for immunohistochemistry included PGP9.5 (Abcam, Cambridge, UK) and nNOS (Abcam, Cambridge, UK). The secondary antibody used was HRP-Polymer Rabbit anti-Mouse IgG (Boster Biotech, Wuhan, China).

Black and red carbon suspensions were prepared as follows: acacia gum (100 g) was added to 800 mL of water and boiled until transparent. Then the solution was mixed with black or red carbon powder (50 g) and boiled three times. After cooling, each solution was diluted with water to 1000 mL and then stored at 4 °C. The solutions were agitated prior to use.

EA treatment

After the constipation model was successfully established, the constipated mice were randomly subdivided into two groups ($n = 6$ for each group): the model group, which remained untreated, and the EA group, which received EA at ST 37. EA stimulation was applied by two pairs of stainless steel needles (0.25 mm in diameter) inserted bilaterally at ST 37 (2 mm lateral to the anterior tubercle of the tibia and 6 mm below the knee joint) [19]. After insertion into the acupoint of constipated mice, the needles were stimulated by an EA apparatus (#HANS-100A, Nan Jing Ji Sheng Medical Treatment Science and Technology Co., China). Electrical stimulus intensity was set at 1 mA with a frequency of 2-15Hz. The stimulation was delivered for 15 min a day for 3 days.

Measurement of intestinal function

After 12 h of fasting, mice were intragastrically administrated a suspension of black carbon (0.3 mL) and killed 10 min later via cervical dislocation. The section of intestine extending from the pylorus to the ileocecal valve was removed. The full length of the intestinal tract as well as the propulsive distance of black carbon in the tract was measured under a tension-free state, and the ratio of the propulsive distance to the length of the intestinal tract was determined for all groups. Additionally, after 12 h of fasting, another group of mice were given a red carbon suspension (0.3 mL), and the time required to defecate the first stool pellet containing the red indicator was recorded.

Tissue preparation and immunohistochemistry

At the end of the experiment, small intestine (jejunum and ileum) and proximal colon tissue specimens were removed after 12 h of fasting. Segments approximately 1 cm in length were opened along the mesenteric border, and immediately fixed by immersion in 4 % paraformaldehyde for 24 h. Then the samples were processed for paraffin embedding in vacuum and cut at a thickness of 10 μm for immunohistochemistry.

Sections were deparaffinized in xylene and hydrated in a graded solution of ethanol. Activity of endogenous peroxidases was blocked with 3 % hydrogen peroxide. Sections were sequentially incubated in 3 % hydrogen peroxide and blocked with 5 % bovine serum albumin (BSA) for 30 min at 37 °C. The primary antibodies (Abcam, Cambridge, UK) for PGP9.5 (1:1000) and nNOS (1:800) were applied to the sections and each specimen was incubated in a moist chamber overnight at 4 °C, and then washed for three times in 0.01 mol/L phosphate-buffered saline (PBS; pH 7.2). After that, the slides were incubated with horseradish peroxidase (HRP)-Polymer Rabbit anti-Mouse IgG(Boster Biotech, Wuhan, China) for 90 min at 37 °C, then incubated in 3,3-diaminobenzidine (DAB) solution for 2-5 min. Specificity of the antibody was confirmed by negative control staining in the absence of primary antibody treatment. Two observers evaluated the slides using an Olympus FV500 optical microscope (Olympus, Tokyo, Japan). Positive immunostaining was evaluated at 5 random visual fields at a magnification of 400. The mean density of positive expression was assessed using image analysis software (Image Pro Plus 6.0).

Statistical analysis

Data were expressed as mean ± standard error Statistical analysis was conducted using SPSS 17.0 software with one-way analysis of variance. Data were compared using the

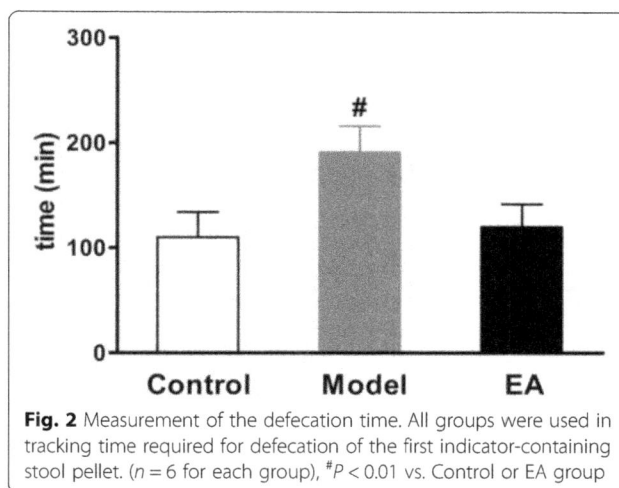

Fig. 2 Measurement of the defecation time. All groups were used in tracking time required for defecation of the first indicator-containing stool pellet. ($n = 6$ for each group), $^{\#}P < 0.01$ vs. Control or EA group

Student Newman Keuls post-hoc test. Differences where $P < 0.05$ were considered to be statistically significant.

Results

Effects of EA stimulation on small intestine function

Carbon intestinal propulsion experiments showed the distances by which black carbon was propelled decreased in constipation models compared to control group (Fig. 1a, $P < 0.05$). After EA treatment, carbon propulsion rates significantly increased, and did not differ from control group values (Fig. 1b).

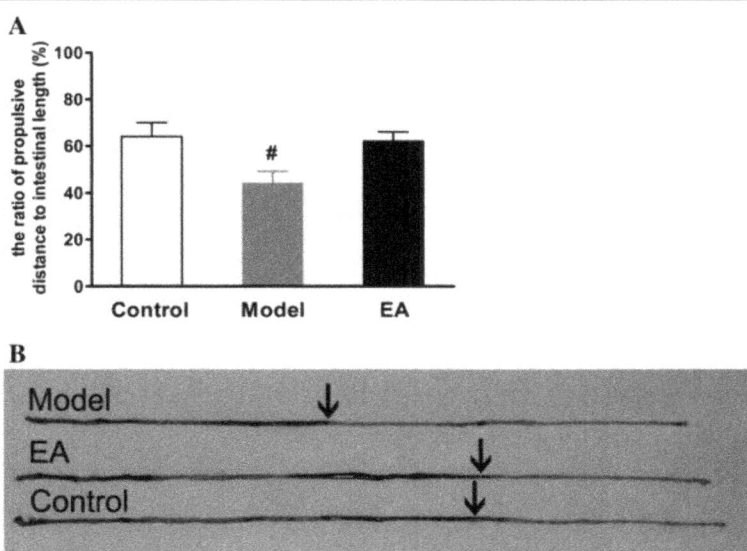

Fig. 1 Measurement of carbon propulsion rate. **a**: All groups were used in the intestinal propulsion experiment. The distances traveled by black carbon significantly increased in the EA group compared to the Model group. **b**: Examples of intestine and black carbon trace for all three groups. ($n = 6$ for each group), $^{\#}P < 0.05$ vs. Control or EA group

Effects of EA stimulation on defecation time

In this experiment, the defecation time was prolonged in constipation models compared to control group, as would be expected. After EA stimulation treatment, defecation time significantly decreased compared to constipation models and almost returned to normal (Fig. 2).

Effect of EA on total neuronal PGP9.5 protein expression

Immunohistochemical staining revealed that the number of PGP9.5-positive cells in the constipation model was markedly decreased compared with the control group in the small intestine and proximal colon. After EA treatment, the protein expression of PGP9.5 was significantly increased compared to constipation models in jejunum (Fig. 3a, b, c), ileum (Fig. 3e, f, g) and proximal colon (Fig. 3i, j, k), but there was no difference compared with the control group, respectively (Fig. 3d, h, l).

Effects of constipation and EA stimulation on nNOS protein expression

Statistical analysis indicated that the expression of nNOS in constipation models were increased compared with the control group in the in jejunum, ileum and proximal colon. After EA at ST 37, the expression of nNOS was significantly decreased compared to constipation models in jejunum (Fig. 4a, b, c), ileum (Fig. 4e, f, g) and proximal colon (Fig. 4i, j, k), almost returned to normal levels

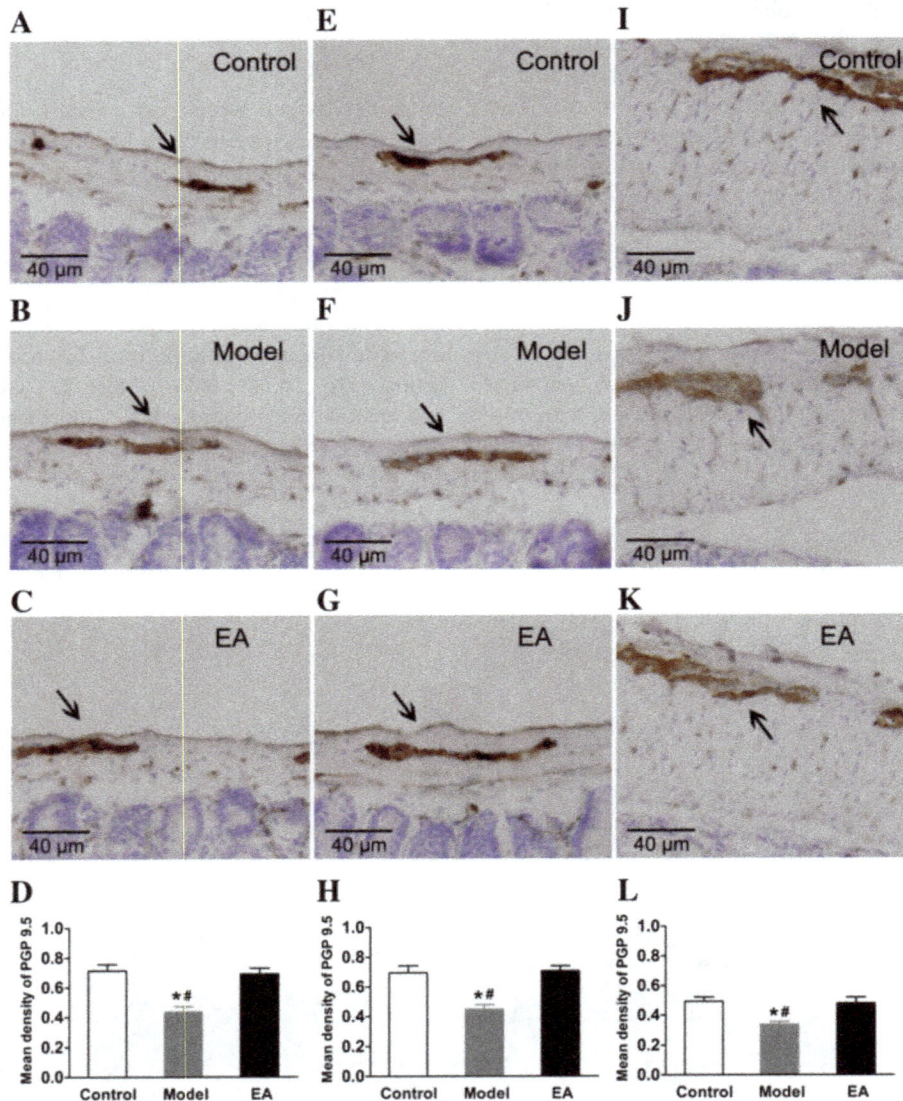

Fig. 3 Effects on total neurons-PGP9.5 protein expression in immunohistochemical staining. Tissue with brown granular deposits indicate positive immunostaining (arrows) Scale bar: 40 μm, magnification: ×400. **a**, **b**, **c**: In jejunum; **e**, **f**, **g**: In ileum; **i**, **j**, **k**: In proximal colon; **d**, **h**, **l**: Comparison of the mean density of PGP9.5-positive expression, respectively. *P < 0.01 vs. Control group; #P < 0.05 vs. EA group, n = 5 for each group

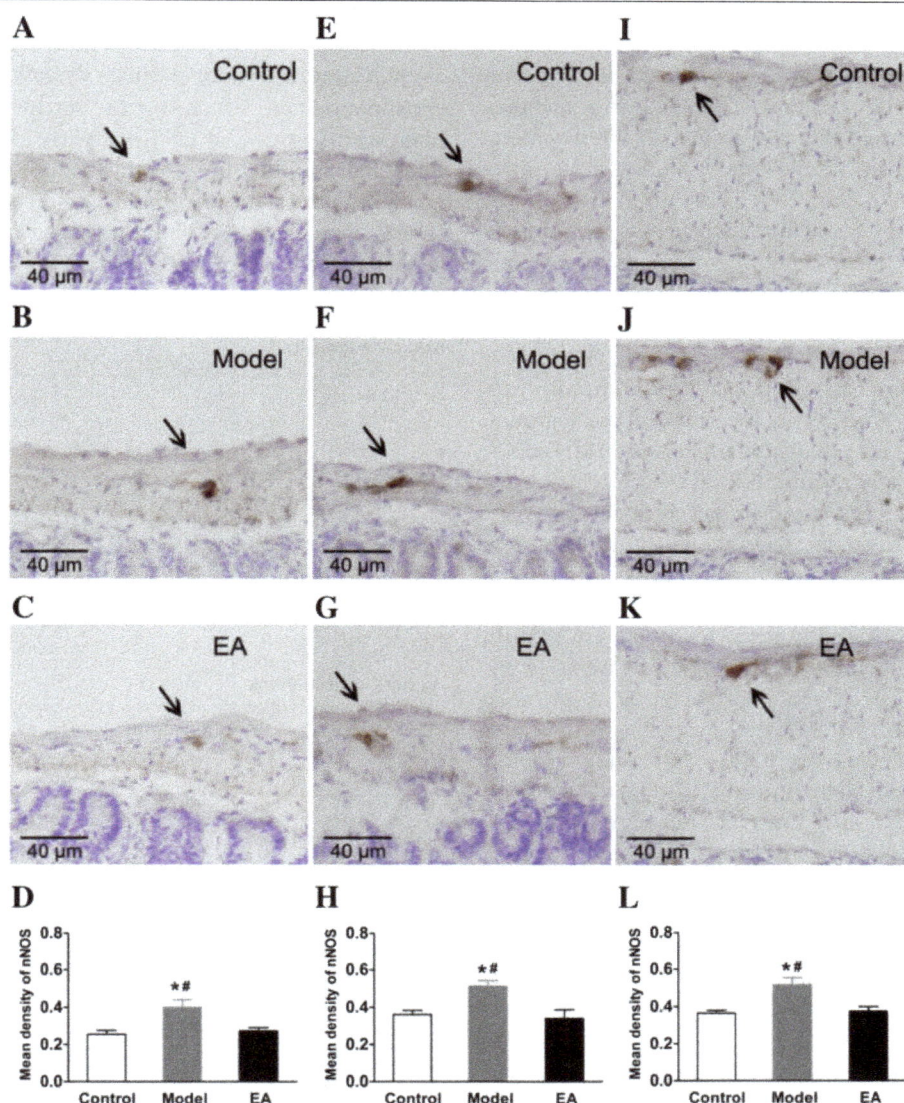

Fig. 4 Effects on nNOS expression in immunohistochemical staining. Tissue with brown granular deposits indicate positive immunostaining (arrows) Scale bar: 40 μm, magnification: ×400. **a, b, c**: In jejunum; **e, f, g**: In ileum; **i, j, k**: In proximal colon; **d, h, l**: Comparison of the mean density of nNOS-positive expression, respectively. *$P < 0.01$ vs. Control group; #$P < 0.05$ vs. EA group, $n = 5$ for each group

and there was no difference compared with the control group, respectively (Fig. 4d, h, l).

Discussion

Acupuncture is beneficial as an alternative treatment for the management of gastrointestinal functional disorders, including constipation, diarrhea and irritable bowel syndrome [20–22]. Although acupuncture has been used as an appropriate adjunct treatment for GI dysfunction disorders, the underlying mechanisms of EA on the ENS have not been well studied.

In this study, the results indicate that EA at ST 37 improved impaired intestine functions, accelerating GI motility. Acupuncture is recognized to have regionally specific effects [23]. ST 37 is located in the hind limb, and some studies have demonstrated that acupuncture at the hind limb increases GI motility [24]. In clinical treatment, ST 37 can improve GI motility and alleviate symptoms, which is effective for treating constipation [25, 26]. Previous research has focused on the effects of acupuncture on central and peripheral neural pathways; EA stimulation of points on the abdomen can influence sympathetic nerves to the GI tract, while points in the four limbs can influence parasympathetic nerves [27, 28]. Parasympathetic nerves can promote GI peristalsis, while sympathetic nerves inhibit GI movement [29]. Accordingly, the effect of stimulation at ST 37 support these previous results. Stimulation at ST 37 may increase the parasympathetic-sympathetic balance and promote GI movement. As the ENS plays an important role in the GI motility, we hypothesized that the ENS could participate in EA stimulation of GI function. The ENS is a complex network of neurons and glia that resides in the myenteric and submucosal plexus of the bowel, and controls many aspects of bowel function [30]. The myenteric plexus, located between longitudinal and circular muscle, primarily controls muscle contraction and relaxation [31]. Therefore, ENS defects may underlie common GI motility problems such as constipation.

Our previous study indicated that irritation with ice-cold saline caused changes in the ENS in the jejunum, ileum and proximal colonic myenteric plexus [18]. Indeed, immunohistochemistry results showed the protein expression of PGP9.5 after EA stimulation was significantly increased compared to constipation models in the jejunum, ileum and proximal colon myenteric plexus. PGP9.5 is a neuron-specific protein, which can be used to accurately locate enteric neurons and indicate ENS function [32]. In this study, our results indicated that EA may improve enteric neurons and repair the impaired ENS. A previous study found that EA at ST 36 (Zusanli), which is also located in the hind limb, can induce regeneration of lost enteric neurons in a diabetic model [33]. Thus, the enteric neurons in the ENS are likely to be affected by EA stimulation. As we know, abnormal activity of the ENS can have significant effects on the functions of the digestive tract, and many diseases illustrate essential roles of the ENS [34, 35]. In our opinion, EA ameliorates intestinal motility impairment through both central and peripheral neural pathways, which works in concert with the ENS.

Furthermore, the expression of neuronal nitric oxide synthase (nNOS) in the constipation model was significantly increased compared with the control group, and returned to almost normal after EA treatment. In the ENS, nitric oxide (NO) is a major inhibitory neurotransmitter, and is synthesized by neuronal NOS [29]. It has been suggested that, in the ENS, structural abnormalities of the myenteric and submucosal plexus and an abnormal neurotransmitter content have been considered to be responsible for primary chronic constipation [36]. Studies on different parts of the intestine reveal the participation of NO in the regulation of spontaneous contractions, such as colonic contractile activity [37, 38]. We concluded from our experiments that increased NO in the myenteric plexus might reduce intestinal motility, and be closely related to the development of constipation. In our view, EA at ST 37 can restore the balance of inhibitory neurotransmitters of the enteric neurons, leading to improvement of the impaired ENS function.

Conclusion

In summary, EA stimulation at ST 37 is capable of ameliorating intestinal motility dysfunction in a mouse constipation model, and can partly restor e enteric neuron function. The ENS can participate in changes in intestinal motility by affecting inhibitory neurons. EA could effects on internal organs, and restore the homeostatic balance via central and peripheral neural pathways working in concert with the ENS.

Acknowledgments
We thank Qian Li (Nanjing University of Chinese Medicine) for experimental instruction.

Funding
This work was supported by the National Key Basic Research Program (973 Program, No. 2011CB505206), the National Natural Science Foundation of China (Nos. 81202744, 81373749, 81574071), and the People Programme (Marie Curie Actions) of the European Union's Seventh Framework Programme under REA grant agreement No: PIRSES-GA-2013–612589.

Authors' contributions
Conceived and designed the experiments: CL. Performed the experiments: CL, KW. Wrote the paper: CL. Manuscript editing: ZY BX. All authors read and approved the final manuscript.

Authors' information
Chao Liang, Ph.D candidate, Major Research Direction: basic research of acupuncture treatment.

Competing interests
The authors declare that they have no competing interests.

Author details
[1]Nanjing University of Chinese Medicine, Nanjing 210046, Jiangsu Province, China. [2]Xi'an Traditional Chinese Medicine Brain Disease Hospital, Xi'an 710000, China.

References
1. Park HJ, Jarrett M, Cain K, Heitkemper M. Psychological distress and GI symptoms are related to severity of bloating in women with irritable bowel syndrome. Res Nurs Health. 2008;31(2):98–107.
2. Choung RS, Locke GR 3rd, Zinsmeister AR, Schleck CD, Talley NJ. Psychosocial distress and somatic symptoms in community subjects with irritable bowel syndrome: a psychological component is the rule. Am J Gastroenterol. 2009;104(7):1772–9.
3. Bittencourt AF, Martins JR, Logullo L, Shiroma G, Horie L, Ortolani MC, et al. Constipation is more frequent than diarrhea in patients fed exclusively by enteral nutrition: results of an observational study. Nutr Clin Pract. 2012;27(4):533–9.
4. Na JR, Oh KN, Park SU, Bae D, Choi EJ, Jung MA, et al. The laxative effects of Maesil (Prunus mume Siebold & Zucc.) on constipation induced by a low-fibre diet in a rat model. Int J Food Sci Nutr. 2013;64(3):333–45.
5. McCarberg BH. Overview and treatment of opioid-induced constipation. Postgrad Med. 2013;125(4):7–17.

6. Chiarelli P, Brown W, McElduff P. Constipation in Australian women: prevalence and associated factors. Int Urogynecol J Pelvic Floor Dysfunct. 2000;11(2):71–8.

7. Liu Z, Liu J, Zhao Y, Cai Y, He L, Xu H, et al. The efficacy and safety study of electro-acupuncture for severe chronic functional constipation: study protocol for a multicenter, randomized, controlled trial. Trials. 2013;14:176.

8. Xiong F, Wang Y, Li SQ, Tian M, Zheng CH, Huang GY. Clinical study of electro-acupuncture treatment with different intensities for functional constipation patients. J Huazhong Univ Sci Technolog Med Sci. 2014;34(5):775–81.

9. Xu X, Zheng C, Zhang M, Wang W, Huang G. A randomized controlled trial of acupuncture to treat functional constipation: design and protocol. BMC Complement Altern Med. 2014;14:423.

10. Chen DP, Xiong YJ, Tang ZY, Yao QY, Ye DM, Liu SS, et al. Characteristics of deslanoside-induced modulation on jejunal contractility. World J Gastroenterol. 2012;18(41):5889–96.

11. Yang X, Xi TF, Li YX, Wang HH, Qin Y, Zhang JP, et al. Oxytocin decreases colonic motility of cold water stressed rats via oxytocin receptors. World J Gastroenterol. 2014;20(31):10886–94.

12. Zhu X, Liu Z, Qu H, Niu W, Gao L, Wang Y,et al. The effect and mechanism of electroacupuncture at LI11 and ST37 on constipation in a rat model. Acupunct Med. 2016;34(3):194–200.

13. Qin QG, Gao XY, Liu K, Yu XC, Li L, Wang HP, et al. Acupuncture at heterotopic acupoints enhances jejunal motility in constipated and diarrheic rats. World J Gastroenterol. 2014;20(48):18271–8.

14. Inanç BB. A new theory on the evaluation of traditional chinese acupuncture mechanisms from the latest medical scientific point of view. Acupunct Electrother Res. 2015;40(3):189–204.

15. Fabrin S, Soares N, Pezarezi Yoshimura D, Hallak Regalo SC, Donizetti Verri E, de Freitas Vianna JR, et al. Effects of acupuncture at the Yintang and the Chengjiang acupoints on cardiac arrhythmias and neurocardiogenic syncope in emergency first aid. J Acupunct Meridian Stud. 2016;9(1):26–30.

16. Zhao C, Bao C, Li J, Zhu Y, Wang S, Yang L, et al. Moxibustion and acupuncture ameliorate Crohn's disease by regulating the balance between Th17 and Treg cells in the intestinal mucosa. Evid Based Complement Alternat Med. 2015;2015:938054.

17. Iwa M, Matsushima M, Nakade Y, Pappas TN, Fujimiya M, Takahashi T. Electroacupuncture at ST-36 accelerates colonic motility and transit in freely moving conscious rats. Am J Physiol Gastrointest Liver Physiol. 2006;290(2):G285–92.

18. Liang C, Wang KY, Yu Z, Xu B. Development of a novel mouse constipation model. World J Gastroenterol. 2016;22(9):2799–810.

19. Wang SJ, Yang HY, Xu GS. Acupuncture alleviates colorectal hypersensitivity and correlates with the regulatory mechanism of TrpV1 and p-ERK. Evid Based Complement Alternat Med. 2012;2012:483123.

20. Li Y, Zheng H, Zeng F, Zhou SY, Zhong F, Zheng HB, et al. Use acupuncture to treat functional constipation: study protocol for a randomized controlled trial. Trials. 2012;13:104.

21. Sun JH, Wu XL, Xia C, Xu LZ, Pei LX, Li H, et al. Clinical evaluation of Soothing Gan and invigorating Pi acupuncture treatment on diarrhea-predominant irritable bowel syndrome. Chin J Integr Med. 2011;17(10):780–5.

22. MacPherson H, Bland M, Bloor K, Cox H, Geddes D, Kang'ombe A, et al. Acupuncture for irritable bowel syndrome: a protocol for a pragmatic randomised controlled trial. BMC Gastroenterol. 2010;10:63.

23. Kaptchuk TJ. Acupuncture: theory, efficacy, and practice. Ann Intern Med. 2002;136(5):374–83.

24. Tada H, Fujita M, Harris M, Tatewaki M, Nakagawa K, Yamamura T, et al. Neural mechanism of acupuncture-induced gastric relaxations in rats. Dig Dis Sci. 2003;48(1):59–68.

25. Zhenzhong L, Xiaojun Y, Weijun T, Yuehua C, Jie S, Jimeng Z, et al. Comparative effect of electroacupuncture and moxibustion on the expression of substance P and vasoactive intestinal peptide in patients with irritable bowel syndrome. J Tradit Chin Med. 2015;35(4):402–10.

26. Chen CY, Ke MD, Kuo CD, Huang CH, Hsueh YH, Chen JR. The influence of electro-acupuncture stimulation to female constipation patients. Am J Chin Med. 2013;41(2):301–13.

27. Noguchi E. Acupuncture regulates gut motility and secretion via nerve reflexes. Auton Neurosci. 2010;156(1-2):15–8.

28. Li YQ, Zhu B, Rong PJ, Ben H, Li YH. Neural mechanism of acupuncture-modulated gastric motility. World J Gastroenterol. 2007;13(5):709–16.

29. Furness JB. The enteric nervous system and neurogastroenterology. Nat Rev Gastroenterol Hepatol. 2012;9(5):286–94.

30. Heanue TA, Pachnis V. Enteric nervous system development and Hirschsprung's disease: advances in genetic and stem cell studies. Nat Rev Neurosci. 2007;8(6):466–79.

31. Furness JB, Callaghan BP, Rivera LR, Cho HJ. The enteric nervous system and gastrointestinal innervation: integrated local and central control. Adv Exp Med Biol. 2014;817:39–71.

32. Sidebotham EL, Woodward MN, Kenny SE, Lloyd DA, Vaillant CR, Edgar DH. Assessment of protein gene product 9.5 as a marker of neural crest-derived precursor cells in the developing enteric nervous system. Pediatr Surg Int. 2001;17(4):304–7.

33. Du F, Wang L, Qian W, Liu S. Loss of enteric neurons accompanied by decreased expression of GDNF and PI3K/Akt pathway in diabetic rats. Neurogastroenterol Motil. 2009;21(11):1229–e114.

34. Matsuda NM, Miller SM, Evora PR. The chronic gastrointestinal manifestations of Chagas disease. Clinics (Sao Paulo). 2009;64(12):1219–24.

35. Di Nardo G, Blandizzi C, Volta U, Colucci R, Stanghellini V, Barbara G, et al. Review article: molecular, pathological and therapeutic features of human enteric neuropathies. Aliment Pharmacol Ther. 2008;28(1):25–42.

36. Wedel T, Roblick U, Gleiss J, Ott V, Eggers R, Kühnel W, et al. Disorders of intestinal innervation as a possible cause for chronic constipation. Zentralbl Chir. 1999;124(9):796–803.

37. Boeckxstaens GE, Hirsch DP, Kodde A, Moojen TM, Blackshaw A, Tytgat GN, et al. Activation of an adrenergic and vagally-mediated NANC pathway in surgery-induced fundic relaxation in the rat. Neurogastroenterol Motil. 1999; 11(6):467-74.

38. Lies B, Beck K, Keppler J, Saur D, Groneberg D, Friebe A. Nitrergic signalling via interstitial cells of Cajal regulates motor activity in murine colon. J Physiol. 2015;593(20):4589–601.

15

How do medical students engaging in elective courses on acupuncture and homeopathy differ from unselected students?

Alexandra Jocham[1], Levente Kriston[2], Pascal O. Berberat[3], Antonius Schneider[1] and Klaus Linde[1*] (iD)

Abstract

Background: We aimed to investigate whether students at German medical schools participating in elective courses on acupuncture and homeopathy differ from an unselected group of students regarding attitudes and personality traits.

Methods: Elective courses on acupuncture and homeopathy in the academic half-year 2013/14 all over Germany were identified and participants invited to fill in a questionnaire including nineteen questions on attitudes towards Complementary and Alternative Medicine (CAM), orientation towards science, care and status orientation, and a short validated instrument (Big-Five-Inventory-10) to measure personality traits (extraversion, neuroticism, openness, conscientiousness, and agreeableness). Participants of a mandatory family medicine course at one university served as unselected control group.

Results: Two hundred twenty and 113 students from elective courses on acupuncture and homeopathy, respectively, and 315 control students participated (response rate 93%). Students participating in elective courses had much more positive attitudes towards CAM, somewhat lower science and status orientation, and somewhat higher care orientation than control group students (all p-values for three-group comparisons < 0.001). There were no differences between the three groups regarding personality traits with the exception of lower values for agreeableness in controls ($p = 0.009$).

Conclusions: The findings of this study show that attitudes of students participating in elective courses on acupuncture or homeopathy at German medical schools differ to a considerable degree from the attitudes of unselected students.

Keywords: Complementary and alternative medicine, Medical education, Attitudes, Personality traits

Background

The US National Centre of Complementary and Integrative Health pragmatically defines Complementary and Alternative Medicine (CAM) "as a group of diverse medical and health care interventions, practices, products, or disciplines that are not generally considered part of conventional medicine" [1]. From the perspective of skeptical scientists most CAM therapies lack plausibility and a convincing proof of efficacy beyond placebo effects [2]. Yet, the use of CAM therapies is not only widespread in

the general population in many industrialized countries [3, 4] but also considerable among physicians, particularly those working in primary care [5, 6]. Given the wide use of CAM it makes sense that medical students learn about the basic principles, risks and state of the evidence on the most important therapies in order to be able to give competent advice to their patients [7]. However, it has been criticized that many CAM courses at medical schools go beyond a critical introduction and actually teach basics how such therapies can be practiced in a rather uncritical manner [8].

In Germany, the use of CAM methods is popular among physicians working in ambulatory care [6] and a number of medical schools offer courses on these

* Correspondence: klaus.linde@tum.de
[1]Institute of General Practice, Klinikum rechts der Isar, Technical University of Munich, Orleansstrasse 47, 81667 Munich, Germany
Full list of author information is available at the end of the article

subjects [9]. Two therapies which are very widely used are acupuncture and homeopathy [6]. Acupuncture originates from China and involves the insertion of thin needles at specific points of the body to stimulate self-healing. A considerable body of evidence of suggests that acupuncture is likely to be effective in practice for a number of conditions. Yet, correct placement of the needles seems to have limited relevance (e.g. [10]) challenging important tenets of acupuncture. Homeopathy uses highly diluted remedies of agents claimed to cause similar symptoms to those seen in the patient when given in high dose. Many scientists consider homeopathy highly implausible (e.g. [2]) and the interpretation of the available placebo-controlled trials ranges from carefully positive [11] to proving that homeopathy does not work [12].

A number of studies have investigated the attitudes of medical students towards CAM therapies (e.g. [13, 14]), but we are not aware of any studies comparing characteristics and views of students actually engaging in elective courses on such therapies to those of "average" students. Such comparisons are important to understand whether students engaging in CAM are distinct groups. Therefore, we aimed to investigate whether students at German medical schools participating in elective courses on acupuncture and homeopathy differ from an unselected group of students regarding attitudes towards CAM, science, care and status orientation, and personality traits. In addition, we tried to identify classes of students showing similar patterns of attitudes across groups.

Methods

Study design, target populations and sampling procedures

The study was a cross-sectional, quantitative, exploratory, anonymous survey. Three groups of students were investigated: an acupuncture, a homeopathy and a control group. The target populations for the acupuncture and homeopathy groups were all medical students participating in an elective course on this subject in the academic half-year 2013/14 at a German medical school. The target population for the control group were all medical students in the same time period in Germany.

To identify all relevant courses on acupuncture (including also courses on traditional Chinese medicine in general) and homeopathy, inquiries were made to faculties and student representatives at all 37 German medical schools. Furthermore, a foundation (Carstens- Stiftung, Essen) and a professional society (German Medical Acupuncture Society) supporting elective courses across Germany provided lists of courses. In summer 2013, contact persons of identified courses were informed about the planned survey and invited to participate, if a course was planned for the half-year 2013/14. Contact persons agreeing to participate then received questionnaires, a short summary for introducing the survey to students, a sheet for documenting the number of questionnaires handed out and collected, and a prepared envelope for sending the material back to the researchers. Participation was voluntary.

The optimal control group would have consisted of a nation-wide random sample of medical students. However, given the limited resources for our study, the lack of a central nation-wide register of medical students and the low likelihood of obtaining high response rates from 37 medical schools, we chose to use a convenience sample. Within a mandatory course on family medicine at the Technical University Munich in November 2013 all participants were invited to fill in the questionnaire. All medical students have to participate in this family medicine course; most do so in their fourth study year (academic half-years 7 or 8), a minority of students at an earlier or later stage.

Questionnaire

The questionnaire consisted of two modules: module 1 (two pages) for all participants and module 2 (two pages) for students participating in acupuncture and homeopathy courses only. Module 2 included open questions about motives and closed questions about personal experiences, influence of the personal environment and attitudes directly related to the course topic. This paper focuses on methods and findings from module 1; details of the methods and findings for module 2 will be reported elsewhere.

Module 1 had three parts. The first part consisted of 19 statements (see Additional file 1: Table S1 for exact wording) aiming to measure attitudes considered potentially relevant for choosing elective courses or not. Agreement to statements was rated on a 5-point Likert-scale ranging from full agreement (coded as 2) to complete disagreement (coded as −2). Originally, we had assigned the 19 statements to six domains to be summarized in scores. However, confirmatory factor analysis did not completely confirm our postulated factor structure, thus minor modifications for scoring were necessary (see Additional file 2 Digital Content 2 for details). The instrument measured the following scales:

1. "CAM orientation" (a second-order scale consisting of four subscales):
   a. "CAM interest" (two statements; internal consistency quantified with Crohnbach's $\alpha = 0.88$) addressed the general interest in CAM;
   b. "positive attitudes towards acupuncture" (three statements; $\alpha = 0.78$) the interest in acupuncture, belief in its efficacy and personal experience with it;
   c. "positive attitudes towards homeopathy" (three statements; $\alpha = 0.80$) the interest in homeopathy, belief in its efficacy and, personal experience with it;

d. and "beyond science" (four statements; $\alpha = 0.58$) agreement to statements indicating an orientation deviating from a scientific view or expressing a critical view of conventional medicine;

2. "Science orientation" (two statements; $\alpha = 0.68$) attitudes towards a scientific view of medicine;

3. "Care orientation" (three statements; $\alpha = 0.61$) the willingness to care for others and empathy;

4. "Status orientation" (two statements; $\alpha = 0.79$) the relevance of status motives for choosing to study medicine.

The second part of module 1 consisted of the Big-Five-Inventory-10 (BFI-10), a short, validated questionnaire to investigate personality traits [15]. The Big-Five is a widely examined theory of five broad dimensions to describe the human personality. The five factors are extraversion, neuroticism, openness to experience, conscientiousness, and agreeableness. The third part of module 1 documented sociodemographic and study- or career-related characteristics.

Statistics

The study was exploratory (hypothesis-generating). Basic analyses were performed with SPSS 23 software (Armonk, NY). We explored differences between all three groups using the Chi^2-test (nominal data), the Kruskal-Wallis-test (ordinal data) and ANOVA (summary scales). Pairwise comparisons were done using Fisher's exact test, the Chi^2-test, the Mann–Whitney U-test, or the Student t-test. Given the large number of p-values calculated these should primarily be interpreted as a reading aid. We did not adjust for multiple testing. The structure of the attitude measure was investigated with confirmatory factor analysis in Mplus 7.2 (see Additional file 3 for details). Participants were classified into homogeneous classes by latent profile analysis. Latent profile analyses (LPA) aim at the grouping of individuals into distinct classes based on response patterns to a defined set of items, so that individuals within a class are more similar than individuals between classes. Usually models with an increasing number of classes are tested and the one with best balance between model fit and parsimony is selected. It is an exploratory procedure with a probabilistic allocation of individuals to classes (rather than setting a deterministic group membership, like, for example, in k-means cluster analysis). We used responses to the 19 attitude statements as input for the LPA. Although previous confirmatory factor analysis revealed a theoretically reasonable factorial structure of the statements, hierarchical factor or scale scores cannot be satisfactorily dealt with in LPA, so that we used the individual items. To express the results, however, we used scale scores due to higher comprehensibility and consistency with rest of the study report. We used a

robust maximum likelihood estimator in Mplus 7.2 with 10,000 initial stage random starts, 50 initial stage iterations, and 50 final stage optimizations. Residual correlations between items (i.e., item-correlations within classes) were set to zero. Fit indices did not completely agree regarding the best model. Models with a higher number of classes than three were not significantly better than models with one less class (likelihood ratio tests), but the information criteria suggested that a model with a higher number of classes is necessary. Both the Akaike information criterion and the sample-size adjusted Bayesian information criterion (lower values favorable) decreased continuously with a higher number of classes, while the Bayesian information criterion had a minimum at the model with 6 classes. As the entropy and the size of the smallest class were both favorable of this class, we decided to retain this model for further analyses.

Results

Information on acupuncture and homeopathy courses could be obtained for 34 (92%) of the 37 medical schools contacted. A total of 18 acupuncture courses were offered at 15 medical schools (41% of 37, assuming that there were no courses at the three medical schools for which no information could be obtained) during the study period. At further four (11%) medical schools acupuncture courses were sometimes offered, but not in the study period. At 10 medical schools (27%) a total of 13 homeopathy courses were offered in the study period (further four (11%) had no current offer). Filled-in questionnaires were obtained from 16 acupuncture (89% of courses offered) and 12 homeopathy courses (92%). A total of 220 questionnaires from acupuncture courses and 113 questionnaires from homeopathy courses could be included in the analysis. In 24 of the 28 participating courses the number of questionnaires handed out was documented; the response rate here was 94%. In the mandatory family medicine course serving as control 315 of 344 (92%) of the registered participants filled in the questionnaire.

Students participating in acupuncture or homeopathy courses tended to be slightly more often female and older in spite of having studied for a slightly shorter time compared to students in the control group (Table 1). Results of the final secondary school examinations were significantly worse in the acupuncture and homeopathy group compared to the control group. Furthermore, students from these groups had more often completed another professional education and had more often a clear idea in which medical area to specialize. In particular, the proportion aiming to specialize in family medicine was higher and the proportion aiming to specialize in surgery was lower than in the control group. A total of 27 (9%) students in the control group reported that they

Table 1 Characteristics of participants. Values are absolute frequencies (percentages) or medians (25th and 75th percentile)

Variable (n missing)	Acupuncture (n = 220)	Homeopathy (n = 113)	Control (n = 315)	p-value global (pairwise)
Female (9)	161 (73%)	87 (77%)	202 (66%)	.05 (–/*/-)
Age (12)	24 (23, 27)	24 (22, 28)	23 (22, 25)	.005 (**/–/–)
Half-years at medical school (12)	7 (5, 9)	7 (3, 9)	7 (7, 8)	.04 (–/*/*/)
Score secondary school[a] (28)	1.7 (1.3, 2.3)	1.6 (1.3, 2.0)	1.4 (1.2, 1.6)	<.001 (**/**/-)
Professional training before medical school (9)	69 (31%)	40 (35%)	53 (17%)	<.001 (**/**/-)
Knows planned type of specialization (10) Among those knowing specialization	115 (52%)	63 (56%)	130 (43%)	.015 (*/*/-)
- family medicine	29 (25%)	30 (48%)	19 (15%)	<.001 (–/**/*)
- surgery	13 (11%)	3 (5%)	33 (25%)	.001 (*/*/-)
- internal medicine	13 (11%)	6 (10%)	23 (18%)	.19 (–/–/-)

p-values for three-group comparisons from Kruskal-Wallis-tests and Pearson-Chi^2-tests; p-values for pairwise comparisons from Fisher's exact tests and Mann–Whitney-U-tests: – $p \geq .05$; * $p = .002$ to $p = .049$; ** $p \leq .001$ (order: first position - acupuncture vs. control, second position - homeopathy vs. control; third position - acupuncture vs. homeopathy)
[a]scores for final examinations at German secondary schools qualifying for university can vary between 0.7 (best score) and 6 (worst score)

had participated or were currently participating in an elective course on acupuncture (6%) or/and homeopathy (4%).

There were statistically significant ($p < 0.001$) differences between the groups for the scores for all four main attitude factors (Fig. 1; see Additional file 1 for answers to all individual items and scores). As expected, participants in elective courses on average had positive views towards CAM while control students tended to be neutral to slightly negative on average. The majority of participants considered science important, yet summary scores among acupuncture and homeopathy students were lower than among students in the control group. Care orientation was high in all three groups, but participants of homeopathy courses had the highest scores and control group students the lowest scores. Status motives had a very limited role as reasons for studying medicine among participants of acupuncture and homeopathy courses while they were more important in the control group.

When the four sub-scales contributing to the main factor "CAM orientation" were analysed separately, there were also major differences between the three groups (Fig. 2). The general interest in CAM was similar among acupuncture and homeopathy students and much higher than in the control group. However, the attitude towards the specific complementary therapy chosen as elective course was much more positive than for the complementary therapy not chosen. Agreement to statements indicating an orientation deviating from a scientific view or expressing a critical view of conventional medicine ("beyond science") was limited also among students participating in the elective courses, yet considerably higher than among control group students.

There were no differences between the three groups regarding personality traits with the exception of lower values for agreeableness in controls ($p = 0.009$; see Additional file 3: Figure S4).

Latent profile analysis suggested six classes of students (see Table 2 and Fig. 3). Absolute differences between classes were very pronounced for CAM attitudes and relatively small for science, care and status orientation. Class 1 (comprising 28% of control group students and only two students in elective courses) was characterized by a rather distinct "anti-CAM orientation", a strong scientific orientation, and – compared to the other classes - a lower care and a higher status orientation. Class 5 students (24% of acupuncture, 26% of homeopathy and 6% on control group students) can be considered antagonists to class 1 students, as they have a strong CAM, comparably low science, strong care and low status orientation. Class 2 students (comprising 11% of acupuncture, 19% of homeopathy students and 36% of control students) tended to be neutral regarding CAM, had a relatively strong science orientation and were in the middle regarding care and status orientation. Class 3 students (11% of acupuncture, 43% of homeopathy and 9% of control students) had positive attitudes towards CAM in general and homeopathy, but were neutral towards acupuncture, had comparably low science orientation, high care and low status orientation. Instead, among class 4 students (41% of acupuncture, 12% of homeopathy and 8% of control students) attitudes towards acupuncture were quite positive, but neutral regarding general CAM interest, negative towards homeopathy, and these students had a comparably high science orientation. The relative small class 6 (11% of acupuncture, none of homeopathy and 13% of control group students) has a quite unique pattern with rather positive attitudes towards acupuncture and science, but low care and high status orientation. With respect to personality traits class 5 students scored particularly high on openness and conscientiousness, and class 1

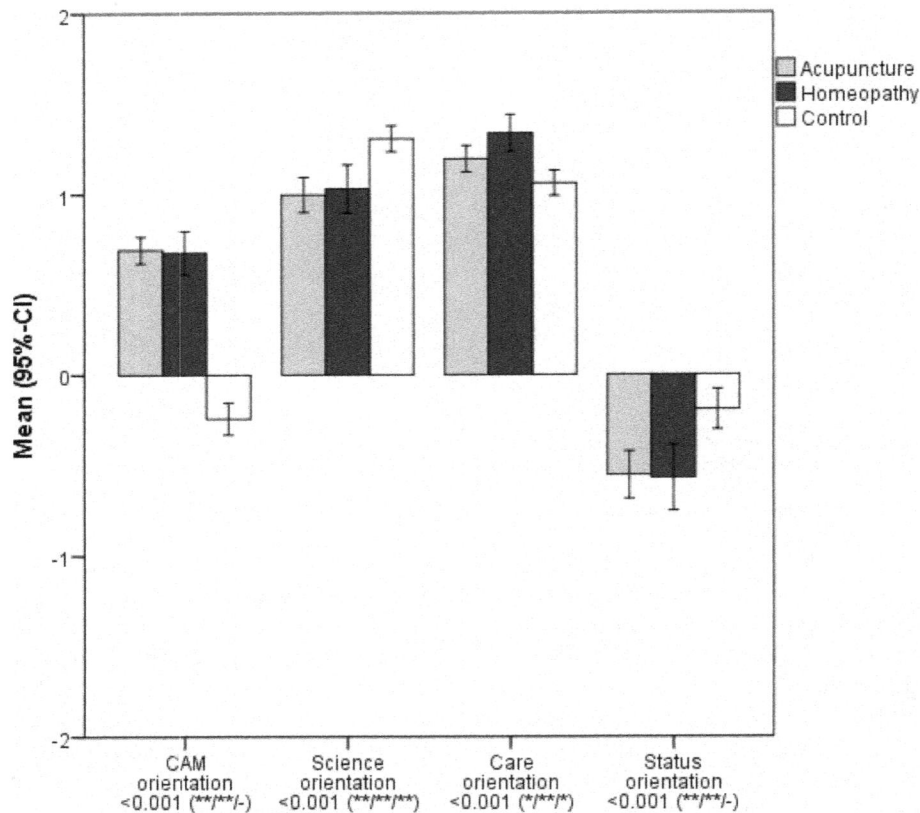

Fig. 1 Means (95% confidence intervals) for the four main factors CAM orientation, science orientation, care orientation and status orientation. Higher values indicated stronger agreement. *p*-values for three-group comparisons from ANOVA (significance levels for pairwise comparisons from Student t-tests: − p ≥ 0.05; * *p* =0.002 to *p* =0.049; ** p ≤ 0.001; order: first position - acupuncture vs. control, second position - homeopathy vs. control; third position - acupuncture vs. homeopathy)

students particularly low on agreeableness (results not shown).

Discussion

Compared to an unselected control group, students participating in elective courses on acupuncture and homeopathy at German medical schools had on average more positive attitudes towards CAM, considered science less important, had stronger care and lower status orientation, and scored higher on the personality trait agreeableness. Yet, attitudes towards CAM varied much more than science, care and status orientation. If we assume that attitudes of our control group students are broadly representative, it might be expected that about a quarter of German medical students has positive attitudes towards CAM (classes 3, 4 and 5 in Table 2), are at least partly critical about science, and have a high care and a low status motivation. Another quarter (class 1) has strong scientific orientation, is very skeptical about CAM, has lower care and higher status orientation, and scores lower on the personality trait agreeableness. About half of the students (classes 2 and 6) might be

expected to be neutral towards CAM, rather scientifically oriented but also to some extent open to heretic views, and have slightly lower care and stronger status orientation than CAM proponents.

To the best of our knowledge, our survey is the first comparing attitudes and personality traits of students participating in elective courses on acupuncture or homeopathy and unselected medical students. The large sample size allowed the reliable detection of relevant differences. The nationwide sampling and the high response rate make it likely that our results give a realistic and representative picture of students participating in such elective courses. An important shortcoming is that we cannot be certain that our control group is representative of German medical students. Compared to many other countries the ranking of universities is much less pronounced in Germany and when choosing a university its reputation is only a secondary criterion [16]. Yet, medical students from the Technical University of Munich compare well with those from other universities regarding the proportion passing the final examination and completing their study in time [17]. Furthermore,

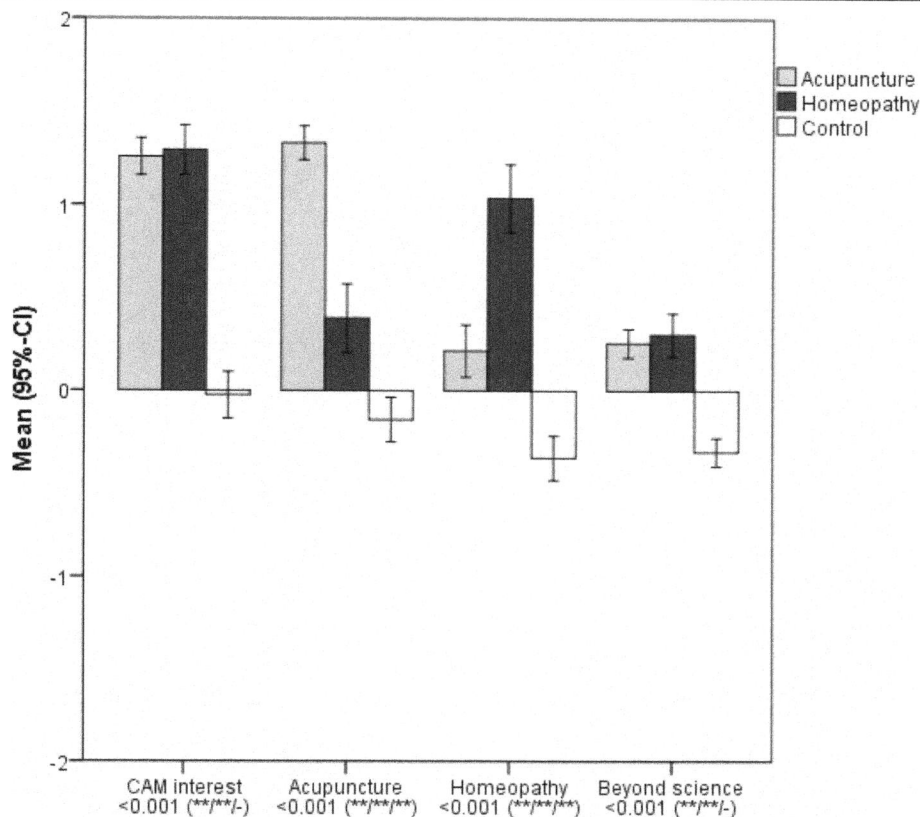

Fig. 2 Means (95% confidence intervals) for the four factors CAM interest, acupuncture, homeopathy, and beyond science contributing to the main factor CAM orientation. Higher values indicated stronger agreement. See legend of Fig. 1 for further details

for reasons of feasibility our scales for measuring CAM, care and status orientation mostly consist of only two to three items. The individual statements were developed mainly to differentiate the three groups. Our data-driven classification (latent profile analysis) was performed post-hoc with a strictly exploratory approach. Yet, we consider it an interesting part of our work as it allows to postulate some hypotheses regarding patterns of attitudes among (German) medical students.

Multiple studies have shown that medical students in general have positive attitudes towards science (e.g. [18–21]). While the majority of participants of elective CAM courses in our study held positive views about science, too, agreement to the two statements was significantly lower than among participants in the control group. Croatian surveys among students and doctors also found a negative correlation between attitudes towards CAM and science [18, 22]. However, the ratings on our beyond science scale suggest

Table 2 Results of the latent profile analysis per group. Values are absolute frequencies (percentages)

Class – class characteristics (compared to other classes)	Acupuncture (n = 220)	Homeopathy (n = 113)	Control (n = 315)	Total (n = 648)
1 – CAM negative, science high, care low, status high	2 (1%)	-	**89 (28%)**	91 (14%)
2 – CAM neutral, science high & care & status moderate	25 (11%)	22 (19%)	**114 (36%)**	161 (25%)
3 – CAM interest strong/Acupuncture moderate/Homeopathy positive, science low, care high, status low	24 (11%)	**49 (43%)**	28 (9%)	101 (16%)
4 – CAM interest strong/Acupuncture positive/Homeopathy neutral, science & care and status moderate	**91 (41%)**	13 (12%)	26 (8%)	130 (20%)
5 – CAM interest strong, science low, care high, status low	**53 (24%)**	**29 (26%)**	18 (6%)	100 (15%)
6 – CAM interest neutral/Acupuncture positive/Homeopathy negative, science moderate, care low, status high	25 (11%)	-	40 (13%)	65 (10%)

Bold data indicate the two most frequent classes per group, respectively

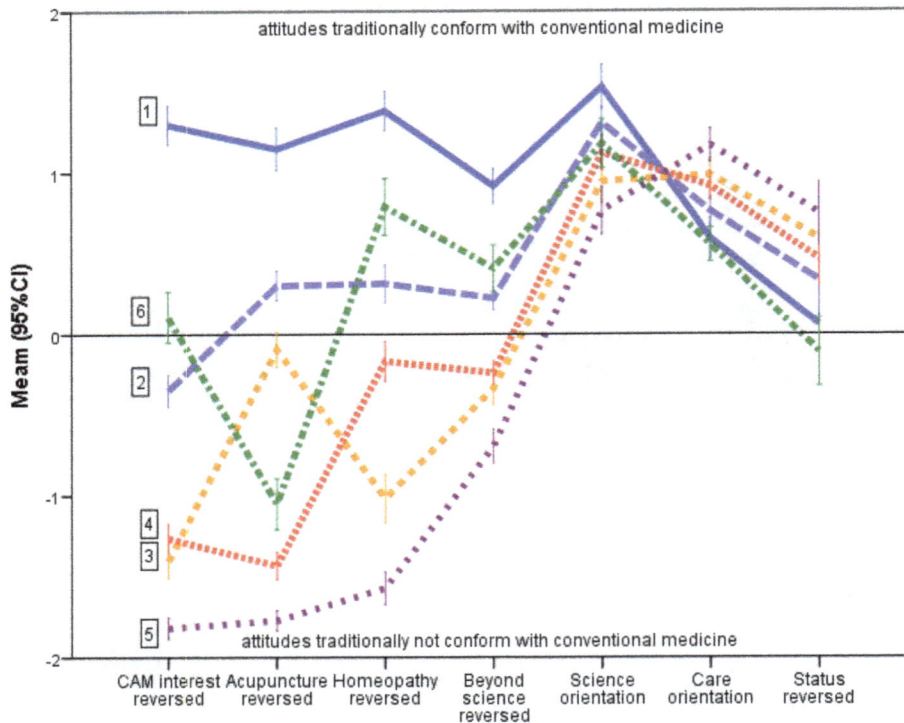

Fig. 3 Means (95% confidence intervals) for attitudes according to classes (class number in boxes) identified by latent profile analysis. Note that some scales have been reversed for better graphical separation of classes. The scales CAM interest, Acupuncture, Homeopathy, Beyond Science and Status (orientation) were reversed with positive values now indicating attitudes traditionally conform with conventional medicine academically and negative values attitudes traditionally not conform with conventional medicine

that even many control group students share the view that a purely biomedical scientific approach alone might not be sufficient. For example, 37% agreed to the statement that "conventional medicine does not grasp the patient entirely" and further 37% were uncertain. Also other studies have shown that many medical students are open to more or less non-conventional views [19, 21]. We are not aware of other studies investigating the association of attitudes towards CAM and care or status orientation. Yet, it is an interesting finding that students open to CAM tend to have a somewhat higher care orientation and are more often interested in specializing in family medicine. Competency models for general practice emphasize empathy and perspective taking as key domains [23].

In our study, we did not investigate the contents of the elective courses. Based on what we know from personal contacts we assume that course instructors often are providers of the respective therapy. It seems likely that therapies are taught in a rather "positive" manner and it is unclear whether the courses include a critical discussion of the scientific debates relating to CAM. To what extent and how CAM is taught within the mandatory basic curriculum at German medical schools is unclear but likely to be minimal [9]. The somewhat science-sceptic attitude of many participants in elective CAM courses is a matter of concern. We

think our findings provide support for the demand that a critical discussion of the scientific basis of the respective therapy should be a mandatory part in elective CAM courses at medical schools. For the basic curriculum, CAM might be an interesting theme for discussing what is scientific in medicine, what is not, where important limitations are, and where demarcations are professionally inevitable. For example, it has been argued that CAM can serve as a "mirror image" helping to understand scientific reasoning [24]. Discussing CAM examples when teaching evidence-based medicine makes clear how prior beliefs and mechanistic theories shape the interpretation of data [25, 26]. They also make understandable that although placebo *effects* are seen as positive in clinical practice when they are associated with active treatments, placebo *interventions* or interventions without "specific" effects pose major ethical and professional problems [27, 28]. Understanding how a CAM therapy in a specific situation might better address the subjective needs of patients [29] can help to understand fundamental limitations of how modern medical practice approaches the patient [30].

Conclusion

In conclusion, the findings of our study show that attitudes of students participating in elective courses on acupuncture or homeopathy at German medical schools differ to a considerable degree from the attitudes of unselected students. Further empirical studies using well-validated, comprehensive scales investigating associations between attitudes and personality traits are desirable to investigate whether our findings can be confirmed and whether they apply to other countries.

Additional files

Additional file 1: Table S1. Agreement to individual statements and summary scales to the 19 questions of module 1, part 1. Values are means (standard deviations = SD) or absolute frequencies (valid percentages).

Additional file 2: Confirmatory factor analysis of the attitude measure.

Additional file 3: Figure S4. Means (95% confidence intervals) for Big Five personality traits.

Acknowledgements
We thank all course organizers and students participating in the survey.

Funding
There was no external funding for the study. AJ performed the survey for her MD thesis at the Technical University Munich, Germany, and received a personal stipend by the Karl und Veronica Carstens-Stiftung, Essen for writing up her thesis.

Authors' contribution
Conception and design: AJ, POB, AS, KL. Data collection and data entry: AJ. Statistical analysis: AJ, LK, KL. Drafting of the manuscript: KL. Interpretation, revision and approval of the manuscript: All authors.

Competing interests
The authors declare that they have no competing interests.

Author details
[1]Institute of General Practice, Klinikum rechts der Isar, Technical University of Munich, Orleansstrasse 47, 81667 Munich, Germany. [2]Department of Medical Psychology, University Medical Center Hamburg-Eppendorf, Hamburg, Germany. [3]TUM Medical Education Center, TUM School of Medicine, Technical University of Munich, Munich, Germany.

References
1. NIH National Center for Complementary and Integrative Health. Website – introduction. https://nccih.nih.gov/about/plans/2011/introduction.htm. Accessed 13 Sept 2016.
2. Singh S, Ernst E. Trick or treatment: the undeniable facts about alternative medicine. New York and London: WW Norton & Co; 2009.
3. Nahin RL, Barnes PM, Stussman BJ, Bloom B. Costs of Complementary and Alternative Medicine (CAM) and Frequency of Visits to CAM Practitioners: United States, 2007. National Health Statistics Reports; no: 18. Hyattsville: National Center for Health Statistics; 2009.
4. Eardley S, Bishop FL, Prescott P, Cardini F, Brinkhaus B, Santos-Rey K, Vas J, von Ammon K, Hegyi G, Dragan S, Uehleke B, Fønnebø V, Lewith G. A systematic literature review of complementary and alternative medicine prevalence in EU. Forsch Komplementmed. 2012;19 Suppl 2:18–28.

5. Astin JA, Marie A, Pelletier KR, Hansen E, Haskell WL. A review of the incorporation of complementary and alternative medicine by mainstream physicians. Arch Intern Med. 1998;158:2303–10.
6. Linde K, Alscher A, Friedrichs C, Wagenpfeil S, Karsch-Völk M, Schneider A. Belief in and use of complementary therapies among family physicians, internists and orthopaedists in Germany - cross-sectional survey. Fam Pract. 2015;32:62–8.
7. Gaster B, Unterborn JN, Scott RB, Schneeweiss R. What should students learn about complementary and alternative medicine? Acad Med. 2007;82:934–8.
8. Marcus DM. An evaluation of the evidence in "evidence-based" integrative medicine programs. Acad Med. 2009;84:1229–34.
9. Brinkhaus B, Witt CM, Jena S, Bockelbrink A, Ortiz M, Willich SN. Integration of complementary and alternative medicine into medical schools in Austria, Germany and Switzerland-results of a cross-sectional study. Wien Med Wochenschr. 2011;161:32–43.
10. Vickers AJ, Cronin AM, Maschino AC, Lewith G, MacPherson H, Foster NE, Sherman KJ, Witt CM, Linde K. Acupuncture Trialists' Collaboration. Acupuncture for chronic pain: individual patient data meta-analysis. Arch Intern Med. 2012;172:1444–53.
11. Mathie RT, Lloyd SM, Legg LA, Clausen J, Moss S, Davidson JR, Ford I. Randomised placebo-controlled trials of individualised homeopathic treatment: systematic review and meta-analysis. Syst Rev. 2014;3:142.
12. Anonymous. Lancet. 2005;366:690.
13. Furnham A, McGill C. Medical students' attitudes about complementary and alternative medicine. J Altern Complement Med. 2003;9:275–84.
14. Abbott RB, Hui KK, Hays RD, Mandel J, Goldstein M, Winegarden B, Glaser D, Brunton L. Medical student attitudes toward complementary, alternative and integrative medicine. Evid Based Complement Alternat Med. 2011;2011:985243. doi:10.1093/ecam/nep195.
15. Rammstedt B, John O. Measuring personality in one minute or less: A 10-item short version of the Big Five Inventory in English and German. J Res Pers. 2007;41:203–12.
16. EDU-CON. Umfrage: Studienfach ist wichtiger als die Stadt. https://www.berlin.de/special/jobs-und-ausbildung/uni-und-studium/news/2217073-999260-umfrage-studienfach-ist-wichtiger-als-di.html. Accessed 10 Nov 2016.
17. CHE Hochschulranking 2016/17. http://ranking.zeit.de/che2016/de/. Accessed 10 Nov 2016.
18. Dogas Z, Kardum G, Mirić L, Sevo V, Tolić T, Ursić A, Vasiljević P, Zekić S. Attitudes towards science and alternative medicine of medical, economics and business, and electrical engineering students in Split. Croatia Croat Med J. 2003;44:75–9.
19. Pruskil S, Burgwinkel P, Georg W, Keil T, Kiessling C. Medical students' attitudes towards science and involvement in research activities: a comparative study with students from a reformed and a traditional curriculum. Med Teach. 2009;31:e254–259.
20. Kaderli R, Burghardt L, Hansali C, Businger A. Students' view of evidence-based medicine: a survey in Switzerland. Arch Clin Exp Surg. 2012;1:34–40.
21. Plaisant O, Stephens S, Apaydin N, Courtois R, Lignier B, Loukas M, Moxham B. Medical students' attitudes towards science and gross anatomy, and the relationship to personality. J Anat. 2014;224:261–9.
22. Rogulj ZM, Baloevic E, Dogas Z, Kardum G, Hren D, Marusic A, Marusic M. Family medicine practice and research: survey of physicians' attitudes towards scientific research in a post-communist transition country. Wien Klin Wochenschr. 2007;119:164–9.
23. Patterson F, Tavabie A, Denney M, Kerrin M, Ashworth V, Koczwara A, MacLeod S. A new competency model for general practice: implications for selection, training, and careers. Br J Gen Pract. 2013;63:e331–338.
24. Vandenbroucke JP, de Craen AJ. Alternative medicine: a 'mirror image' for scientific reasoning in conventional medicine. Ann Intern Med. 2001;135:507–13.
25. Pandolfi M, Carreras G. The faulty statistics of complementary alternative medicine (CAM). Eur J Intern Med. 2014;25:607–9.
26. Rutten L, Mathie RT, Fisher P, Goossens M, van Wassenhoven M. Plausibility and evidence: the case of homeopathy. Med Health Care Philos. 2013;16:525–32.
27. Linde K, Fässler M, Meissner K. Placebo interventions, placebo effects and clinical practice. Phil Trans R Soc B. 2011;366:1905–12.
28. Sullivan MD. Placebo controls and epistemic control in orthodox medicine. J Med Philos. 1993;18:213–31.
29. Schmacke N, Müller V, Stamer M. What is it about homeopathy that patients value? And what can family medicine learn from this? Qual Prim Care. 2014;22:17–24.
30. Agledahl KM, Gulbrandsen P, Førde R, Wifstad Å. Courteous but not curious: how doctors' politeness masks their existential neglect. A qualitative study of video-recorded patient consultations. J Med Ethics. 2011;37:650–4.

16

Effect of catgut implantation at acupoints for the treatment of allergic rhinitis

Xinrong Li[1†], Yang Liu[1†], Qinxiu Zhang[1*], Nan Xiang[2], Miao He[2], Juan Zhong[2], Qing Chen[2] and Xiaopei Wang[1]

Abstract

Background: The effect and safety of catgut implantation at acupoints o treat allergic rhinitis (ICD-10 code J30.4) remain controversial. Here, we used a sham catgut implantation group to determine whether catgut implantation at acupoints is an effective and safe treatment for allergic rhinitis.

Methods: A randomized double-blind clinical trial, with parallel groups was conducted. Skin prick and puncture test (SPT) was performed to confirm the diagnosis before enrollment. The participants received two sessions of treatments of active or sham catgut implantation at acupoints (once every two weeks) with a follow-up phase of 8 weeks. The visual analogue scale (VAS) and Rhinoconjunctivitis Quality of Life Questionnaire (RQLQ) were used to determine the severity of allergic rhinitis. The use of anti-allergic medication was used as a secondary indicator. The incidence of adverse events was also recorded and analyzed.

Results: An improvement of the VAS and RQLQ scores was observed in both the active and sham-controlled group sat four and eight weeks after the treatment in the self-control analysis. Comparison revealed no significant difference between the treatment and sham-controlled groups until 8 weeks after the 2-week treatment regimen ($t = -2.424$, $P = 0.017$). However, the RQLQ scores significantly differed between the two groups after 4 weeks of treatment completion ($t = -2.045$, $P = 0.05$) and this difference lasted until the end of 8-week follow-up ($t = -2.246$, $P = 0.033$). Throughout the treatment regimen, none of the participants took any relief medication, and no severe adverse events occurred.

Conclusion: Our findings suggest that catgut implantation at acupoints is an effective and safe method for symptomatic treatment of allergic rhinitis.

Trial registration: Chinese Clinical Trial Registry ChiCTR-TRC-12002191 (Date of Registration: 2012-05-09)

Keywords: Allergic rhinitis, Catgut implantation at acupoints, Randomized controlled trial

Background

Allergic rhinitis (ICD-10 code J30.4) is a symptomatic disorder of the nose triggered by allergens such as house dust mites, pet dander, or pollen. Allergic rhinitis has become a major health problem worldwide and affects a substantial number of people. The Allergic rhinitis and its impact on asthma (ARIA)2008 document estimated that over 600 million patients from all countries, all

ethnic groups, and of all ages suffer from AR [1]. An epidemiological study in 11 major Chinese cities reported that the prevalence of allergic rhinitis has increased to 24.6 % in 2007 [2]. Although allergic rhinitis comprises the classic symptoms of sneezing, rhinorrhea, and nasal obstruction, it is associated with impairments of patient function in day-to-day life. Patients with allergic rhinitis may also suffer from sleep disorders, emotional problems, and impairment in activities and social functioning [3].

Pharmaceutical care is an optimal strategy for the management of allergic rhinitis. A stepwise medical treatment was proposed in the ARIA workshop report

* Correspondence: zhqinxiu@163.com

†Equal contributors

[1]Department of Otorhinolaryngology, Head and Neck Surgery of the Teaching Hospital of Chengdu University of Traditional Chinese Medicine, Chengdu, Sichuan Province 610072, People's Republic of China

Full list of author information is available at the end of the article

[1]. However, not all the patients' symptoms can be controlled with pharmacological treatment. Treatment based on guidelines is not effective in all patients [4]. Around one-third of patients with moderate/severe symptoms are uncontrolled despite optimal pharmacologic treatment [1]. Complementary/alternative treatment is now being extensively used for allergic rhinitis and appears to yield satisfactory results [5]. Among these interventions, acupuncture is widely accepted as an easily available and affordable treatment choice in China and other countries, to relieve the symptoms of AR [6–10]. Catgut implantation at acupoints is a subtype of acupuncture. In this treatment, approximately 1- to 1.5-cm-long catgut is embedded in the acupoint by a special needle. The catgut can be completely absorbed by the tissue in 2–4 weeks. Then, the continuous stimulation caused by the catgut at the acupoint produces a therapeutic effect. Therefore, catgut implantation at acupoints may help treat chronic diseases such as AR [11–13].

We carried out a systematic review in order to assess the effectiveness and the possible adverse effects of catgut implantation at acupoints for allergic rhinitis [14]. In this review, due to the methodological shortcomings and risk of bias of the included trials, limited evidence showed that catgut implantation can be used to treat allergic rhinitis. There is an urgent need for robust randomized clinical trials (RCTs) with high quality and larger sample size in this field.

Therefore, we undertook a randomized, double-blind, large-scale study to evaluate the effectiveness of catgut implantation in adults with allergic rhinitis. This study has been approved by the Sichuan Regional Ethics Review Committee on Traditional Chinese Medicine (ethics approval number, 2012KL-002). The work reported in this article has been registered with an identifier (ChiCTR-TRC-12002191) by the Chinese Clinical Trial Registry.

Methods

A detailed description of this double-blinded randomized clinical trial with two parallel groups (described as "treatment group" or "sham-controlled group" respectively) has been previously published [15]. This study protocol followed the guidelines for clinical research on acupuncture (WHO Regional Publication, Western Pacific Series No.15, 1995) and both the recommendations of Consolidated Standard of Reporting Trials [16] and Standards for Reporting Interventions in Clinical Trials of Acupuncture [17]. The protocol was approved by the Sichuan Regional Ethics Review Committee on Traditional Chinese Medicine, and the ethics approval number of 2012KL-002. The work reported in this article was registered with an identifier (ChiCTR-TRC-12002191) by Chinese Clinical Trial Registry.

Participant inclusion criteria

The clinical diagnostic criteria published by ARIA in 2008 [1] was used to assess the eligibility for participation with AR in this study. The diagnosis of allergic rhinitis was based upon the concordance between a typical history of allergic symptoms and diagnostic tests. Typical symptoms of allergic rhinitis included rhinorrhea, sneezing, nasal obstruction, and pruritus. Prick and puncture tests were used for the diagnosis of specific allergies. Subjects were included if they met the following inclusion criteria:

(1) Patients aged between 18–70 years
(2) Those not participating in any other clinical trial
(3) Those with no previous experience of catgut implantation at acupoints
(4) Those who provide written informed consent
(5) Those presenting with typical symptoms of AR, such as rhinorrhea, sneezing, nasal obstruction, and pruritus. These symptoms should last more than one hour on most days.
Some patients may have ocular symptoms due to outdoor allergens.
(6) Those with positive skin prick and puncture test performed by trained health professionals. Standardized vaccine (Alutard SQ, ALK- Abelló, Denmark) was used in the prick and puncture test. Oral H1-antihistamines are not permitted before the skin test. Skin prick tests should be read at the peak of their reaction by measuring the wheal and flare approximately 15 min after the performance of the test.

Exclusion criteria

Patients with any of the following conditions were excluded:

(1) Pregnant women or women who were ready to conceive in the past six months, or lactating women
(2) Patients who were receiving immune therapy
(3) Patients with other allergic diseases such as bronchial asthma or allergic purpura
(4) Patients with nasal polyposis
(5) Patients with heterologous protein allergy
(6) Patients with other organic disorders such as AIDS, vascular malformation, hypertension, hematologic diseases, diabetes mellitus, malignant tumor, or mental disorders

Recruitment

Participants were enrolled either by the recruiting hospital when they came to our otorhinolaryngology clinics to seek therapy or by the printed recruitment posters in the hospital and the campus of Chengdu University of

Traditional Chinese Medicine. Patients who satisfied the inclusion criteria and were willing to participate in the trial were recruited.

Randomization and blinding

A random allocation sequence was generated by Excel (Microsoft Office) random number generator (Microsoft, USA). Patients were assigned to either the real catgut implantation group or the sham-controlled one in 1:1 ratio by computer program. The random numbers were sealed in opaque envelopes. Participant who met the inclusion criteria was asked to pickup one of the envelopes. They were randomized into either the study or control groups depending on the random number that was in the envelope. At the same time, the corresponding randomization information of the participant was collected, which included the participant's name in Pinyin format, the participant's numerical birthday and gender. All this information was recorded in duplicate and sealed in opaque envelopes. These opaque envelopes were preserved separately by the principal investigator and the primary sponsor. The envelopes were all kept intact until the blinding was removed. Participants, researchers, and study physicians who interviewed and recruited patients were blinded to the group assignments. For the sake of the specialty of the treatment of acupuncture, the acupuncturists were not blinded during the study. However, they were allowed to neither communicate with the participants about the treatment nor participate in the assessment of study outcomes.

The two groups were designated A (real treatment group) and B (sham-controlled group) in the medical records and case report forms. All information was locked out and saved in a database. Blind exposure was not provided until the statistical analysis was complete. Then two opaque envelopes containing the random allocation tables were unsealed by the principal investigator and the primary sponsor simultaneously to determine which groups the participants belonged to.

Procedures

A total of 128 participants who were found eligible for inclusion and provided their written informed consents to participant in the study wereassigned into one of the two study arms according to the random numbers of computer-generated allocation sequences, including the sham-control group consisting of patients who would receive a placebo treatment. After completing the baseline measures, both groups received real or sham catgut implantation at acupoints once per two weeks. Each patient had 2 treatment weeks and 8 weeks of follow-up. Figure 1 illustrates the flowchart of this study. The intervention was designed according to the documentary records in the ancient books and was consistent with both the Standards

for Reporting Interventions in Controlled Trials of Acupuncture (STRICTA) guidelines for the performance of acupuncture studies [18] and the World Health Organization (WHO) standard acupuncture point locations in the Western Pacific Region Geneva (WHO,2008) [19]. Both the real and sham catgut implantation was performed by the same acupuncturist throughout the study. Acupuncturists should have undergone at least 8 years of acupuncture training and be qualified TCM doctors.

Intervention

Five acupoints were selected for this research on the basis of our previous study [20]. For the first treatment, three acupoints were used for each patient. They were Yingxiang (LI20), Yintang(EX-HN3), and Hegu(LI4). For the second treatment, Zusanli(ST36) and Quchi(LI11) were chosen (Fig. 2). The acupoints were the same in both the treatment groups. All the treatments were performed by the same registered acupuncturists to ensure participant blinding and consistency of treatment.

To locate the acupoint [21]:

Hegu (LI4): abduct thumb and index figure, the point is located at the middle point between the web and the junction of the first and second metacarpal bones.
Quchi (LI11): with the elbow flexed, the point is located at the end of the cubital crease.
Yingxiang (LI20): in the nasolabial groove, beside the midpoint of the lateral border of the ala nasi.
Yintang (EX-HN3): on the forehead, at the midpoint between the eyebrows.
Zusanli (ST36): on the anteriolateral side of the lower leg, 3 cun inferior to Dubi (ST35), one finger breadth (middle finger) lateral to the anterior crest of the tibia. (Dubi-ST35: with the knee flexed, the point is located on the knee, in the depression internal to the patella and the patellar ligament.)

Participants received one session of real or sham catgut implantation at acupoints once every two weeks. Subjects were advised to lie supine. The pulse rate, blood pressure, and oxygen saturation were monitored routinely during the procedure as a precautionary measure. In both groups, swabs with 75 % alcohol and dry sterile cotton wool were used when withdrawing the needles. Pre-sterilized disposable needles (9#, Hanjiang Guoxiang Medical Appliance Factory, Yangzhou, China) and catguts (000, Pudong Jinhuan Medical Products Co., Ltd., Shanghai, China) were used for the treatment. For Yintang (EX-HN3), the needle was inserted to a depth of 1.0 cm downward to the nose in a horizontal direction with respect to the skin. For Yingxiang(IL20), the penetration was 2.0 cm in an oblique direction along the nasolabial sulcus towards the root of the nose with

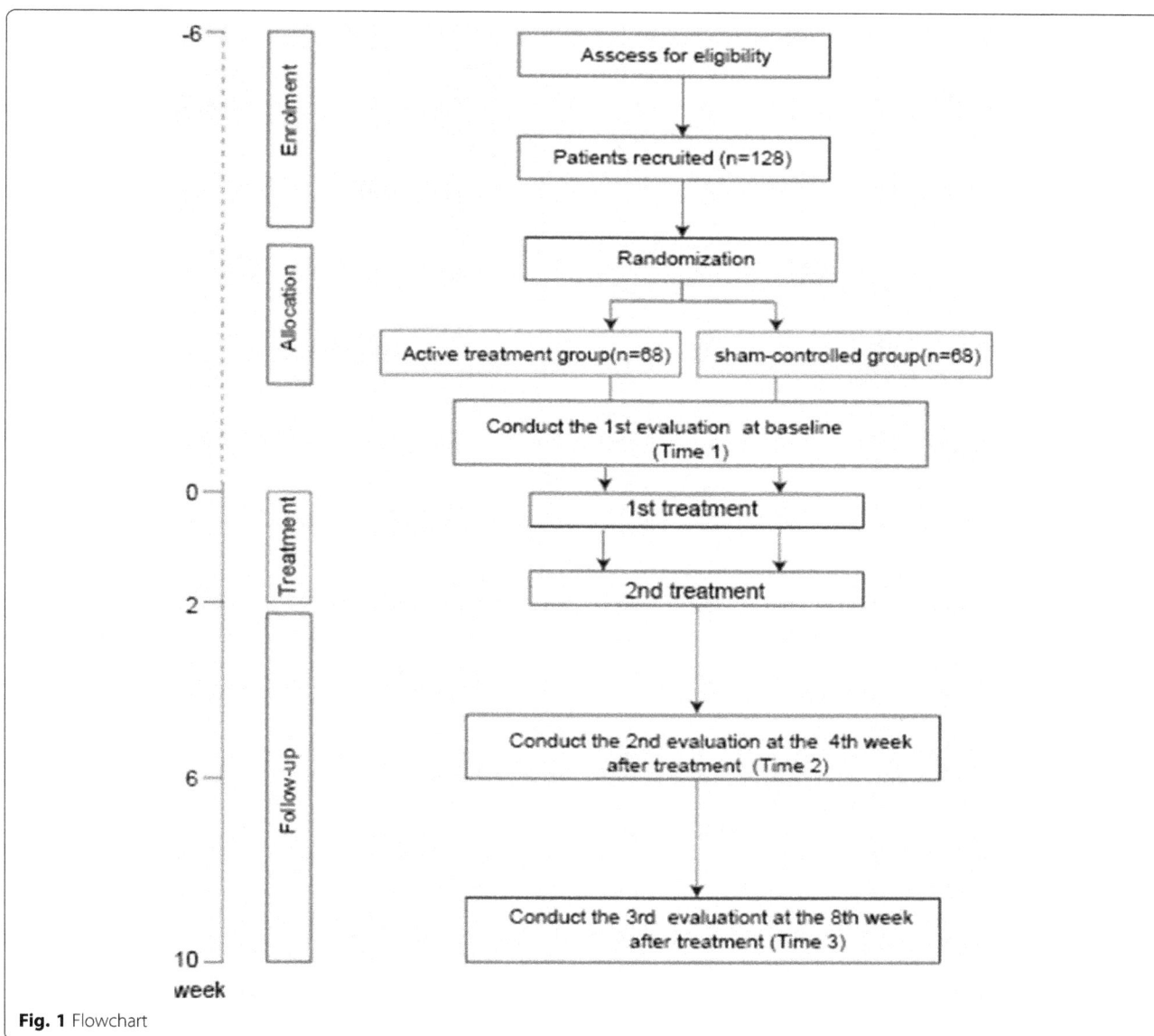

Fig. 1 Flowchart

respect to the skin. For Hegu, Zusanli, and Quchi, the penetration was 2.5 cm, and carried out in a perpendicular direction with respect to the skin (Table 1). Twirling, lifting, and thrusting of the needle were performed. After treatment, the skin of the acupoints should not be touched with water or any cosmetics for three days.

Needle used for catgut implantation was made up of two parts: the internal blunt stylet and the external cannula with a sharp pinhead which ensured that the cannula could puncture the skin. These two parts made the needle similar to a kind of trocar. In real catgut embedding, the internal stylet should be withdrawn from the cannula for about 1.5 cm. Then a 2- to 3-mm catgut was placed into the cannula from the side of the pinhead. When the needle is inserted into the acupoints with

proper depth, the catgut was pushed into the tissue of the acupoint by the stylet (Figs. 3 and 4).

For sham catgut implantation, the whole therapeutic procedure was the same as that in the real group, with the same acupoints, the same needles, and the standard techniques. However, only the sham treatment group did not contain catgut was not present in the cannula in the sham treatment. Without the catgut embedded in acupoints, patients in this group received just the stimulus of needling. To ensure the blinding, acupuncturists were instructed not to communicate with the participants throughout the duration of the treatment.

In both groups, patients were permitted to use chlorpheniramine when needed. The use of chlorpheniramine (dosage, frequency, and period of treatment) should be recorded as relief medicine scores.

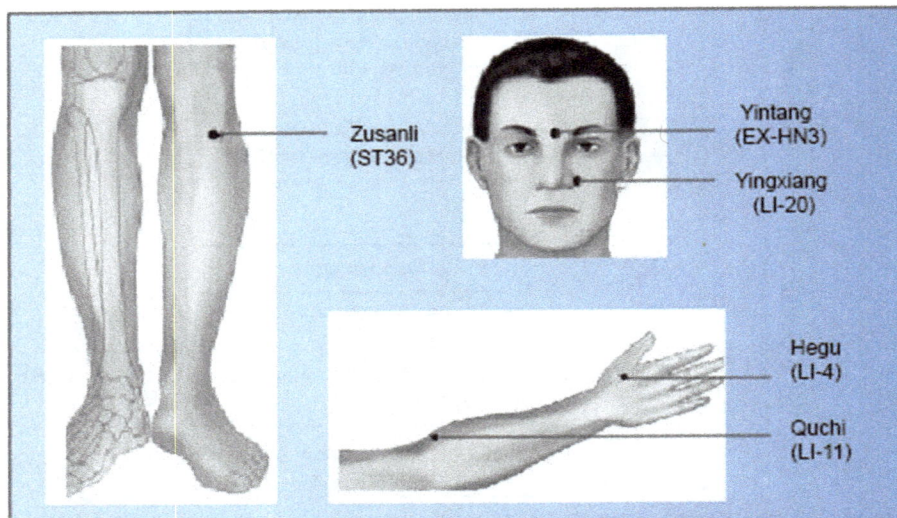

Fig. 2 Locations of selected acupoints (for both of the groups)

Clinical evaluation

Primary outcome

Visual analogue scale (VAS) [22] and Rhinoconjunctivitis Quality of Life Questionnaire (RQLQ) [23, 24] were used to evaluate the severity of the symptoms of allergic rhinitis at week 0 (baseline) and at weeks 2 and 8. In VAS, the influence of the presenting symptoms of allergic rhinitis on each participant was evaluated. The symptoms were classified as mild, moderate, or severe based on the total VAS score (0–10 cm: mild, VAS 0–3; moderate, VAS 3.1–7; severe, VAS 7.1–10).

RQLQ was also used to assess the disease-associated problems of the participants in seven aspects of daily life: activities, sleep, non-nose/eye symptoms, practical problems, nasal symptoms, nose symptoms, and emotional symptoms. The score of each of the item was graded into 0–6. The total score of the seven items was calculated for every participant at baseline and at weeks 4 and 10.

Secondary outcome

Relief medication scores and adverse events were evaluated as the secondary outcome. Participants were asked to complete diaries in the baseline and every two weeks after randomization. In the diaries, the participants

recorded if H_1-blocker (chlorpheniramine) had been taken during the treatment period, including the dosage and time of medication. In addition, adverse events (e.g., numbness, hematoma, local infection of the acupuncture sites, headache, fainting, and serious pain) were also recorded during the treatment and follow-up phases.

Statistical analysis

The sample size was estimated from equations and our preliminary study. An improvement of no less than 25 % of the treatment group compared with the sham-controlled one was suggested. With participants recruited in the two groups in a 1:1 ratio, the following formula was used to estimate sample size [25]:

$$n_1 = n_2 = \left[\frac{Z_\alpha\sqrt{2\pi_c(1-\pi_c)} + Z_\beta\sqrt{\pi_1(1-\pi_1) + \pi_2(1-\pi_2)}}{\pi_1-\pi_2} \right]^2$$

In the formula, n_1 and n_2 represent the sample size of each group. π_1 and π_2 are the overall rates of each sample. $\pi_c = (\pi_1 + \pi_2)/2$, $\alpha = 0.05$, $Z_{0.05} = 1{,}96$, $\beta = 0.10$, $Z_{0.10} = 1.282$. Statistical analysis was performed using 5 % significance and 90 % power, resulting in an estimated 64 patients per group.

Table 1 Acupoints and manipulation in both the real and sham groups

Weeks for treatment	Acupoints	Angle and direction	Depth
Week 1	Yintang(EX-HN3) (unilateral)	Downward to the nose in a horizontal direction with respect to the shin	1.0 cm
	Yingxiang(LI20) (both)	In an oblique direction along the nasolabial sulcus towards the root of nose with respect to the skin	2.0 cm
	Hegu(LI4) (both)	Perpendicular direction with respect to the skin	2.5 cm
Week 2	Zusanli(ST36) (both)	Perpendicular with respect to the skin	2.5 cm
	Quchi(IL11) (both)	Perpendicular direction with respect to the skin	2.5 cm

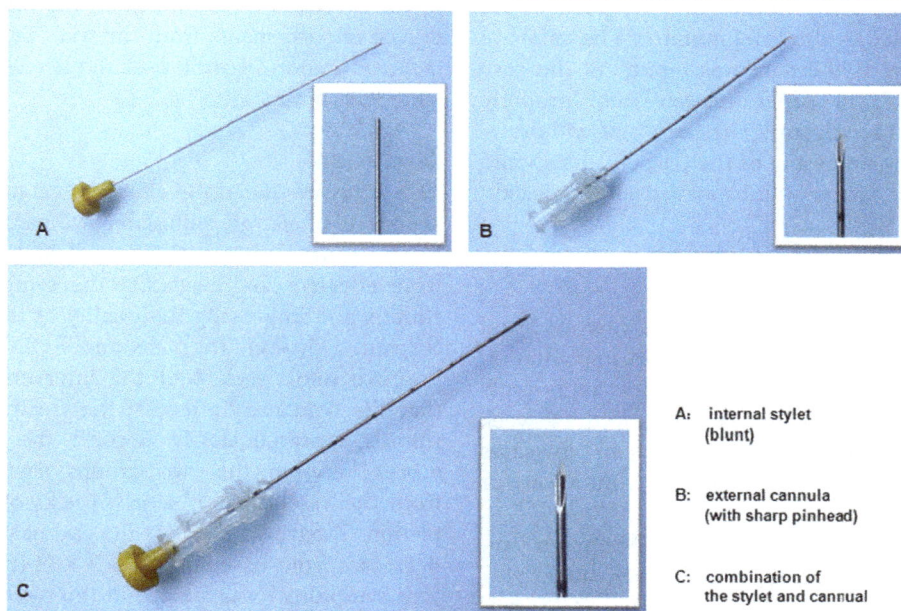

Fig. 3 Needle used for the treatment

A: internal stylet
      (blunt)

B: external cannula
      (with sharp pinhead)

C: combination of
      the stylet and cannual

To assess the baseline characteristics of the two groups, unpaired t test or x^2 test was used. In comparing the efficacy of real catgut implantation with the sham one, the chi-square test was used for analysis of categorical data. Measurement data were analyzed using the independent sample test or Kruskal-Wallis H Test. For non-normally distributed data, Wilcoxon rank-sum test was used. Statistical analysis was performed with SPSS software version 19 (SPSS Inc., Illinois) and the values were considered statistically significant at $P < 0.05$. Statistical analysis was carried out in a blinded manner by qualified statisticians.

An intention-to-treat (ITT) analysis of the results was conducted based on the initial treatment assignment. Participants who strayed from the protocol (for instance, by not adhering to the prescribed intervention, or by withdrawing from the study due to adverse event or other reasons) should still be kept in the analysis. The missing data were supplemented with those obtained recently before the participant was lost to follow-up. A complete outcome data was performed for all randomized subjects.

Patient safety

Before randomization, the participants were asked to take routine blood, urine, liver function, blood glucose, and kidney function tests to exclude any related serious illness. When any adverse effect occurred, proper medical treatment should be given as soon as possible.

Quality control

All acupuncturists were experienced in the technique for catgut implantation, and how to deal with adverse events. The acupuncturists also received training on how to communicate with participants and how to keep them blind to the treatment throughout the trial.

In order to maintain the quality of this trial, audits were conducted regularly on compliance with standard

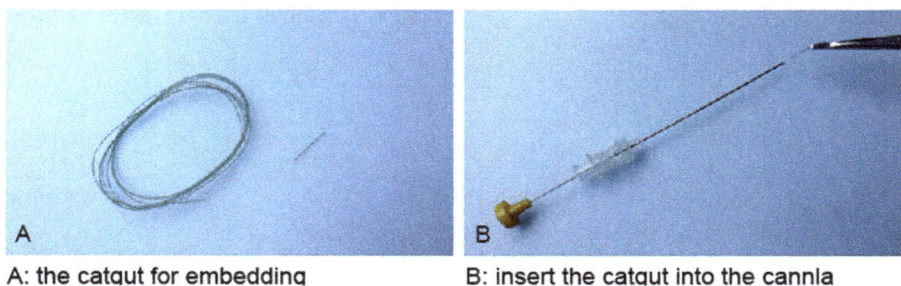

A: the catgut for embedding

B: insert the catgut into the cannla

Fig. 4 Insert the catgut into the cannula of the needle

operation procedures every week, and the reports of the audits were presented to the chief monitor. The database was locked as soon as the data was input. All the case report forms (CRF) in paper version were properly maintained by the investigator. The reason of withdrawing or loss of follow-up of any of the participants should be clarified, and the rate should be statistically analyzed.

Results

Participant characteristics at baseline

A total of 128 participants with AR were recruited and randomly assigned to the active catgut implantation group or the sham-controlled group in a 1:1 ratio. Only two of the patients were unable to complete the 2-week treatment. In the follow-up period, another six cases dropped out. The main reasons for the withdrawals or dropouts are listed in Table 2.

No significant differences were identified between subjects in either group regarding age, gender, underlying health status, RQLQ score, VAS score and TCM syndrome type on baseline (Table 3)

Primary outcome

For the analysis based on VAS scores, the difference between the treatment group and the sham-controlled group was not significant until 8 weeks after the 2-week treatment regimen ($t = -2.424$, $P = 0.017$; Table 4). However, the RQLQ scores between the two groups after 2 weeks of treatment completion significantly differed ($t = -2.045$, $P = 0.05$), and this difference could be observed until the end of the 8-week follow-up ($t = -2.246$, $P = 0.033$).

In the self-control study, the efficacy of the active treatment and sham groups was evaluated. The results indicated a significant improvement in the VAS and RQLQ scores of both the groups at weeks 4 and 8 after the treatment regimen when compared with the respective baseline scores. These differences are illustrated in Table 5.

Secondary outcome

None of the participants took H_1 blockers (chlorpheniramine) as relief medicine.

No adverse events occurred that necessitated withdrawal of participants from the trial. The reported events included minor discomfort at the needling sites and subcutaneous induration (Table 6).

Discussion

This study evaluated the effects of catgut implantation at acupoints of allergic rhinitis in two parallel samples. The results showed that both the real and sham treatments were effective for alleviating the symptoms of allergic rhinitis and improving the quality of the life of the participant. However, the VAS and RQLQ scores did not improve until week 4 of the interventions, suggesting that the regulatory effect of the treatments for allergic rhinitis appeared slowly. Second, the VAS and RQLQ scores between the two groups significantly differed from the baseline after 4 or 8 weeks of treatment completion. Twelve weeks after the end of the treatment, the decreases from baseline in the TNSS (total score for the four symptoms) was greater in the treatment group than in the sham group. The improvement in the TNSS and RQLQ with treatment and the persistence of the effect appear to be the most clinically significant findings of the study.

To our knowledge, no other randomized controlled trial of catgut implantation has been reported in English, although many recent reports in Chinese literatures have reported the efficacy of this intervention for allergic rhinitis. Catgut implantation is a subtype of acupuncture that can extend the sensation of needling because of the persistent stimulus to acupoints caused by the embedded catgut. Furthermore, catgut implantation has an effect which is similar to pricking blood therapy. It was found to have a therapeutic effect for chronic diseases by dredging the channels, invigorating the pulse, and regulating the qi and blood. Our study demonstrates positive outcomes of both active and sham catgut implantation for allergic rhinitis. Although no catgut was embedded in the acupoints in the patients receiving sham treatment, the penetrating of the needles produces a therapeutic stimulation similar to that in conventional acupuncture. The external diameter of the needle (9#) used in the treatment is approximately 0.9 mm, which is larger than that used in acupuncture. The thicker the

Table 2 Reasons for withdrawal or dropout

	Group A (Active treatment group)		Group B (Sham-controlled group)	
	Patients lost to follow-up	Reason	Patients lost to follow-up	Reason
During treatment (weeks 0–2)	1	Not adhering to the prescribed intervention	1	Not adhering to the prescribed intervention
During follow-up (weeks 2–10)	2	Too busy to complete follow-up	1	Too busy to complete follow-up
	1	Admitted to the hospital for appendectomy	2	Went abroad for business or tour

Table 3 Subject characteristics

	Group A (Active treatment group)	Group B (Sham-controlled group)	Statistics	P value
Age (years)	36.112 ± 11.495	38.083 ± 12.106	T = 1.047	0.297
Gender[a] (males/female)	29/35	36/28	x^2=1.532	0.216
Weight (kg)	60.391 ± 9.407	59.817 ± 8.697	t = 0.177	0.860
Height (cm)[b]	166.031 ± 6.575	164.752 ± 6.731	U = 1854.5	0.356
Pulse (beats/min)[b]	75.828 ± 6.870	77.297 ± 6.004	U = 1788.000	0.214
EO (10^9/L)[b]	0.201 ± 0.132	0.195 ± 0.139	U = 1952.000	0.647
AST (U/L)	28.141 ± 7.322	29.672 ± 9.952	t = −0.991	0.324
ALT (U/L)	21.656 ± 6.393	23.125 ± 6.646	t = −1.274	0.205
BUN (mmol/L)[b]	4.572 ± 1.540	4.988 ± 1.325	U = 1804.000	0.245
Crea (μmol/L)[b]	53.367 ± 11.068	56.094 ± 9.018	U = 1726.520	0.125
RQLQ score	83.933 ± 10.076	88.801 ± 8.872	t = −1.405	0.171
VAS score[b]	7.036 ± 1.839	6.648 ± 1.379	U = 1739.500	0.136
TCM syndrome type[a] (number of patients)			x^2=1.030	0.794
Insufficiency of the Spleen-qi[a]	25	23	–	–
Insufficiency of the Lung-qi[a]	23	26	–	–
Insufficiency of the Kidney-yang[a]	9	6	–	–
Retention of the Pathogenic Heat of the Lung[a]	7	9	–	–

RQLQ Rhinitis Quality of Life Questionnaire, VAS Visual Analogue Scale
For each variable except gender and TCM syndrome type, the values are expressed as the means ± SD
[a]Chi-square test
[b]Wilcoxon rank-sum test for the non-normally distributed data
The categories without [a] or [b] were analyzed with t test

needle, the greater is the intensity of stimulation. Therefore, the participants in the controlled group received both the acupuncture stimulus and pricking blood therapy. This might explain the improved scores of VAS and RQLQ in the sham-controlled group. However, the improvements in the sham group were inferior at weeks 4 and 8 after treatment compared to the treatment group. This difference might be due to the slow but lasting stimulation of catgut implanted at the acupoints.

Deciding on an appropriate control procedure for clinical studies on catgut implantation at acupoints is a particular challenge. For the clinical trial of acupuncture, two approaches for sham-controlled treatment have been to use non-penetrating needles [26, 27] or needles inserted shallowly 1–2 cm away from the defined acupoints [28, 29]. Based on the special structure of the

needle for catgut implantation, we found that the best approach for the sham treatment was to insert needles at the same acupoints with the same acupuncture manipulation but without embedding catgut. The difference between the two groups depended on whether or not the catgut was embedded. Consistent with the findings of our previous study on catgut implantation for allergic rhinitis, we found that the participants could be blind adequately by this approach. The sham treatment may have unspecific physiological effects of needling or just have placebo effects. In both groups, minor and minimal adverse events occurred only in a few cases, none of which were serious and did not result in participant withdrawal from the trial.

In our study, five acupoints were chosen for the treatment: Yintang (EX-HN3), Yingxiang (LI20),Zusanli (ST36),

Table 4 Results on RQLQ and total VAS scores between the two groups (means ± SD)

	Total VAS score			RQLQ score		
	T1	T2	T3	T1	T2	T3
Treatment group (n = 64)	7.036 ± 1.839	5.302 ± 1.86	3.75 ± 1.93	83.933 ± 10.076	78.67 ± 8.57	73.73 ± 10.48
Sham-controlled group (n = 64)	6.648 ± 1.379	5.204 ± 1.72	4.535 ± 1.724	88.801 ± 8.872	84.471 ± 6.883	79.807 ± 6.221
Statistical analysis	U = 1739.500	t =0.324	t = −2.424	t = −1.405	t = −2.045	t = −2.246
P value	0.136	0.751	0.017	0.171	0.050	0.033

T1, baseline at subject recruitment
T2, 2 weeks after intervention
T3, 8 weeks after intervention

Table 5 Efficacy of the active and sham-controlled groups in the self-control study

		Group A		GroupB	
		VAS	RQLQ	VAS	RQLQ
T2-T1	Statistical t value	9.887	4.314	12.599	5.951
	P value	$P < 0.001$	0.001	$P < 0.001$	$P < 0.001$
T3-T1	Statistical t value	13.153	6.287	13.659	5.892
	P value	$P < 0.001$	$P < 0.001$	$P < 0.001$	$P < 0.001$

T1, baseline at subject recruitment
T2, 4 weeks after intervention
T3, 8 weeks after intervention

Hegu (LI4), and Quchi (LI11). The selection of acupoints was guided by Chinese traditional medicinal theory. In traditional acupuncture theories, allergic rhinitis is stated as Biqiu, which is in close correlation with the Taiyin lung meridian of hand and Yangming large intestine meridian of hand. Thus, the most frequently used specific acupoints for these two meridians would be selected in this trial according to a previous review of ancient and modern literature. The ancient Chinese also believed that Yangming is a meridian abundant of blood and Qi and is the acquired foundation. Four of the five acupoints selected in the study are on the Yangming Meridian, namely, Yingxiang (LI20),Zusanli (ST36), Hegu(LI4), and Quchi (LI11). Hegu(LI4) is the source-point of the large intestine meridian of the hand. Qi of the visceral is input at this point. Based on the theory in TCM, the lung opens at the nose and the large intestine which are interior-exteriorly related. Therefore, Yingxiang (LI20) and Hegu (LI4) are important acupoints for improving lung air (qi) deficiency syndrome. Zusanli (ST36) and Quchi(LI11) are sea points of Yangming large intestine meridian of the hand and Yangming stomach meridian of the foot. These acupoints are used to fortify the spleen and replenish the Qi. At the same time, stimulation of these points could reinforce earth to generate metal and regulate asthenia-cold in the remission stage of allergic rhinitis.

On the other hand, the nose is an orifice with lucid Yangin traditional Chinese medicine. Lucid Yang is confluent at the acupoints of Yingxiang (LI20) and Yintang(EX-HN3). These two acupoints are on the median line of the face and play an important role in

clearing the nasal passages. In addition, Yingxiang (LI20) is considered a specific point on the Yangming large intestine meridian of the hand. In our previous trial, it has been suggested that symptoms of allergic rhinitis could be effectively alleviated by embedding catgut at these acupoints.

Not many studies have investigated the mechanism of catgut implantation at acupoints. We explored the probable mechanism focusing on neurogenic inflammation. Some studies have demonstrated that nerve stimulation could induce leukocyte activation and plasma extravasation, which is termed neurogenic inflammation [30, 31]. Based on this theory, we speculated that catgut implantation at acupoints might stimulate the sensory nerve and regulate the neuropeptide-mediated airway smooth muscle constriction and decrease vascular permeability of the nose. Our results showed that there was significant decrease in neuropeptides such as substance P (SP), neurokinin A (NKA), and calcitonin gene-related peptide (CGRP) in the nasal mucosa of catgut implantation group [32]. Hematoxylin-eosinstaining (HE) staining revealed that edema of the nasal mucosa was alleviated and the number of inflammatory cells decreased in the treatment group. This might be a preliminary attempt to understand the mechanism of acupuncture with catgut in the treatment of allergic rhinitis. Further studies are needed to elucidate the effective relationship stimulation for this treatment.

In our study, participants were permitted to take chlorpheniramine as relief medicine when they considered it necessary. As a first-generation oral H1-antihistamine, chlorpheniramine has been used to treat allergic diseases for a long time. In recent decades, it has not been recommended as the first-line medicine for allergic rhinitis as second-generation drugs are available and because of its sedative and anticholinergic effects. In our study, we desired to use short-acting relief medication that would not have a lasting effect and would only last until the participant could endure the symptoms of allergic rhinitis and stopped taking the medicine. Compared with other first-generation H1-antihistamines, chlorpheniramine has the weakest influence on the central nervous system and cardiovascular system. Furthermore, the peak concentration of this drug in plasma is

Table 6 Reported events associated with real and sham treatment participants

Group	Cases	Adverse events	Degree	Measurement	Prognosis of the adverse events
Group A	3	Subcutaneous induration the size of a grain of rice at Yingxiang(LI20) or Yintang(EX-HN3)	Mild	Hot-wet compression at the acupoint	The subcutaneous induration gradually disappeared 2–4weeks after the treatment
	1	Ache in the leg after catgut implantation at Zusanli(ST36)	Mild	Hot-wet compression was applied at the acupoint 24 h after the treatment	Cured
Group B	3	Ache in the leg after catgut implantation at Zusanli(ST36)	Mild to moderate	Hot-wet compression was applied at the acupoint 24 h after the treatment	Cured

reached in2.8 ± 0.8 h. The effect lasts 18–24 h. On the other hand, a longer duration of action-persistence of clinical effects could be found in second-generation antihistamines. In order to minimize the effect of the drug on the study participants, we selected chlorpheniramine as the drug of choice. For participant safety, they were advised not to drive or work at heights or engage in work involving attention to detail after taking the drug.

Although relief medicine was available as a rescue method, none of the participants took medication to relieve their symptoms. For most of the participants, the mean VAS score ranged from 5.2–8.9. In weeks 4 and 8 after treatment, within-group comparison revealed this score decreased significantly, which indicated that both real and sham catgut implantation were effective. Therefore, we believe this is why few participants sought to take relief medication during the treatment period.

There are many topics in clinical studies on allergic rhinitis. According to the severity of the disease, a stepwise treatment was proposed in the ARIA workshop, which include oral H1-antihistamines, antileukotrienes, intranasal glucocorticosteroids, intranasal H1-blocker, decongestant, specific immunotherapy, and so on. However due to the complexity of AR pathogenesis, multiple risk factors, pharmacologic treatment is not effective in all patients. Around one third of patients with moderate/severe symptoms are uncontrolled despite optimal pharmacologic treatment and some still have severe symptoms [1].

Catgut implantation at acupoints is one of the external therapies of TCM, which tries to stimulate certain portions of the body by mechanism stimulation. In fact, external therapy is also based on the differentiation of a symptom-complex and the principle behind this treatment is to invigorate or strengthen the automatic regulation capacity of the body through the meridians and collaterals.

Although the external therapy is totally different from conventional medicine, these two types of treatment should respect and complement each other. Zhou [33] integrated catgut implantation at acupoints with Loratadine tablet and Budesonide nasal spray to treat several allergic rhinitis. The result indicated a long-term improvement of severity of symptoms and signs of allergic rhinitis by the therapy. But there are various risks of biases of this trial, high level evidence could not be obtained.

Well-designed RCTs needed be conducted to provide a definitive answer for the combination therapy.

From the long-term perspective, delaying the occurrence and progression of AR and establishing an efficient and practical prevention and control system is the focus of the future AR research in the world. Possible future research direction of integrating TCM with western

medication may provide a new space for the development of therapy against AR.

Although this is the first robust randomized, double-blinded large-scale clinical trial of catgut implantation at acupoints for allergic rhinitis, there are still some limitations. First, only two sessions of treatments were administrated. The duration of treatment using acupuncture with catgut is unknown. Thus, it is possible that shorter durations could have a similar effect, and that longer use of the treatment or repeated treatments may enhance the outcome, although further studies are required to verify this. Second, all participants in this study were followed up for only eight weeks. Our result just revealed a short-term efficacy of catgut implantation at acupoints for allergic rhinitis. Further research is still needed.

Conclusion
Based on the efficacy of improving the VAS and RQLQ scores of allergic rhinitis and minor adverse events, we concluded that catgut implantation at acupoints may provide an effective and safe option for the symptomatic treatment of allergic rhinitis. This study might be the first to present good clinical evidence of this treatment in allergic rhinitis.

Acknowledgements
We would like to thank Prof. DY Wang, from the Yong Loo Lin School of Medicine, National University of Singapore, for his advice in the study design. Also, the authors would like to acknowledge the helpful comments from the reviewers.

Funding
This trial was financially supported by National Natural Science Foundation of China (No.81273985, No.81473523 and No.81603492), Doctoral Fund of Ministry of Education of China (No.20125132110011), Primary Funding Source: Ministry of Science and Technology of the People's Republic of China through the Twelfth Five-Year National Science and Technology Pillar Program(No. 2015BAI04B00). The funding agent plays no role in study design, data collection, data analyses, data interpretation, or writing of the report.

Authors' contributions
XRL, YL, QXZ and JZ designed the study, conducted the questionnaire interview, and selected the subjects. XRL YL and NX wrote the manuscript. JZ, XPW, MH and QC developed the computational methods for pattern differentiation, performed the statistical analysis. All authors read and approved the final version of the manuscript.

Competing interests
The authors declare that they have no competing interests.

Author details
[1]Department of Otorhinolaryngology, Head and Neck Surgery of the Teaching Hospital of Chengdu University of Traditional Chinese Medicine, Chengdu, Sichuan Province 610072, People's Republic of China. [2]Chengdu University of Traditional Chinese Medicine, Chengdu, Sichuan Province 610072, People's Republic of China.

References
1. Bousquet J, Khaltaev N, Cruz AA, Denburg J, Fokkens WJ, Togias A, Zuberbier T, Baena-Cagnani CE, Canonica GW, van Weel C, Agache I, Aït-Khaled N, Bachert C, Blaiss MS, Bonini S, Boulet LP, Bousquet PJ, Camargos P, Carlsen KH, Chen Y, Custovic A, Dahl R, Demoly P, Douagui H, Durham SR, Gerth van Wijk R, Kalayci O, Kaliner MA, Kim YY, Kowalski ML, et al. Allergic rhinitis and its impact on asthma(ARIA) 2008. Allergy. 2008;63(Suppl.86):8–160.
2. Zhen D. Nasal mucosal hyperreactive rhinopathy. In: Weijia K, Liang Z, Geng X, Bingquan W, Anzhou T, editors. Otorhinolaryngology-Head and neck surgery. Chapter 2. 2nd ed. Beijing: People's Medical Publishing House; 2010. p. 288.
3. Juniper EF, Thompson AK, Ferrie PJ, Roberts JN. Validation of the standardized version of the rhinoconjunctivitis quality of life questionnaire. J Allergy Clin Immunol. 1999;104:364–9.
4. Bousquet J, Lund VJ, van Cauwenberge P, Bremard-Oury C, Mounedji N, Stevens MT, El-Akkad T. Implementation of guidelines for seasonal allergic rhinitis: A randomized controlled trial. Allergy. 2003;58:733–41.
5. Kung YY, Chen YC, Hwang SJ, Chen TJ, Chen FP. The prescriptions frequencies and patterns of Chinese herbal medicine for allergic rhinitis in Taiwan. Allergy. 2006;61:1316–8.
6. Xue CC, English R, Zhang JJ, Da Costa C, Li CG. Effect of acupuncture in the treatment of seasonal allergic rhinitis: A randomized controlled clinical trial. Am J Chin Med. 2002;30:1–11.
7. Ortiz M, Witt CM, Binting S, Helmreich C, Hummelsberger J, Pfab F, Wullinger M, Irnich D, Linde K, Niggemann B, Willich SN, Brinkhaus B. A randomised multicentre trial of acupuncture in patients with seasonal allergic rhinitis–trial intervention including physician and treatment characteristics. BMC Complement Altern Med. 2014;14:128.
8. Ernst E. Acupuncture for persistent allergic rhinitis: A randomised, sham-controlled trial. Med J Aust. 2008;188:64.
9. Magnusson AL, Rita EB. The effect of acupuncture on allergic rhinitis: A randomized controlled clinical trial. Am J Chin Med. 2004;32:105–15.
10. Brinkhaus B, Witt CM, Jena S, Liecker B, Weqscheider K, Willich SN. Acupuncture in patients with allergic rhinitis: A pragmatic randomized trial. Ann Allergy Asthma Immunol. 2008;101:535–43.
11. Zhou K. Clinical obseraviton for catgut implantation at acupoints combined with moxibustion for treatment of allergic rhinitis. Clin J Tradit Chin Med. 2011;23:599–600.
12. Zhu Y, Wang YM, Du Y. Obseraviton for the therapy of catgut implantation at dorsal acupoints combined with cupping glass for 36 cases with allergic rhinitis. Hebei J Tradit Chin Med. 2009;31:422–3.
13. Guo YQ, Chen LY, Zhang SP. Comparison of short-term therapeutic effects of acupoint catgut embedding and crude herb moxibustion on allergic rhinitis. Chin Acupunct Moxibustion. 2004;24:16–8.
14. Xin-rong LI, Qin-xiu Z, Min L, Qing C, Yang L, Zhen-dong Z. Catgut implantation at acupoints for allergic rhinitis: a systematic review. Chin J Integr Med. 2014;20:235–40.
15. Li X, Zhang Q, Jiang L, Li T, Liu M, Liu H, Wang X, Zhang F. Clinical effect of catgut implantation at acupoints for allergic rhinitis: Study protocol for a randomized controlled trial. Trials. 2013;14:12. doi:10.1186/1745-6215-14-12.
16. Moher D, Hopewell S, Schulz KF, Montori V, Gøtzsche PC, Devereaux PJ, Elbourne D, Egger M, Altman DG. Consolidated standards of reporting trials group. Consort 2010 explanation and elaboration: Updated guidelines for reporting parallel group randomised trials. J Clin Epidemiol. 2010;63:e1–37.
17. MacPherson H, Altman DG, Hammerschlag R, Youping L, Taixiang W, White A, Moher A, on behalf of the STRICTA Revision Group. Revised standards for reporting interventions in clinical trials of acupuncture (STRICTA): extending the consort statement. J Altern Complement Med. 2010;16:ST1–ST14.
18. MacPherson H, White A, Cummings M, Jobst KA, Rose K, Niemtzow RC. Standards for Reporting Interventions in Controlled Trials of Acupuncture: The STRICTA Recommendations. J Altern Complement Med. 2002;8:85–9.
19. World Health Organization. WHO Standard acupuncture point locations in the Western Pacific Region. Geneva: WHO; 2008.
20. Huanxing L, Qingxiu Z, Derong J. Effect of catgut implantation at acupoints for allergic rhinitis in onset period. Chin J Otorhinolaryngol Integr Med. 2012;20:118–9.
21. Wang L, Sherry L, Liu L, Zhang J, Maholoda A, Jiang J. Diagram of Chinese acupoints. 1st ed. Nanjing: Phoenix Science Press of Jiangsu; 2006.
22. Bousquet PJ, Combescure C, Neukirch F, Klossek JM, Méchin H, Daures JP, Bousquet J. Visual analog scales can assess the severity of rhinitis graded according to arir guidelines. Allergy. 2007;62:367–72.
23. Roberts G, Mylonopoulou M, Hurley C, Lack G. Impairment in quality of life is directly related to the level of allergen exposure and allergic airway inflammation. Clin Exp Allergy. 2005;35:1295–300.
24. Juniper EF, Guyatt GH. Development and testing of a new measure of health status for clinical trials in rhinoconjunctivitis. Clin Exp Allergy. 1991;21:77–83.
25. Jiahong L, Xiuhua G. Medical statistics. 2nd ed. Beijing: Science Press; 2011.
26. Streitberger K, Kleinhenz J. Introducing a placebo needle into acupuncture research. Lancet. 1998;352:364–5.
27. McManus CA, Schnyer RN, Kong J, Nguyen LT, Hyun Nam B, Goldman R, Stason WB, Kaptchuk TJ. Sham acupuncture devices - practical advice for researchers. Acupuncture in Medicine. 2007;25:36–40.
28. Xue CC, An X, Cheung TP, Da Costa C, Lenon GB, Thien FC, Story DF. Acupuncture for persistent allergic rhinitis: A randomised, sham-controlled trial. Med J Aust. 2007;187:337–41.
29. Dincer F, Linde K. Sham interventions in randomized clinical trials of acupuncture — a review. Complement Ther Med. 2003;11:235–42.
30. Umeno E, Nadel JA, McDonald DM. Neurogenic inflammation of the rat trachea: fate of neutrophils that adhere to venules. J Appl Physiol. 1990;69:2131–6.
31. McDonald DM. Neurogenic inflammation in the rat trachea. I. changes in venules, leucocytes and epithelial cells. J Neurocytol. 1988;17:583–603.
32. Li XR, Zhang QX, Wang XP, Liu Y, Chen Q, Zhong ZD. Effects of catgut implantation at acupoint of face on regulating nasal mucosa neurogenic inflammation of rats with allergic rhinitis. China J Tradit Chin Med Pharm. 2014;29:2587–90.
33. Zhou WJ, Qin GD, Peng QH, Mo L, Liang ZC, Hou T. Catgut implantation at acupoints for patients with moderate/severe allergic rhinitis. Jiangxi J Tradit Chin Med. 2012;354:46–7.

17

A pilot randomized controlled trial of acupuncture at the *Si Guan Xue* for cancer pain

To-Yi Lam[1], Li-Ming Lu[2], Wai-Man Ling[3] and Li-Zhu Lin[1*]

Abstracts

Background: Pain is a common symptom in cancer patients. Acupuncture is a suggested treatment for a wide range of clinical conditions, usually for its beneficial effects on pain control. *Si guan xue* (the four points) have been widely used in clinical practice, and has shown that it is highly effective, effective in obtaining *qi*, shows strong acupuncture stimulation, and is simple to manipulate and safe to use. Therefore, the aim of this study is to test the protocol and safety of acupuncture at the *si guan xue* in the management of cancer pain.

Methods: This is a single-blind, randomized controlled pilot trial. 42 patients with moderate to severe cancer pain were randomly assigned to three different arms with seven sessions of treatment; that is, treatment arm 1 (the *si guan xue* arm, $n = 14$), treatment arm 2 (the *si guan xue* plus commonly used acupoints arm, $n = 14$) and the control arm (the commonly used acupoints arm $n = 14$). Primary outcomes included acupuncture relieving cancer pain, and patients' subjective improvement as measured by the Patient Global Impression of Change (PGIC). Secondary outcomes included the scores of the European Organization for Research and Treatment of Cancer Quality of Life Questionnaire-Core 30 (EORTC QLQ-C30) and Karnofsky's Performance Status (KPS).

Results: The analysis showed that the cancer pain reduction in treatment arm 2 was most prominent on day 5 when compared with the control arm ($P<0.05$). There was no difference in the scores of PGIC, EORTC QLQ-C30 or KPS among the three groups ($P>0.05$). Furthermore, no serious adverse events were observed.

Conclusions: These results indicate that acupuncture at the *si guan xue* plus commonly used acupoints tends to be effective in reducing cancer pain. However, the sample size was small, and a future multi-centre study with a larger sample size is warranted.

Trial registration: ChiCTR-IOR-15007471 (Retroactively registered on 28 NOV 2015)

Keywords: Acupuncture, *Si guan Xue*, Cancer pain, Randomized controlled trial

Background

Cancer is one of the world's leading causes of death. According to recent reports, 12.7 million people diagnosed with cancer in 2008, and 7.6 million people died of it, accounting for 13% of all the deaths. It has been predicted that the total number of cancer deaths worldwide will increase from 13% in 2007 to 45% in 2030. For newly developed countries, the number is expected to increase from 11.3 million in 2007 to 15.5 million in 2030 [1].

Pain is a common cancer symptom. According to the World Health Organization (WHO) in 1995, there are 24.6 million cancer patients worldwide, 20% to 30% of whom suffer from various levels of pain. Although the three-step analgesic ladder of the WHO has been widely used, there is still a paucity of effective pain controls for many cancer patients, especially those in advanced stages of the disease. Many of these patients need to use analgesics such as opioids which act on the central nervous system. However, they may cause serious side effects, including nausea, vomiting, constipation, dryness

* Correspondence: lizhulin903@139.com
[1]Department of Oncology, Guangzhou University of Chinese Medicine, Guangzhou 510405, China
Full list of author information is available at the end of the article

of mouth, urinary retention, sleep disturbance, confusion, hallucinations, or even respiratory distress. They can give rise to intolerance among patients and coping difficulty for their families [2, 3].

Acupuncture is recommended for a wide range of clinical conditions. In particular, it has beneficial effects on pain control, and more importantly is safe to use. The benefits of acupuncture include rapid onset of analgesic effect, long sustained remission, ease of application, no risk of drug dependence or addiction, and by and large the absence of serious side effects [4].

Si guan xue is a unique combination of acupoints for acupuncture. It was first described in the "Twelve of the original nine-pin, *Lingshu*." It pointed out that "there are five *zang* and six *fu*. The six *fu* come from twelve original *fu*. The original twelve come from the *si* (four) *guan*. The *si guan* treat the five *zang*." Then Yang Jizhou, a famous Chinese Medicine Practitioner of the Ming Dynasty added that, "the *si guan* are *Taichong* (LR3) and

Hegu (LI4)" [5]. The combination of these acupoints has the important effect of communicating the *yin* and *yang*, *zang* and *fu*, superior and inferior parts of the human body, and the *qi* and blood, and thus complementing each other. The *si guan xue* are widely used clinically. They have high treatment efficacy, easily get to the *qi*, are simple to manipulate, and safe to use [6, 7]. Their clinical use and efficacy for many clinical conditions are worthy of further studies. Therefore, this pilot study aims at testing the safety of acupuncture at the *si guan xue* in the management of cancer pain and informing the protocol for a larger study.

Methods

Settings and subjects

A pilot randomized clinical trial was conducted in the Department of Oncology at the First Affiliated Hospital of Guangzhou University of Chinese Medicine and at the OncWell Integrated Cancer Centre in Hong Kong.

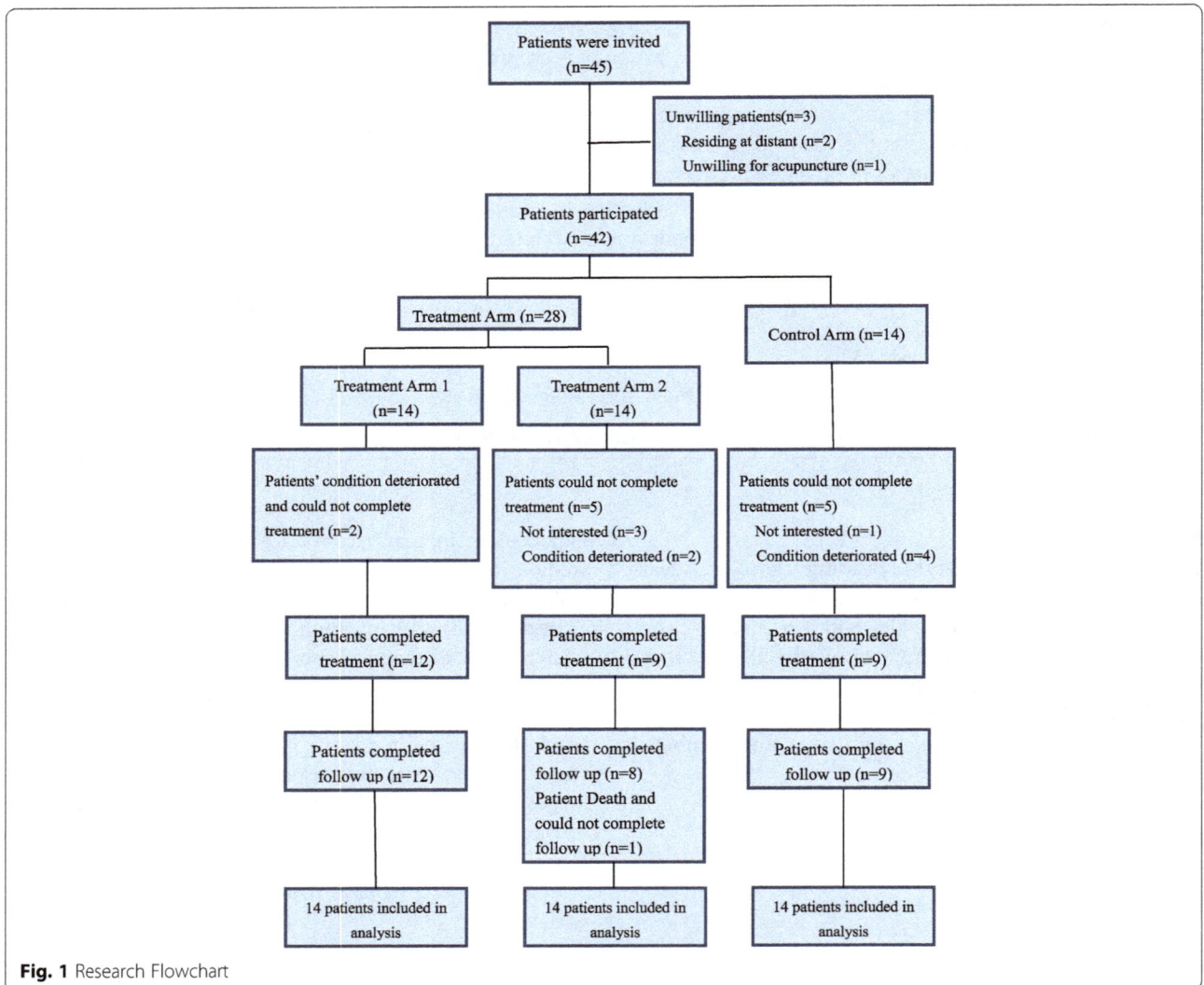

Fig. 1 Research Flowchart

The trial lasted from May 2012 to February 2014. The study protocol was approved by the Ethics Committee of Hong Kong East Cluster (Reference no.: HKEC-2012-024) before the start of the study. The reporting of the study complied with the requirements of the CONSORT 2010 statement [8].

Patients who fulfilled the following criteria were recruited into this study: (1) having advanced cancer with cancer pain as the chief complaint; (2) no chemotherapy or radiotherapy within one month before the study; (3) men or women aged 18 years or above; (4) levels of conscious to the extent that he/she could evaluate and report on their pain; (5) life expectancy of three months or above; and (6) capability of giving informed consent. Those with the following conditions were excluded: (1) pain was unrelated to cancer; (2) inability to report his/her pain accurately; (3) mental illness or lack capacity; (4) children or pregnant/lactating women; (5) other

Table 1 Baseline characteristics of patients (*n* = 45)

General Information	All patients	Participants		Unwilling participants
		Mainland China	Hong Kong	Hong Kong
Sex				
Male	20 (47.62)	15 (50)	5 (41.67)	0 (0)
Female	22 (52.38)	15 (50)	7 (58.33)	3 (100)
Age				
Average	57.59	56	59.17	78.33
Range	24–91	24–79	42–91	74–82
Marital status				
Single	2 (4.76)	0 (0)	2 (16.67)	0 (0)
Married	38 (90.48)	30 (100)	8 (66.66)	2 (67)
Widowed	2 (4.76)	0 (0)	2 (16.67)	1 (33)
Education				
Illiteracy	8 (19.05)	6 (20)	2 (16.67)	1 (33)
Primary school	13 (30.95)	12 (30)	1 (8.33)	1 (33)
Secondary school	2 (4.76)	2 (6.67)	0 (0)	0 (0)
High school	14 (33.33)	9 (30)	5 (41.67)	1 (33)
University or above	5 (11.91)	1 (3.33)	4 (33.33)	0 (0)
Primary Disease Site				
Head and neck	5 (11.9)	1 (3.33)	4 (33.33)	1 (33)
Lung	12 (28.57)	11 (36.67)	1 (8.33)	1 (33)
Breast	3 (7.14)	1 (3.33)	2 (16.67)	0 (0)
Gynecological	6 (14.29)	5 (16.67)	1 (8.33)	0 (0)
Liver	5 (11.9)	5 (16.67)	0 (0)	0 (0)
Upper GI (Esophagus, stomach and spleen)	5 (11.9)	3 (10)	2 (16.67)	0 (0)
Lower GI(Colon)	3 (7.14)	2 (6.67)	1 (8.33)	0 (0)
Other	3 (7.14)	2 (6.67)	1 (8.33)	1 (33)
Stage of cancer				
III	5 (11.9)	1 (3.33)	4 (33.33)	0 (0)
IV	37 (88.1)	29 (96.67)	8 (66.67)	3 (100)
Other chronic diseases	26 (61.9)	20 (66.67)	6 (50)	2 (67)
Level of pain				
Average	5.81	5.9	5.58	7
Range	2–8	2–8	5–8	5–8
KPS score				
Average	70	69	72.5	70
Range	40–90	40–90	60–80	60–80

Table 2 Use of analgesics in the three study arms

Use or not	Arm 1 (n = 14)	Control arm (n = 14)	Arm 2 (n = 14)	P-value
Yes	10	6	7	0.287
No	4	8	7	

serious diseases; (6) unwillingness to cooperate or give informed consent [9–13].

Randomization and blinding

A computer program was used to randomize the participants [14]. The study coordinator was responsible for allocating the randomization codes that indicated the arms into the sequentially numbered and sealed envelopes. These envelopes were concealed from the investigators. In this pilot study, neither the investigators nor the participants were blinded, however the analyst was blinded.

Treatment procedures

The Chinese Medicine style of acupuncture was used. Acupuncture was conducted by two qualified Chinese Medicine Practitioners with nine and twelve years of experience in clinical practice, and three and ten years of acupuncture experience respectively. Both have bachelor's and master's degrees in Chinese Medicine related fields (one of whose master's degrees is in acupuncture), and are well trained in acupuncture. A course of acupuncture with seven treatment sessions, delivered either daily or on alternating days, was given to the patients in the three arms. The standards of the study complied with the requirements of the Checklist for items in the Standards for Reporting Interventions in Clinical Trials of Acupuncture (STRICTA) 2010 [15].

Theoretical basis for using acupuncture to treat cancer pain

The design of our acupuncture treatment protocol was based on traditional Chinese Medicine theory. Pathophysiology of cancer pain, based on Western Medicine, did not affect the formulation of acupuncture interventions in this

Table 3 Types of analgesics used in the three study arms

Drugs	Arm 1 (n = 14)	Control arm (n = 14)	Arm 2 (n = 14)
Morphine	0	3	2
Oxycodone	3	1	3
Fentanyl patch	3	3	4
Celecoxib	2	1	1
Tramadol	2	0	0
Carbamazepine	0	2	1
Meloxicam	0	1	0

Note: P = 0.513

Table 4 Distribution of pain sites

Pain sites	Number of sites		
	All	Mainland China	Hong Kong
Head	2	0	2
Neck and shoulder	10	2	8
Upper limb	8	1	7
Upper back	12	8	4
Lower back	10	8	2
Chest	8	5	3
Upper abdomen	7	5	2
Lower abdomen	8	5	3
Lower limb	20	11	9
Other	5	2	3

study. According to the Chinese medical diagnosis, diseases can be conceptualized as conditions of deficiency or strength. The former refers to the insufficiency of *qi* and blood, *ying* and *yang*, *zang fu* etc., whereas the latter implies a surplus of *qi* and blood. The normal circulation of *qi* and blood in the meridians requires warming by *yang*, moisturizing by *yin*, promotion by *qi* and the nourishment by blood. Deficiency of these elements leads to the malnutrition of *zang fu*, and then the pain. Deficiency is more prominent in advanced cancer patients [16, 17]. The *si guan xue* have been considered to have an important effect on communicating the *yin* and *yang*, *zang* and *fu*, superior and inferior parts of the human body, as well as the *qi* and blood. They thus complement each other. Hence, we hypothesized that *si guan xue* would enhance the treatment effects of the commonly used acupoints.

The choice of Acupoints

There were two treatment arms in the study. Treatment arm 1 used only the *si guan xue*, whereas treatment arm 2 used the *si guan xue* in combination with a set of

Table 5 NRS on the level of pain over the previous 24 h

Level of pain	All patients	Mainland China	Hong Kong
Average of most severe pain	7.48	7.87	6.5
Range	3–10	5–10	3–9
Average number of severe pain outbursts	4.74	4.3	5.83
Range	0–9	1–8	0–9
Average range of slightest pain	3.1	2.93	3.5
Range	0–8	0–7	0–8
Average pain	5.62	5.73	5.33
Range	3–8	3–8	3–8
Average current pain	5.8	5.9	5.58
Range	0–9	1–8	0–9

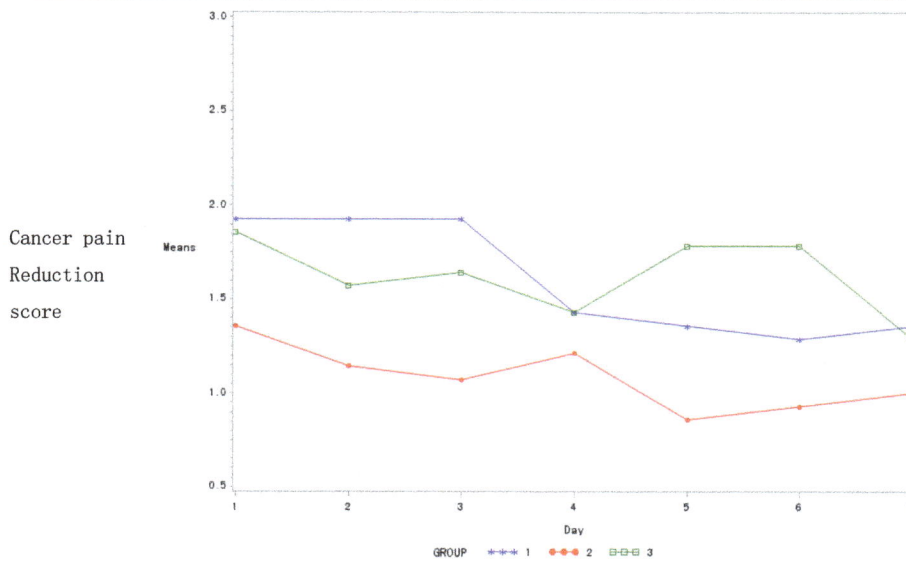

Fig. 2 Changes of pain reduction scores in the three study arms. (Group 1: Treatment arm 1; Group 2: Control group; Group 3: Treatment Arm 2)

commonly used acupoints. This set of commonly used acupoints, including *Neiguan* (PC6), *Zusanli* (ST36) and *Sanyinjiao* (SP6), were chosen according to a previous extensive literature review [18–32]. They also constituted the control arm of the pilot study. All these acupoints, especially those located below the elbow and knee joints of the twelve regular meridians, have therapeutic effects on diseases in both the local and the remote regions.

Acupuncture intervention

Single-use acupuncture needles (0.25 x 25 mm or 0.30 x 40 mm) manufactured by MOCM International Development Limited were inserted under the skin at 10-20 mm vertical depth. Then, a reinforcing-reducing method was used to activate the *qi* until the sensation of the arrival of *qi* (numbness, fullness and heaviness) was

reported by patients. Patients were maintained in supine positions with the needles left in situ for 30 min. A course of acupuncture treatment consisted of seven sessions in total, performed either daily or on alternating days. Safety precautions were conducted for the patients before each treatment session to prevent acupuncture related adverse events such as fainting, hematoma, curved needles and broken needles.

Clinical assessment

The primary outcome of the study, the change in pain, was evaluated by two methods. Firstly, it was measured by the pain assessment form with a numeric rating scale (NRS) from 0 to 10 (0 = the best, 10 = the worst) [33]. Secondly, patients' subjective improvement was assessed using the Patient Global Impression of Change (PGIC) [34].

Table 6 Changes of NRS reduction in the three study arms ($\bar{x} \pm SD$)

Time	Arm 1 (n = 14)	Control arm (n = 14)	Arm 2 (n = 14)	P-value
Day 1	1.93 ± 1.21	1.36 ± 1.15	1.86 ± 1.03	0.36
Day 2	1.93 ± 1.14	1.14 ± 0.77	1.57 ± 1.28	0.17
Day 3	1.93 ± 1.14	1.07 ± 1.07	1.64 ± 1.22	0.14
Day 4	1.43 ± 1.16	1.21 ± 0.97	1.43 ± 1.02	0.83
Day 5	1.36 ± 1.01	0.86 ± 0.86	1.79 ± 0.89[a]	0.04
Day 6	1.29 ± 1.14	0.93 ± 0.83	1.79 ± 1.19[a]	0.11
Day 7	1.36 ± 1.08	1.00 ± 1.04	1.29 ± 1.07	0.65
Main effect of time (P-value)*	>0.05			

*There was no interaction between the changing trends in pain reduction scores and intervention factor of the three groups over time
[a]Compared with the control group, the difference in cancer pain reduction scores was statistically significant, P<0.05

Secondary outcomes included the scores determined by the European Organization for Research and Treatment of Cancer Quality of Life Questionnaire-Core 30 (EORTC QLQ-C30) [35] and the Karnofsky's Performance Status (KPS). Three sets of EORTC QLQ-C30 were completed by the participants; that is, before the start of the study, after completing the 7th acupuncture treatment, and during the follow-up visit 2 weeks after the treatment. KPS was assessed on each follow-up visit.

Statistical analysis

The analyses were performed on the intention-to-treat population, defined as the participants who had completed baseline assessment and at least one evaluation after treatment. A repeated measures design approach was adopted to compare the treatment outcomes (the score of cancer pain reduction, Global Health Scale, Functional Scale, Symptom Scale and KPS) over time between the three groups. A model was established for performing longitudinal data analysis to explore the intervention effect and the time effect. Among-group differences at each measure time point were further examined using Analysis of Variance (ANOVA). Categorical variables, including categorical baseline variables and incidence of adverse events, were analyzed using a Chi-square (χ^2) or Fisher Exact test. Statistical significance was defined as a two-tailed $P < 0.05$. Statistical analysis was performed by SPSS 20.0 (IBM SPSS Inc., Armonk, New York, USA) and SAS 9.2 software (SAS Institute Inc., Cary, USA).

Results
Baseline characteristics

1. General Information on the Accrued Patients

From May 2012 to February 2014, 45 cancer patients were screened. 3 refused to participate in this study because of geographical reasons or unwillingness to accept acupuncture. 42 participants (30 on the Mainland and 12 in Hong Kong) were randomly assigned to the three study arms with 14 in each of them (Fig. 1). 30 (71.4%) participants completed planned course of treatment. However, since all participants finished at least 2 sessions of treatment and at least 2 evaluations after treatment, they were all included in the data analysis.

Baseline characteristics of the patients are listed in Table 1. There were 20 men and 22 women. For patients

Table 7 PGIC scores in the three study arms ($\overline{x} \pm SD$)

Time	Arm 1 (n = 14)	Control arm (n = 14)	Arm 2 (n = 14)	P-value
Day 7	2.42 ± 0.79	2.64 ± 0.67	2.56 ± 0.53	0.74

Table 8 Global health score and changes in the three study arms ($\overline{x} \pm SD$)

Time	Arm 1 (n = 14)	Control arm (n = 14)	Arm 2 (n = 14)	P-value
Baseline	39.88 ± 19.39	32.74 ± 18.90	35.12 ± 15.04	0.57
Day 7	50.60 ± 17.13	44.64 ± 20.83	48.81 ± 16.62	0.68
Follow up	50.60 ± 19.47	45.24 ± 16.89	46.43 ± 18.98	0.73
Main effect of time (P-value)*	<0.05			

*There was no interaction between the changing trends in Global Health scores and the three groups' intervention factors over time

on the Mainland, the majority had their primary cancer disease in the lung ($n = 11$), while it was in the head or neck for those in Hong Kong ($n = 4$). Most of the patients had stage IV cancer ($n = 37$), and some had been suffering from another chronic disease as well ($n = 26$) (Table 1). Before the acupuncture, the mean of pain score was 5.81, which was a moderate level of pain [33]. KPS was 70%, indicating that they could have lived independently, but could not have maintained normal activities or work [36]. Moreover, the use of analgesics was recorded for all accrued patients. There was no statistically significant difference in analgesic use among the three study arms ($P > 0.05$) (Tables 2 and 3).

Information on pain patients before treatment

The number of pain sites for each participant ranged from 1 to 7. There were 90 pain sites in total. Most were located on the lower limbs ($n = 20$) (Table 4). The average NRS pain score over the previous 24 h before acupuncture was 5.62. Nonetheless, the average NRS score for the most severe pain was as high as 7.48, which was defined as "severe" according to the NRS. The occurrence of this severe NRS pain score was 4.74 on average. The average for even the slightest NRS pain score was 3.1 (Table 5). The average NRS pain score right before acupuncture was 5.8, a moderate level of pain [33].

Table 9 Functional scale score and changes in the three study arms ($\overline{x} \pm SD$)

Time	Arm 1 (n = 14)	Control arm (n = 14)	Arm 2 (n = 14)	P-value
Baseline	90.29 ± 4.00#	87.24 ± 3.89	88.60 ± 3.56	0.12
Day 7	91.56 ± 4.94	89.21 ± 4.16	90.35 ± 4.10	0.38
Follow up	90.79 ± 4.85	89.78 ± 3.53	90.48 ± 4.27	0.81
Main effect of time (P-value)*	<0.05			

*There was no interaction between the changing trends of Functional scale scores and the three groups' intervention factors over time

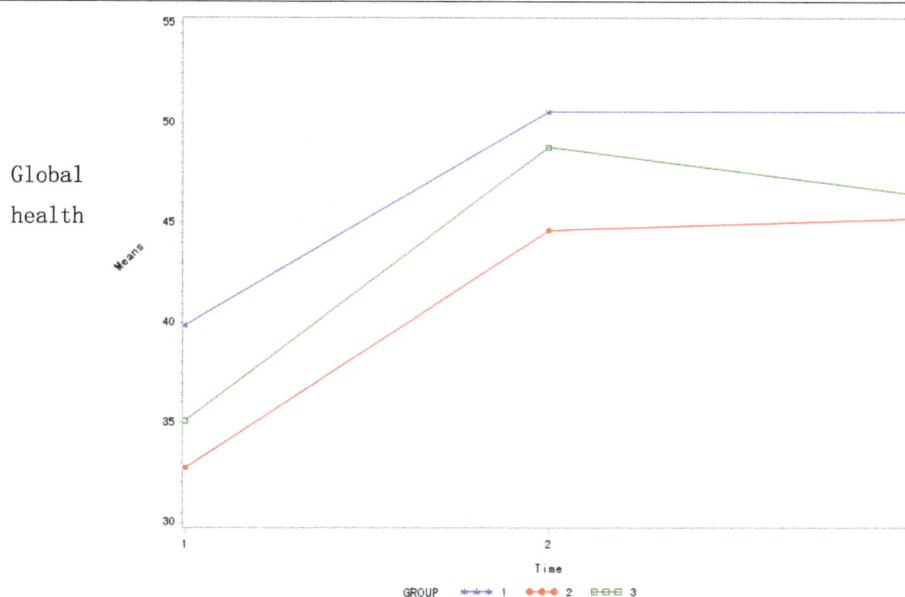

Fig. 3 Global health scores and changes among the 3 groups. (Group 1: Treatment arm 1; Group 2: Control group; Group 3: Treatment Arm 2)

Primary outcome

According to analysis of the seven treatment sessions, the magnitude of pain score reduction tended to decrease in both treatment arm 1 and control arm, while it increased in treatment arm 2 (Fig. 2). For the among-group comparisons at each time point, there was a statistically significant improvement in the pain score in treatment arm 2 on the fifth day of treatment (Table 6) ($P<0.05$). There was no difference among the three groups observed in a repeated measures design approach.

On the other hand, for the patients' perception of the overall improvement, the results of PGIC measurement across the three arms revealed that the difference in their PGIC scores was not statistically significant ($P > 0.05$) (Table 7).

Secondary outcomes

Both the Global Health Scale and the Functional Scale increased during the treatment course (Tables 8, 9 and Fig. 3), whereas the Symptom Scale decreased (Table 10). However, there was no statistically significant difference found across the three arms in all the EORTC QLQ-C30 domains ($P > 0.05$). Additionally, no difference between the three groups was observed in a repeated measures design approach.

The KPS score of the three arms showed an increasing trend during the treatment course, but the difference across the three arms was not statistically significant ($P>0.05$) (Table 11 and Fig. 4).

Safety analysis

The safety of acupuncture, including acupuncture related fainting, hematoma, curved and broken needles was also examined in the pilot study. Throughout the study period, no serious acupuncture-related adverse events occurred. There was only one reported episode of mild local bruising, at one acupuncture site, which was successfully managed with direct digital pressure administered by the practitioner.

Discussion

Acupuncture may be useful in controlling the pain experienced by many cancer patients. It is a complementary and conservative therapy that balances the flow of vital energy, and in turn helps to relieve pain. It is an analgesic adjunctive method for cancer patients that is worthy of additional high quality studies [37–39].

Because of the small sample size, this pilot study mainly intends to examine the preliminary effects of the

Table 10 Symptom scale score and changes in the three study arms ($\overline{x} \pm SD$)

Time	Arm 1 (n = 14)	Control arm (n = 14)	Arm 2 (n = 14)	P-value
Baseline	4.46 ± 1.59	5.45 ± 1.88	5.21 ± 1.86	0.32
Day 7	3.36 ± 2.39	3.93 ± 1.90	4.17 ± 1.92	0.57
Follow up	3.72 ± 2.02	3.91 ± 1.78	4.27 ± 2.10	0.28
Main effect of time (P-value)*	<0.05			

*There was no interaction between the changing trends of Symptom scale scores and the three groups' intervention factors over time

Table 11 KPS score and changes in the three study arms ($\bar{x} \pm SD$)

Time	Arm 1 (n = 14)	Control arm (n = 14)	Arm 2 (n = 14)	P-value
Day 1	70.00 ± 15.19	72.86 ± 13.83	67.14 ± 9.14	0.51
Day 2	70.00 ± 15.19	72.86 ± 13.83	67.14 ± 9.14	0.51
Day 3	70.00 ± 15.19	73.57 ± 13.36	67.86 ± 9.75	0.51
Day 4	70.00 ± 15.19	73.57 ± 13.36	68.57 ± 9.49	0.57
Day 5	70.71 ± 14.92	73.57 ± 13.36	68.57 ± 9.49	0.59
Day 6	70.71 ± 14.92	73.57 ± 13.36	68.57 ± 9.49	0.59
Day 7	70.71 ± 14.92	73.57 ± 13.36	68.57 ± 9.49	0.59
Main effect of time (P-value)*	<0.05			

*There was no interaction between the changing trends of the KPS scores and the three groups' intervention factors over time

acupuncture protocol using the *si guan xue* for cancer pain management for a larger study and its safety. The primary outcomes were the trend of acupuncture in relieving cancer pain and patients' subjective improvement as measured by the PGIC. Secondary outcomes were patients' well-being as determined by the EORTC QLQ-C30 and the KPS. According to the data analysis, the effect of pain relief tended to decrease in treatment arm 1 (*si guan xue* only) and the control arm (commonly used acupoints only). However, it increased in treatment arm 2 (a combination of *si guan xue* and commonly used acupoints), especially on the fifth day of treatment. This phenomenon reflects the fact that acupuncture treatment takes time to accumulate and exert its analgesic effect, which is consistent with the clinical experience of our routine practice [40]. On the other hand, although the trend of analgesic effect was still observed on days 6 and 7, it was not statistically significant. This may be due to the sample size of the pilot study, which is too small to detect any sustained effect.

Also, it revealed that either the acupuncture at *si guan xue* or commonly used acupoints are effective in reducing cancer pain, but that the combination of these two appears to further enhance pain reduction. Thus, this seemed to be a better acupuncture protocol for cancer pain management. There are several possible explanations for this enhanced effect. Firstly, a special technique of acupuncture was used in treatment arm 2. The *si guan xue* was opened first before regulating the commonly used acupoints. It had been recognized that this technique could produce a stronger clinical effect [41, 42]. Secondly, previous studies had suggested that acupuncture at the *si guan xue* could activate the *qi*, replenish the vital substances of the body and strengthen the visceral organs [6, 7]. Thirdly, several other studies have also supported the claim that acupuncture at the *si guan xue* could give rise to sedative, antispasmodic and analgesic effects. Thus, the use of the *si guan xue* would be more effective in controlling cancer pain [43, 44]. Though it was limited to patients with liver cancer, there has been one randomized controlled study of acupuncture at the *si guan xue*. It enrolled 86 patients and revealed that acupuncture achieved a better control on cancer pain than codeine treatment [45]. The results of our pilot study are not only consistent with these previous findings, but also reveal that the beneficial effect on cancer pain is applicable to other cancer-related diseases.

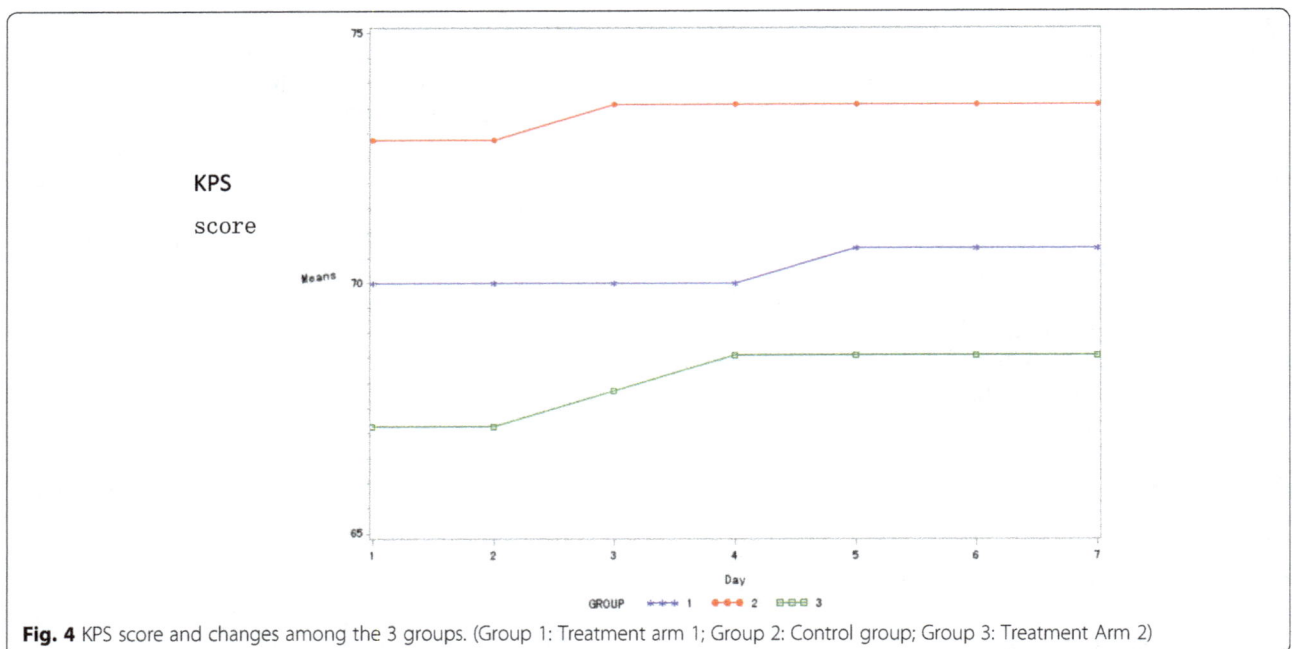

Fig. 4 KPS score and changes among the 3 groups. (Group 1: Treatment arm 1; Group 2: Control group; Group 3: Treatment Arm 2)

There was no statistically significant difference found across the three arms in the PGIC, EORTC QLQ-C30, and KPS scores ($P>0.05$). A possible explanation is that the treatment and evaluation period was too short to reveal the full effect of the acupuncture. However, these clinical outcomes might require longer observation times to see improvement, as documented by these scores. Therefore, the clinicians should contemplate the appropriate duration of acupuncture treatment for cancer pain. A course of 14 acupuncture sessions, or at least 2 weeks of treatment is needed for better management of this problem [40, 46]. In addition, the small sample size is another possible factor accounting for the negative results in the above outcomes.

Limitations of the pilot study

As mentioned above, the main limitation of this study was the small sample size, which was inadequate to confirm the efficacy of acupuncture in the management of cancer pain. Moreover, the treatment and observation time were too short to reveal the full effect of the acupuncture. Seven patients even requested to continue their acupuncture treatment upon completion of the study. This may reflect the fact that acupuncture at the *si guan xue* helps to control their cancer pain and improve their quality of life, but a longer treatment course remains more desirable.

Conclusion

The results of this pilot study indicate that acupuncture at the *si guan xue* plus commonly used acupoints tends to be effective in reducing cancer pain. It may also be beneficial in controlling cancer pain in advanced cancer patients. The use and addition of the *si guan xue* in acupuncture for cancer pain has also been found to be feasible and manageable. Although no firm conclusions can be drawn from such an under-powered study, it did show a trend towards an improvement in cancer pain scores. Therefore, further large scale and multi-centre randomized controlled trials of the *si guan xue* plus commonly used acupoints are warranted to confirm its treatment efficacy.

Acknowledgements
Not applicable.

Funding
There is no external funding for this study. The authors have no financial relationships to disclose.

Authors' contributions
TYL and LZL designed and led the entire study. TYL and LML analyzed and interpreted the patient data for generating the study results. TYL and WML drafted the manuscript. All authors read and approved the final manuscript.

Competing interests
The authors declare that they have no competing interests.

Author details
[1]Department of Oncology, Guangzhou University of Chinese Medicine, Guangzhou 510405, China. [2]The Second Affiliated Hospital of Guangzhou University of Chinese Medicine, Guangdong Provincial Hospital of Chinese Medicine, Guangzhou 510120, China. [3]Department of Clinical Oncology, Pamela Youde Nethersole Eastern Hospital, 3 Lok Man Road, Chai Wan, Hong Kong.

References
1. World Health Organization. Is the number of cancer patients in the world increasing or decreasing? http://www.who.int/features/cancer/zh/. Accessed 15 July 2013.
2. Jadad AR, Browman GP. The WHO analgesic ladder for cancer pain management:stepping up the quality of its evaluation. The Journal of the American Medical Association. 1995;274(23):1870–3.
3. Cherny NI. The Management of Cancer Pain. CA-A Cancer Journal for Clinicians. 2000;50(2):72–3.
4. Johnstone PAS, Polston GR, Martin PJ. Integration of acupuncture into the oncology clinic. Palliat Med. 2002;16:235–9.
5. Yin J, Longxiang H, Jizhou Y. The culmination of Acupuncture. Beijing: People's Medical Publishing House. 2010;7:47.
6. Geng T. Meta clinical experience of si guan xue. Journal of Inner Mongolia Traditional Chinese Medicine. 2007;9:49–51.
7. Jing H, Liu C. Clinical application of si guan xue. Journal of Jilin Traditional Chinese Medicine. 2005;25(4):34.
8. Schulz KF, Altman DG, Moher D; CONSORT Group. CONSORT 2010 statement: updated guidelines for reporting parallel group randomised trials. PLoS Med 2010;3;7(3):e1000251.
9. Wang R, Zhu Y, Hongwen J, et al. Investigation of cancer pain treatment in 43 cases [J]. Pharmaceutical Care and Research. 2004;4(3):287–8.
10. Chen H, Jun P. Clinical observation on the efficacy of Integrative treatment of bone metastases pain in 23 cases [J]. Journal of Yunnan Chinese medicine. 2008;29(10):12–3.
11. Wang H, Wang Y-h. Chinese medicine combined with chemotherapy in the treatment of advanced breast cancer bone metastasis pain in 53 cases [J]. Journal of Henan Traditional Chinese Medicine. 2000;15(5):53–4.
12. Chen Y, Danhong W. Integrative medicine metastatic bone pain in 30 cases [J]. Journal of Fujian Traditional Chinese Medicine. 2001;32(5):12.
13. Dong J, Li Q. Clinical observation on the efficacy of Integrative treatment of bone metastases pain in 27 cases [J]. Journal of Henan Medical College. 2010;22(5):575–7.
14. Urbaniak GC,Plous S. Research Randomizer (Version 4.0) [Computer software]. http://www.randomizer.org//form.htm. Accessed 22 December 2011.
15. MacPherson H, Altman DG, Hammerschlag R, et al. Revised standards for reporting interventions in clinical trials of acupuncture (STRICTA): extending the CONSORT statement. PLoS Med. 2010;7(6):e1000261.
16. Liu Z, Liang L. Essentials of Chinese medicine volume 1. New York : Springer-Verlag London Limited. 2009:284–8.
17. Li Y, Wenbin F. Pain caused by healthy qi deficiency and its management with moxibustion. Hong Kong : Proceedings of the International Academic Seminar of Acumoxa in Pain Management. 2009;5:355–8.
18. Zhang W. Acupuncture treatment of cancer pain in 160 cases. Emergency of Chinese Medicine of China. 2008;17(4):543–4.
19. Gao Z, Xiaohuang XBQR, et al. Clinical observation on the efficacy of combination of acupuncture and topical treatment of cancer pain. Practical Journal of Chinese Medicine. 1998;11:7.
20. Jinhua X. The combination of electroacupuncture with the three-step analgesia for the treatment of cancer pain in 15 cases. Shanghai Journal of Acupuncture. 1999;18(5):21.
21. Guiping Chen, Jinhong Yang, Mei Juan Yu, et al. Acupuncture treatment of radiotherapy and chemotherapy gastrointestinal reactions in 44 cases. Chinese acupuncture and moxibustion, 1996,16(7):9.
22. Rong Mu, Qu Bin Zheng, Wei Zhu Yang, et al. Observation on therapeutic effect of acupuncture of Neiguan in complications of interventional treatment on hepatic carcinoma. Chinese Journal of Integrated Chinese and Western Medicine, 1995,16(10):611.

23. Dong W, Yang J. Observation on acupuncture analgesic effect of cancer pain. Practical Journal of Chinese Medicine. 1999;15(7):28.

24. Deng L. Acupuncture treatment of hepatocellular carcinoma after interventional chemotherapy induced hiccups. Shanxi Chinese Medicine. 1997;13(2):42.

25. Yu D. The clinical study of acupuncture of analgesic effect on cancer pain. Chinese acupuncture and moxibustion. 1998;1(18):17.

26. Bian R. The clinical study of acupuncture treatment on cancer pain of stomach cancer. Journal of Chinese Medicine. 1995;36(5):277–80.

27. Wu B, Zhou R, He K. Research status and prospects of acupuncture and moxibustion regulating immunological function. Shanghai Journal of Acupuncture and moxibustion. 1999;18(1):46.

28. Chen X. Clinical and experimental research survey of acupuncture and moxibustion on antitumor effect. Hubei Journal of Chinese Medicine. 1998;5:59.

29. Gao X. Observation on the therapeutic effect and nursing care of acupuncture combined with three step analgesic ladder treatment of cancer pain. Modern Nursing. 2002;8(8):588.

30. Sun YL, Yu LR. Observation on therapeutic effect of needle-retaining method of triple acupuncture in 80 cases of pain due to liver cancer. Chin Acupuc Moxibustion. 2000;21:211–2.

31. Lee H, Schmidt K, Ernst E. Acupuncture for the relief of cancer-related pain:a systematic review. Eur J Pain. 2005;9:437–44.

32. Peng H, Peng FD, Xu L, et al. Efficacy of acupuncture in treatment of cancer pain: a systematic review. Chinese Journal of Integrative Medicine. 2010;8:501–9.

33. National Institutes of Health: Warren Grant Magnuson Clinical Center. Pain Intensity Instruments. http://www.mvltca.net/Presentations/mvltca.pdf, Accessed 01 December 2011.

34. Farrar JT, Young JP Jr, LaMoreaux L, et al. Clinical importance of changes in chronic pain intensity measured on an 11-point numerical pain rating scale. Pain. 2001;94:149–58.

35. EORTC Quality of Life Department. The Chinese version of European Organization for Research and Treatment of Cancer Quality of Life Questionnaire-Core (EORTC QLQ-C30). http://www.eortc.be/home/qol/files/C30/QLQ-C30%20Chinese%20Mandarin%20Simplified.pdf. Accessed 07 Jan 2012.

36. Karnofsky DA, Burchenal JH. The Clinical Evaluation of Chemotherapeutic Agents in Cancer. In: MacLeod CM (Ed). Evaluation of Chemotherapeutic Agents. New York: Columbia University Press, 1949:196.

37. Aung S. The clinical use of acupuncture in oncology : symptom control. Acupunct Med. 1994;12:37–40.

38. Hyangsook Lee, Katja Schmidt, Edzard Ernst. Acupuncture for the relief of cancer-related pain – a systematic review. European Journal of Pain. 2005; 9(4):437–444.

39. Johnstone PA, Polston GR, Niemtzow RC, Martin PJ. Integration of acupuncture into the oncology clinic. Palliat Med. 2002;16(3):235–9.

40. Choi T, Lee MS, Kim T. Acupuncture for the treatment of cancer pain: a systematic review of randomized clinical trials. Support Care Cancer. 2012;20:1147–58.

41. Ming X. Experience on clinical application "si guan xue". Practical Journal of Chinese Medicine. 2006;22(5):300.

42. Jia YJ. Preliminary knowledge on opening of si guan xue. Chinese Medicine of Shanxi. 2008;29(8):1103–4.

43. Geng T. Meta clinical experience on si guan xue. Inner Mongolia Traditional Chinese Medicine. 2007;9:49–51.

44. Jing K, Liu C. Clinical application of si guan xue. J Med. 2005;25(4):34.

45. Hu X, Gu W, Zhou QH. Analgesic efficacy and mechanism of wrist-ankle acupuncture on pain caused by liver cancer. Chinese Journal of Integrative Medicine. 2005;15:131–3.

46. Follwell M, Burman D, Le LW, et al. Phase II study of an outpatient palliative care intervention in patients with metastatic cancer. J Clin Oncol. 2009;27(2):206–13.

18

Effects of acupuncture on nutritional state of patients with stable chronic obstructive pulmonary disease (COPD): re-analysis of COPD acupuncture trial

Masao Suzuki[1,3]* [iD], Shigeo Muro[2], Motonari Fukui[3], Naoto Ishizaki[4], Susumu Sato[5], Tetsuhiro Shiota[6], Kazuo Endo[7], Tomoko Suzuki[1], Tadamichi Mitsuma[1], Michiaki Mishima[8] and Toyohiro Hirai[5]

Abstract

Background: There are an increasing number of evidences that chronic obstructive pulmonary disease (COPD) is a systemic illness and that bodyweight loss is its prominent manifestation. We focused on the nutritional outcomes to find out the effectiveness of acupuncture on nutritional state of COPD patients and on their prognosis in our previous interventional study.

Methods: The present study is re-analysis of our previous interventional study, COPD Acupuncture Trial (CAT) published in 2012. Data from CAT was re-analyzed in terms of nutritional status, inflammatory biomarkers, and prognostic index. Nutritional states were evaluated by the measurements of body weight, body composition, and muscle strength, and the nutritional hematological examination results (retinol-binding protein (RBP), prealbumin (PA), transferrin (Tf), and hemoglobin (Hb) in serum), and inflammation biomarkers such as carboxyhemoglobin (COHb), High sensitivity C-reactive protein (Hs-CRP), Tumor Necrosis Factor-alpha (TNF-α), Interleukin 6 (IL-6), and Serum Amyloid A (SAA) were measured. The BODE index was measured in terms of prognosis. These measurements were compared between the real acupuncture group (RAG) and the placebo acupuncture group (PAG). All data are presented as mean (SD) or mean (95% CI). The difference between baseline and final volumes was compared using analysis of covariance (ANCOVA). Moreover, correlations between nutritional hematological examination scores and inflammation biomarker parameters were assessed using Spearman's rank correlation coefficient.

Results: After 12 weeks, the change in body weight was significantly greater in the RAG compared with the PAG (mean [SD] difference from baseline: 2.5 [0.4] in RAG vs − 0.5 [1.4] in PAG; mean difference between the groups: 3.00, 95% CI, 2.00 to 4.00 with ANCOVA). Patients in RAG also had improvements in the results of nutritional hematological examination (RBP, PA, Tf, Hb), Inflammation biomarkers (TNF-α, IL-6, SAA, Hs-CRP, COHb) and the BODE index.

Conclusion: This study demonstrated some clear evidences that acupuncture can be a useful adjunctive therapy to improve nutritional state of COPD patients.

(Continued on next page)

* Correspondence: masuzuki@fmu.ac.jp
[1]Department of Kampo Medicine, Aizu Medical Center, Fukushima Medical University School of Medicine, 21-2 Maeda, Tanisawa, Kawahigashi, Aizuwakamatsu, Fukushima 969-3492, Japan
[3]Respiratory Disease Center, Kitano Hospital, Tazuke Kofukai Medical Research Institute, 2-4-20 Ohgimachi, Kita-ku, Osaka 530-8480, Japan
Full list of author information is available at the end of the article

(Continued from previous page)

Trial registration: UMIN Clinical Trials Registry (UMIN000001277). Retrospectively registered.

Keywords: COPD, Acupuncture, Nutritional state, Proinflammatory cytokine

Background

There are an increasing number of evidences that chronic obstructive pulmonary disease (COPD) is a systemic illness and that bodyweight loss is its prominent manifestation. Low body mass index (BMI) is closely associated with mortality in COPD [1]; Malnutrition occurs in approximately one-quarter to one-third of patients with moderate to severe COPD [2]; Weight loss may be the result of an increased imbalance in energy expenditure caused by inadequate intake of nutrient. Previous studies have suggested that underweight patients show higher metabolic rate (negative energy balance) [3], lower antioxidant capacity of skeletal muscles [4], and increased systemic inflammation [5], which may be causing weight loss and morbidity. The cachexia associated with COPD was traditionally believed to be more prevalent among those whose airflow limitation was due to predominant emphysema (the "pink puffer" hypothesis) [6].

Previous studies have also shown that patients with COPD exhibit low-grade systemic inflammation which is often associated with significant extra-pulmonary effects, such as cardiovascular abnormalities and skeletal muscle dysfunctions [7]. Gan et al. performed a systematic review of these studies and found that circulating leukocytes, fibrinogen, serum C-reactive protein (CRP) and tumor necrosis factor-alpha (TNF-α) levels were higher in COPD patients than in control subjects [8].

We previously demonstrated that dyspnea and exercise capacity evaluated with Borg scale scores and the 6-min walking distance (6MWD) were markedly improved with acupuncture in a prospective, randomized controlled trial in COPD patients who were receiving standard medication [9]. This study also showed some suggestive results that acupuncture was effective to improve nutritional state of patients.

Therefore, we re-analyzed the data focusing on the nutritional outcomes, inflammatory biomarkers, and oxidative stress which were not fully evaluated in our previous study, to find out the effectiveness of acupuncture on nutritional state of COPD patients and on their prognosis.

Methods

Study design and patients

This is re-analysis study of the data collected in the CAT (COPD Acupuncture Trial) published in 2012 [9]. The study is a randomized, single-blind, placebo-controlled, parallel group study which involved patients with moderate to very severe COPD. Patients with the diagnosis of COPD were eligible for inclusion of the study. All participants met the following criteria: 1) patients who had been diagnosed as stage II, III, or IV COPD, in accordance with the definition and criteria of the Global Initiative for Chronic Obstructive Lung Disease (GOLD) guidelines [10]; 2) patients who were clinically stable with no history of infections or exacerbation of respiratory symptoms, no changes in medication within 3 months preceding the study outset, and no signs of edema; 3) patients who were graded as stage II or higher on the Medical Research Council (MRC) criteria; 4) patients who were able to walk unassisted; 5) patients who had not been receiving pulmonary rehabilitation in the previous 6 months; and 6) outpatients. Patients presenting any evidence of cardiovascular disease, collagen disease, renal failure, thyroid dysfunction, hepatic function disorder, cancer, and severe mental disorders were excluded. This study was performed in accordance with the Declaration of Helsinki and its amendments, and the Guidelines for Good Clinical Practice for Epidemiological Studies and Clinical Research issued by the Japanese Ministry of Health. The Institutional Review Board of Tazuke Kofukai Foundation, Medical Research Institute, Kitano Hospital approved the study, and written informed consents were obtained from each patient. This study was registered with the UMIN Clinical Trials Registry (UMIN000001277).

Intervention

Subjects in the real acupuncture group (RAG) received acupuncture treatment once a week for 12 weeks, in addition to daily medication. Selection of standardized acupuncture points was done in accordance with the past researches on acupuncture for pulmonary dysfunctions [11, 12] and literatures describing traditional prescription of acupuncture points for bronchial asthma and chronic bronchitis, of which the effect on COPD were verified through our clinical experiences over the past 10 years. Also, the importance of acupuncture points close to the respiratory accessory muscles was emphasized in the process of determination of the standardized treatment. The standardized acupuncture points used in the present study were: 1) Zhongfu (LU 1) and 2) Taiyuan (LU 9) in the lung meridian; 3) Futu (LI 18) in the large intestine meridian; 4) Guanyuan (CV 4) and 5) Zhongwan (CV 12) in the conception vessel; 6) Zusanli in stomach meridian 36 (ST 36); 7) Taixi (KI 3) in the kidney meridian; 8) Wangu in the gallbladder meridian (GB12); and 9) Feishu (BL 13), 10) Pishu (BL 20), and 11) Shenshu (BL 23) in the bladder meridian.

A Park sham device, which contains a needle (real or placebo), was used with a guide tube mounted on a base adherent to the skin [13]. The tip of the placebo needles used for the placebo acupuncture group (PAG) were blunt and appeared to be penetrating the skin but actually telescoped back into their handles. The real and placebo needles appear similar and of the same size (0.35 mm × 70 mm, stainless steel, Dong Bang Acupuncture Inc. Korea).

For RAG patients, needles were inserted to a depth ranging from 5 to 25 mm and manually rotated clockwise and counter-clockwise for 3–4 min at each point during 50-min treatment period. No electrical stimulation was performed. Perception of de qi during insertion and/or manipulation was confirmed at every point in the RAG.

The PAG underwent treatment at the same acupuncture points as the RAG. Perception of sensation during treatment sessions in PAG included pricking or poking but no sensation like de qi was reported.

Outcomes

1) Main measurement of nutritional outcome is the change in body weight with Percent Ideal Body Weight (%IBW) of COPD patients after 12 weeks of acupuncture [14, 15]. %IBW was calculated with the following formulas; IBW = (height (m)) [2] × 22, %IBW = (real body weight / IBW) × 100 .

2) Prognosis outcome measurement is the BODE index, which is a multidimensional index that includes four factors that predict the risk of death: BMI (B); degree of air flow obstruction (O); functional dyspnea (D); and exercise capacity (E), assessed by the 6MWD [16].

3) Measurements of body composition are Midupper Arm Circumference (MAC), Triceps Skinfold (TSF) thickness, Scapula Skin folds (SSF) thickness and quadriceps circumference (above patellar 10 cm), all of which were measured except for Arm Muscle Circumference (AMC) which was calculated. Skinfold thickness was measured to assess changes in fat mass using Harpenden skinfold calipers (Holtain) according to its standard methodology [15]. Measurement was performed on the non-dominant hand, and in the case of paralysis, on the non-paralyzed side. Measurer evaluated the average value of the three measurements. The measurement of TSF was performed as follows. Subjects were in a lateral decubitus position, the upper arm was flexed by 90 ° at the elbow joint, a mark was placed at the midpoint between the shoulder bladder projection and the ulnar olecranon projection, the skin 1 cm away from the mark was picked up to so that the fat layer is separated from the muscle, and we measured the thickness by sandwiching the marked part

with caliper. As for the measurement of SSF, with the patients in the lateral decubitus position, the same method as TSF was used at the portion of the shoulder blade lower corner. For MAC, the surroundings of the part marked for TSF was measured with a measuring tape. AMC was calculated by this formula: [AMC(cm) = AC-π × TSF(cm)]. As for the measurement of QC, patient was in supine position, a mark was put at 10 cm above from the upper edge of the patella toward the trunk of the non-dominant or non-paralyzed limb, and the peripheral diameter of the thigh at the mark was measured.

4) Muscle strength was evaluated as a hand grips, and the maximum inspiratory mouth pressure (MIP) and maximum expiratory mouth pressure (MEP) were measured using a standard mouthpiece and a device (Vitaropower KH115, Chest MI Co. Ltd., Tokyo, Japan) according to American Thoracic Society/European Respiratory Society [17].

5) Measurements of Nutritional Hematological Examination and Inflammation Biomarkers

Biochemical tests such as serum retinol-binding protein (RBP), pre-albumin (PA), transferrin (Tf) and hemoglobin (Hb) were measured as nutrition indices, and carboxyhemoglobin (COHb) within arterial blood gas, High sensitivity C-reactive protein (Hs-CRP), Tumor Necrosis Factor-alpha (TNF-α), Interleukin 6 (IL-6), and Serum Amyloid A (SAA) were measured as inflammatory biomarkers. Serum TNF-α, IL-6 and Hs-CRP were measured using commercially available enzyme-linked immunosorbent assay kits (Mitsubishi BCL, inc., Tokyo, Japan).

Statistical analysis

All data are presented as means and SDs or 95% confidence intervals (CI). Analyses of outcome measures were performed according to the Full analysis set. The difference between baseline and final values was compared using analysis of covariance (ANCOVA) with baseline values and age as covariates, and treatment group as the factor of interest.

Correlations between nutritional examination scores and inflammation biomarker parameters were assessed by looking at their changes from baseline to post treatment for each group. Spearman's rank correlation coefficient was calculated. The magnitude of the results was determined by calculating the effect size d. According to Cohen, $d = 0.2$ is a small treatment effect, $d = 0.5$ is a moderate effect, and $d = 0.8$ is a large effect [18].

All main analyses in the present study were carried out with JMP® 11 (SAS Institute Inc., Cary, NC, USA).

In order to avoid bias, the biostatistician performed the statistical analysis with grouping information masked.

Results

Study population

During the period from July 2006 to March 2009, 111 COPD patients were found to meet the inclusion/exclusion criteria. Sixty-eight patients out of these 111 agreed to participate in the study. Of those participants, six were unable to complete the study because they felt it was too difficult to continue (two in the PAG and one in the RAG) and because of acute exacerbation due to respiratory infections (three in the RAG). Baseline characteristics of the patients in each group, are shown in Table 1. All medications remained unchanged through the study period.

Also, no patient had supplement or vitamin newly prescribed by the hospital during 6-month period prior to the study.

Body weight

After 12 weeks of treatment, the body weight increased from 55.5 kg [10.4] to 58.0 kg [10.8] in the RAG. On the other hand, there was no change in the body weight in the PAG before and after the treatment (56.8 kg [13.8] to 56.3 kg [13.0], respectively). The difference in the body weight in the RAG (2.5 [0.4]) was statistically significant compared with that in the PAG (− 0.5 [1.4])

Table 1 Baseline subject characteristics

	PAG (n = 34)	RAG (n = 34)	Mean difference
Sex (M/F)	32/2	31/3	
Age yr	72.5 [7.4]	72.7 [6.8]	0.2
MRC	2.9 [1.1]	3.3 [1.0]	0.4
Body Weight (kg)	56.0 [13.8]	54.6 [10.6]	−1.4
BMI (Kg/m^2)	21.1 [3.9]	21.2 [3.9]	0.1
Brinkman Index	1433.9 [759.8]	1292.5 [526.4]	−141.4
GOLD criteria			
I	0	0	
II	13	6	
III	8	16	
IV	13	12	
	3.0 [0.9]	3.2 [0.7]	0.2
HOT	11	9	
Pulmonary function			
FVC (L)	3.0 [0.7]	2.8 [0.6]	−0.2
FEV$_1$ (L)	1.2 [0.4]	1.0 [0.3]	−0.2
% FEV$_1$(%)	48.0 [16.5]	44.5 [16.3]	−3.5

PAG placebo acupuncture group, RAG real acupuncture group, MRC medical research council, BMI body mass index, GOLD global initiative for chronic obstructive lung disease, HOT home oxygen therapy, FVC forced vital capacity, FEV$_1$ forced expiratory volume in 1 second, % FEV$_1$ forced expiratory volume in 1 second in predicted

(mean difference 3.00, 95% CI 2.00 to 4.00 by ANCOVA) (Table 2, Fig. 1). Improvement in the %IBW found in the RAG was statistically significant compared to that in the PAG. The Cohen's d effect size for the Body weight and %IBW were large(d = 2.87 and d = 1.51), respectively.

BODE index

The BODE index improved from 3.90 (2.38) to 2.70 (1.73) in the RAG. In the PAG, on the other hand, there was no improvement in the BODE index before and after placebo acupuncture treatment (3.28 [2.40] and 3.28 [2.37], respectively). The difference in the BODE index in the RAG (− 1.2 [1.2]) was statistically significant compared with that in the PAG (− 0.03 [1.0]) (mean difference − 1.17, 95% CI -1.55 to − 0.55 by ANCOVA) (Table 2, Fig. 2). The Cohen's d effect size for the BODE index was large(d = 1.06).

Measurements of body composition and muscle strength

Significant improvements in the body composition (MAC, TSF, SSF, quadriceps circumference), and muscle strength (Grip strength, Respiratory muscle strength) were found in the RAG compared to those in the PAG. Only AMC showed no significant improvement (Table 3).

Nutritional hematological examination

Improvements in the nutritional hematological measurements (RBP, PA, Tf, Hg) found in the RAG were statistically significant compared to those in the PAG (Table 4).

Inflammation biomarkers

Decreases in inflammation biomarkers (Hs-CRP, TNF-α, IL-6, SAA, and COHb,) were found in the RAG compared with the PAG (Table 4).

Correlation between nutritional hematological scores and inflammation biomarker parameters

Prealbumin was negatively correlated with Hs-CRP (r = − 0.41, P = 0.049), TNF-α (r = − 0.44, P = 0.042), IL-6 (r = − 0.54, P = 0.010), SAA (r = − 0.44, P = 0.042) and COHb (r = − 0.13, P = 0.318). Tf was negatively correlated with COHb (r = − 0.62, P = 0.001). Weight was negatively correlated with COHb (r = − 0.48, P = 0.0001), Hs-CRP (r = − 0.30, P = 0.18), TNF-α (r = − 0.44, P = 0.041), IL-6 (r = − 0.35, P = 0.11) and SAA (r = − 0.43, P = 0.046) (Table 5) (An additional figure file shows this in more detail (see Additional file 1, Additional file 2, Additional file 3, Additional file 4 and Additional file 5).

Adverse reactions

The following minor adverse reactions were reported by some patients during the study: fatigue (four in the RAG and five in the PAG), subcutaneous hemorrhage (five in the RAG), dizziness (one in the RAG and two in the

Table 2 Changes in the nutritional outcome and prognosis

	Baseline	After 12 weeks	Change from baseline to post treatment measurements	MD	95% CI	Effect size (d)
Main measurement of nutritional outcome						
Body Weight (kg)						
PAG (n 32)	56.8 [13.8]	56.3 [13.0]	−0.5 [1.4]	3.00	2.00, 4.00	2.87
RAG (n 30)	55.5 [10.4]	58.0 [10.8]	2.5 [0.4]			
%IBW: ideal body weight (%)						
PAG (n 32)	96.7 [17.7]	95.9 [16.5]	−0.8 [2.4]	5.20	3.52, 7.00	1.51
RAG (n 30)	98.6 [17.7]	103.0 [18.3]	4.4 [4.3]			
Prognosis outcome measurement						
BODE index						
PAG (n 32)	3.3 [2.4]	3.3 [2.4]	−0.03[1.0]	−1.17	−1.55, −0.55	1.06
RAG (n 30)	3.9 [2.4]	2.7 [1.7]	−1.2 [1.2]			
BMI						
PAG (n 32)	0.5 [0.5]	0.4 [0.5]	−0.1 [1.3]	−0.11		
RAG (n 30)	0.4 [0.5]	0.2 [0.4]	−0.2 [0.5]			
%FEV$_1$						
PAG (n 32)	1.5 [1.1]	1.7 [1.1]	0.2 [0.4]	−0.29		
RAG (n 30)	1.8 [1.0]	1.6 [1.0]	−0.1 [0.6]			
mMRC						
PAG (n 32)	0.9 [1.1]	0.8 [1.1]	−0.1[0.5]	−0.51		
RAG (n 30)	1.2 [1.0]	0.6 [0.8]	−0.6 [0.7]			
6MWD						
PAG (n 32)	0.4 [0.7]	0.4 [0.7]	0.0 [0.3]	−0.30		
RAG (n 30)	0.5 [0.9]	0.3 [0.5]	−0.3 [0.7]			

MD mean difference, *%IBW* ideal body weight (%), *BODE index* BMI (B); degree of air flow obstruction (O); functional dyspnea (D); and exercise capacity (E), assessed by the 6MWD. *BMI* body mass index, *%FEV$_1$* % forced expiratory volume in 1 s, *mMRC* Modified Medical Research Council, *6MWD* 6 minute walk distance

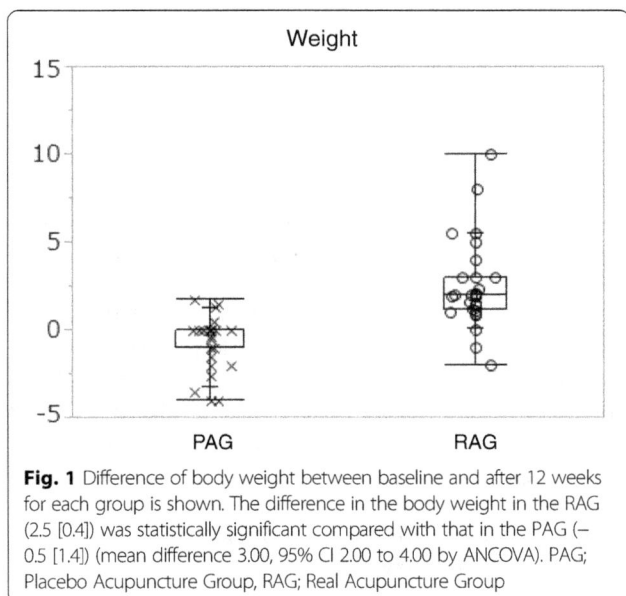

Fig. 1 Difference of body weight between baseline and after 12 weeks for each group is shown. The difference in the body weight in the RAG (2.5 [0.4]) was statistically significant compared with that in the PAG (−0.5 [1.4]) (mean difference 3.00, 95% CI 2.00 to 4.00 by ANCOVA). PAG; Placebo Acupuncture Group, RAG; Real Acupuncture Group

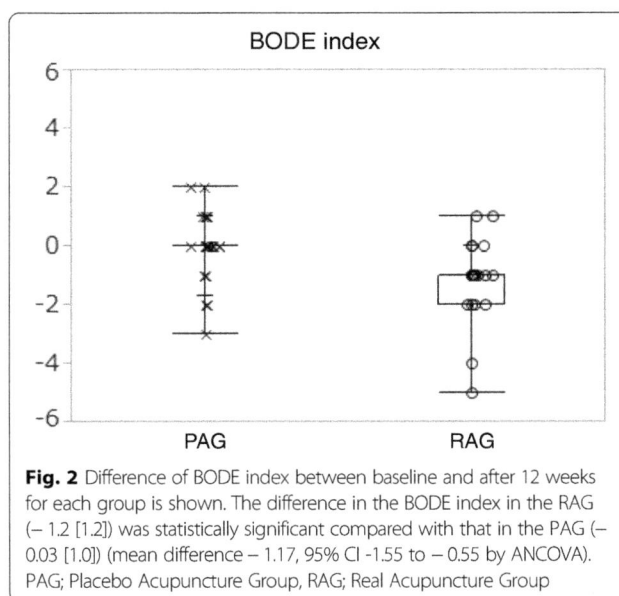

Fig. 2 Difference of BODE index between baseline and after 12 weeks for each group is shown. The difference in the BODE index in the RAG (− 1.2 [1.2]) was statistically significant compared with that in the PAG (−0.03 [1.0]) (mean difference − 1.17, 95% CI -1.55 to − 0.55 by ANCOVA). PAG; Placebo Acupuncture Group, RAG; Real Acupuncture Group

Table 3 Changes in the body composition and muscles strength

	Baseline	After 12 weeks	Change from baseline to post treatment measurements	MD	95% CI	Effect size (d)
Measurements of body composition						
MAC (cm)						
PAG (n 32)	24.3 [3.6]	24.0 [3.6]	− 0.3[1.1]	1.77	1.15, 2.39	1.42
RAG (n 30)	24.7 [3.4]	26.1 [3.9]	1.4 [1.3]			
TSF (mm)						
PAG (n 32)	11.3 [5.5]	9.9 [5.2]	−1.4 [2.5]	5.56	4.10, 7.03	1.92
RAG (n 30)	12.0 [4.9]	16.2 [6.2]	4.2 [3.3]			
AMC (cm)						
PAG (n 32)	20.9 [2.8]	21.0 [2.8]	0.1 [1.0]	0.10	−0.44, 0.64	0.10
RAG (n 30)	21.1 [2.6]	21.3 [2.9]	0.2 [1.1]			
SSF (mm)						
PAG (n 32)	13.4 [5.1]	12.8 [5.2]	−0.6 [2.8]	3.55	2.04, 5.05	1.22
RAG (n 30)	15.9 [5.9]	18.9 [6.3]	3.0 [3.1]			
QC (AP 10 cm) (cm)						
PAG (n 32)	38.3 [4.6]	38.1 [4.6]	−0.2 [0.7]	1.86	1.13, 2.59	1.34
RAG (n 30)	37.9 [4.2]	39.6 [4.6]	1.7 [1.9]			
Muscles strength						
Grip strength (Right) (kg)						
PAG (n 32)	28.9 [6.1]	28.6 [5.5]	−0.3 [2.3]	1.55	0.42, 2.67	0.73
RAG (n 30)	27.5 [6.2]	28.8 [5.9]	1.3 [2.1]			
Grip strength (Left) (kg)						
PAG (n 32)	28.4 [5.4]	27.4 [4.9]	−1.0 [2.5]	1.94	0.73, 3.14	0.85
RAG (n 30)	26.5 [6.4]	27.5 [6.6]	1.0 [2.2]			
Respiratory muscle strength MEP (H_2Ocm)						
PAG (n 32)	63.5 [21.5]	61.8 [22.9]	−1.7 [12.2]	36.09	26.41, 45.77	1.90
RAG (n 30)	59.5 [21.6]	93.9 [32.2]	34.4 [24.3]			
MIP (H_2Ocm)						
PAG (n 32)	56.4 [20.6]	55.4 [19.5]	−1.0 [11.9]	14.83	8.49, 21.16	1.19
RAG (n 30)	60.8 [20.6]	74.6 [15.8]	13.8 [13.0]			

MD mean difference, MAC midupper arm circumference, TSF triceps skinfolds, AMC arm muscle circumference, SSF scapula skinfolds, QC Quadriceps circumference, MEP maximum expiratory mouth pressure, MIP maximum inspiratory mouth pressure

PAG), and needle site pain (five in the RAG). All events were minor reactions and patients recovered in a short time. No serious events due to acupuncture treatment were reported.

Discussion

The present study is the first RCT on acupuncture treatments with precise evaluations of nutritional state and the BODE index of patients with COPD. Previously, we performed a study to evaluate the efficacy of acupuncture on nutritional state and the BODE index with accumulated COPD cases and found significantly improved prognosis in terms of the BODE index comparing before and after 10 weeks of acupuncture [19]. However, since there was no control group, the discussion whether acupuncture was capable of improving symptoms of COPD remained inconclusive.

In the present RCT study, we have found that there are many improvements in nutritional states of the RAG compared to those of the PAG. Above all, body weight increased 2.5 kg on average for the RAG. And there were no patients whose body weight increased in consequence of diseases such as cardiac incompetence or renal insufficiency during the 12 weeks of study period. Therefore, the increase in the body weight, we would say, was brought by improvements of nutritional status caused by acupuncture.

Table 4 Changes in the Nutritional Hematological and Inflammation Biomarkers

	Baseline	After 12 weeks	Change from baseline to post treatment measurements	MD	95% CI	Effect size (d)
Nutritional Hematological						
RBP (mg/dL)						
PAG (n 20)	3.0 [0.7]	3.0 [0.6]	0.02 [0.5]	0.98	0.48, 1.46	1.60
RAG (n 22)	3.3 [1.5]	4.3 [1.3]	1.0 [0.7]			
PA (mg/dL)						
PAG (n 32)	23.4 [3.7]	22.9 [4.6]	−0.5 [2.6]	2.84	0.93, 4.76	0.77
RAG (n 30)	23.0 [4.9]	25.4 [6.7]	2.4 [4.7]			
Tf (mg/dL)						
PAG (n 20)	218.9 [76.6]	208.0 [67.9]	−10.9 [8.8]	54.1	34.53, 71.82	2.94
RAG (n 22)	216.4 [38.1]	259.6 [45.0]	43.2 [24.0]			
Hb (g/dL)						
PAG (n 32)	14.1 [1.1]	13.9 [1.2]	−0.2 [0.9]	0.90	0.54, 1.27	1.17
RAG (n 30)	13.9 [1.6]	14.6 [1.3]	0.7 [0.6]			
Inflammation Biomarkers						
Hs-CRP (ng/mL)						
PAG (n 12)	735.3 [445.6]	717.8 [396.6]	−17.4 [71.7]	− 576.58	− 610.60, −44.23	1.57
RAG (n 10)	1109.3 [437.2]	515.3 [247.6]	− 594.0 [542.4]			
TNF-α (pg/mL)						
PAG (n 12)	2.5 [0.9]	2.8 [1.0]	0.4 [0.8]	−2.09	−2.44, −0.42	1.56
RAG (n 10)	3.3 [1.5]	1.6 [1.2]	−1.7 [1.8]			
IL-6 (pg/mL)						
PAG (n 12)	2.9 [1.0]	3.6 [1.4]	0.7 [1.5]	−2.34	−3.13, −0.87	1.55
RAG (n 10)	3.3 [1.1]	1.7 [1.0]	−1.7 [1.6]			
SAA (μg/mL)						
PAG (n 12)	5.0 [1.7]	5.5 [2.4]	0.5 [1.0]	−2.10	−3.34, −1.02	1.75
RAG (n 10)	4.4 [1.7]	2.7 [0.8]	−1.6 [1.4]			
COHb (%)						
PAG (n 32)	1.4 [1.0]	1.9 [1.1]	0.5 [0.9]	−1.13	−1.51, −0.69	1.10
RAG (n 30)	1.4 [1.2]	0.8 [0.6]	−0.6 [1.1]			

MD mean difference, *RBP* Retinol-Binding Protein, *PA* Pre-Albumin, *Tf* Transferrin, *Hb* Hemoglobin, *Hs-CRP* High sensitivity C-reactive protein, *TNF-α* Tumor Necrosis Factor-alpha, *IL-6* Interleukin 6, *SAA* Serum Amyloid A, *COHb* carboxyhemoglobin

Table 5 Associations among the biomarkers at change from baseline to post treatment

	Weight	%IBW	Hb	Prealbumin	Tf	RBP
COHb	− 0.48+	−0.48+	− 0.25	−0.13	− 0.62+	−0.27
Hs-CRP	−0.30	−0.31	− 0.35	**−0.41+**	0.02	**−0.54+**
TNF-α	**−0.44+**	**−0.44+**	− 0.37	**−0.44+**	0.11	**−0.51+**
IL-6	−0.35	−0.36	**− 0.56+**	**−0.54+**	0.10	**−0.42+**
SAA	**−0.43+**	**−0.43+**	**− 0.55+**	**−0.44+**	0.13	−0.27

Significant associations ($p < 0.05$) are Bold and denoted with cross
COHb Carboxyhemoglobin, *Hs-CRP* High sensitivity C-reactive protein, *TNF-α* Tumor Necrosis Factor-alpha, *IL-6* Interleukin 6, *SAA* Serum Amyloid A, *%IBW* Percent Ideal Body Weight, *Hb* Hemoglobin, *Tf* Transferrin, *RBP* Retinol-Binding Protein

Acupuncture effects on body composition and muscles strength in COPD

Weight loss is one of the main characteristics of advanced COPD, often associated with the increased susceptibility to exacerbations of respiratory symptoms, and considered to be an independent predictor of outcome [1]. Weight loss may involve all of the bodily tissue compartments, nevertheless, loss of skeletal muscle may be particularly important because wasting respiratory muscles leads to the loss of power and endurance [20]. Consequently, in physical examination, their measurements of arm muscle circumference (AMC) and triceps skin fold thickness (TSF) are significantly less than those of the healthy individuals [21].

In our study, although the circumferences of upper arm and thigh and the fat thicknesses of triceps skinfold and scapula skinfold increased significantly in the RAG compared to the PAG, the arm muscle circumference (AMC) which is a substitutional measurement of muscle mass did not show significant increase. Therefore, In the acupuncture group, weight gain of 2.5 kg on average was observed, and this weight gain was considered due to increase in fat mass rather than increase in muscle mass. In addition, it is presumed that the increase in fat mass accompanying acupuncture is related to improvement of appetite and reduction of inflammatory cytokines such as TNF-α and SAA.

At the same time, grip strength and maximum respiratory pressure improved significantly, which implies the recovery of muscle strength. Previous research reported that acupuncture stimulation has effects of relaxing muscle tension and relieving muscle fatigue [22]. Since many COPD patients have tension and fatigue in respiratory muscles and accessory respiratory muscles. Many of the acupuncture points used in this study are corresponding to accessory muscles of respiration. There are smaller pectoral muscle and superior posterior serratus muscle, which are the inspiratory accessory muscles, immediately under the LU1(Zhongfu) and the BL13(Feishu). Beneath the BL20(Pishu) and the BL23(Shenshu) there are inferior posterior serratus muscle and lumbar rectus muscle, which are the expiratory accessory muscles, and under the CV4(Guanyuan) and the CV12(Zhongwan), there is rectus abdominis muscle, which is also the expiratory accessory muscle. The rectus abdominis muscle and the lumbar rectus muscle work together to raise the abdominal pressure to make forced expiration and to hold breath. We considered that acupuncture to respiratory accessory muscles relaxed muscle tone and recovered muscle fatigue, which led to a significant improvement in respiratory muscle strength (MEP/MIP). Considering the contribution of nutritional status to improvement of muscle strength, we believe that acupuncture treatment had the combined effects to improve grip strength and respiratory muscle strength.

In addition, Takaoka et al. reported that when muscle atrophy was recovered by acupuncture in their animal experiment, lowered amount of expression of myostatin gene and increased number of muscle satellite cells were found. Myostatin gene has a function to suppress protein synthesis in muscle to prevent muscle mass to become excessive [23].

The suppression of myostatin gene expression leads to the activation of muscle satellite cells and the facilitation of muscle repair and muscular hypertrophy [24]. Therefore, we speculate that the lowered amount of myostatin gene expression caused by acupuncture led to the activation of muscle protein synthesis due to proliferation of muscle satellite cells; as a result, muscle atrophy was restored and muscle strength was recovered.

Possible mechanism underlying the effect of acupuncture on malnutrition in COPD

Factors of malnutrition in COPD include anorexia and elevated metabolism which is reflected in the increased rest energy expenditure (REE), and factors of REE increase include decrease in ventilation efficiency due to obstructive ventilatory disorder and increase in respiratory muscle workload due to respiratory muscle fatigue [25]. Since patients with COPD often have lowered diaphragm due to hyperinflation of the lungs, intake of food into their stomach pushes up the diaphragm and diaphragmatic breathing is restricted and causes dyspnea. Therefore, such patients tend to avoid aggressive dietary intake and suffer nutritional disorders because of shortage of caloric intake, which leads to weight loss, skeletal muscle weakness, and respiratory muscle atrophy, resulting in easy fatigue of the skeletal muscle. Furthermore, since patients with COPD cannot take sufficient nutrition in spite of their significant energy consumption, they tend to fall into protein energy malnutrition (PEM) state. It has been also reported that the levels of transferrin and prealbumin, which are biomarkers of nutritional condition, of COPD patients are often low [26]. In our preceding study [9], it was found that many patients in the real acupuncture treatment group, compared to the placebo group, had improvement in dyspnea at the time of exertion, obstructive ventilatory impairment, accessory muscle of respiration fatigue and in addition, improvement in shortness of breath accompanying feeding behavior. It is considered that improvement of shortness of breath accompanying acupuncture treatment resulted in not only an increase in dietary intake, but also in a reduction of resting energy consumption which was increased by the disease. Consequently, we infer that improvements in nutritional status reflected in body weight were observed.

In addition, the main neural network that controls the feeding behavior is hypothalamus, but other parts such as paraventricular nucleus, arcuate nucleus, and solitary nucleus in medulla oblongata are also involved in the feeding regulation. ST36, the acupuncture point used in our study has been utilized from ancient times for disorders in gastrointestinal function.

Recent studies have found that acupuncture at ST36 sends stimulus to hypothalamus and solitary nucleus in medulla oblongata and efferently modulates peristalsis of digestive tract via vagus nerve [27, 28]. Therefore, in our study, we considered that acupuncture at ST36 affected the feeding center of the COPD patients and modulated peristalsis of digestive tract, which then led to the increase in the patients' food intake and their better nutritional condition. Improvement in the gastrointestinal functions by acupuncture might have played a role in the increase of the biomarkers of nutritional condition in our trial.

Nutritional biomarkers utilized in our study are the ones generally used to monitor nutritional status of patients with chronic diseases since those biomarkers are sensitive enough to indicate a slight sign of malnutrition. In addition, since each biomarker has its own characteristic half-life period, such as 10–17 h for RBP, 2–4 days for pre-albumin, and 7–10 days for transferrin, it is possible to make a tentative judgment on the duration of malnutrition. In our study, values of each biomarker have been significantly improved in the RAG compared to the PAG, therefore, we considered that the nutritional status has been improved at least 1 week before the examination.

Also, although the number of cases was rather small, it was recognized that inflammatory biomarkers had correlation with body weight and some nutritional biomarkers, therefore, we considered the possibility that the nutritional status was improved with the anti-inflammatory effect of acupuncture. On the other hand, interventional methods such as dietary advice and nutritional therapy for COPD patients, according to meta-analysis, have been found to significantly improve their body weight, fat free mass, maximum respiratory pressure, and grip strength. However, no significant improvements in FEV_1, exercise tolerance, quadriceps muscle strength, or QOL were found [29, 30].

Currently, nutritional therapy including ω-3 fatty acids and ghrelin, which are of much attention recently, is recognized to increase body weight and muscle strength for COPD patients but there has been no fixed consensus on the detailed changes in nutrition and inflammatory biomarkers [31]. Furthermore, the prognosis of COPD patients who had nutritional therapy has not been studied.

Therefore, we consider that acupuncture can be, as our research results indicate, one of the useful methods other than nutritional therapy to improve the nutritional status of COPD patients.

Acupuncture impacts on inflammation in COPD

In our study, inflammatory material or inflammatory cytokine such as COHb, Hs-CRP, SAA, IL-6, TNF-α decreased in the RAG compared to those in the PAG.

It has been reported that unexplained weight loss (muscle wasting and adipose tissue depletion), which is a characteristic feature of advanced COPD, is linked to the systemic inflammation [8]. And bodyweight loss has been linked to the reduction of CRP, TNF-α, IL-1β or IL-6 in most previous studies which considered systemic inflammation in COPD [5]. It has been reported that the functional disorder in skeletal muscle is usually found in COPD due to the wasting of skeletal muscle and change in its quality and the increased level of TNF-α, IL-6, and CRP is related to the lowered muscular strength [32, 33].

Models of anti-inflammatory effects of acupuncture were reviewed by John et al. and summarized to several physiological pathways: hypothalamus-pituitary-adrenal (HPA) axis, sympathetic pathways (via both sympathetic postganglionic neurons and the sympathoadrenal medullary axis), parasympathetic cholinergic pathways, antihistamine effects, down regulation of proinflammatory cytokines (such as TNF-α, IL-1β, IL-6, and IL-10), and suppression of the expression of COX-1, COX-2, and iNOS [34].

The acupuncture points used in this study (CV12(Zhongwanh), ST36(Zusanli), BL20(Pishu)) are traditionally recognized to be effective for the symptoms of the digestive system. ST36, especially, has been used in many basic researches and is the acupuncture point with a lot of clinically accepted evidences. Recent studies have shown that acupuncture stimulation at ST36 could regulate the nerve-endocrine-immune network [35]. Acupuncture stimulation at ST36 can regulate a wide variety of diseases caused by inflammation, and can also modulate TNF-α, IL-1β and IL-6 levels [36, 37].

Also, SAA is an acute phase reactant which corresponds to IL-1, IL-6, TNF-α, etc., and is an amyloidogenic protein, therefore, it is considered that SAA is decreased since IL-6 and TNF-α in the RAG are significantly decreased.

Furthermore, in chronic inflammatory diseases, it is often found that hemoglobin level is low, like in anemia, our study showed that hemoglobin level was improved in the RAG compared to the PAG. John et al. found that erythropoietin level is significantly higher in COPD patients with anemia compared to those without anemia [38]. Also, in COPD patients with anemia, hemoglobin level and erythropoietin level are inversely correlated, which suggests a decrease in hematopoietic response to erythropoietin. Such decrease in hematopoietic response to erythropoietin can be inferred to be caused by increase of inflammatory cytokines such as TNF-α, IL-6, and INF-γ [39]. Consequently, the improvement of hemoglobin level in RAG found in our study implies that the anti-inflammatory effect of acupuncture decreased inflammatory mediators.

Prognosis

Nutritional status is an important determinant of symptoms, disability, and prognosis in COPD, and being underweight can be problematic. The reduction in BMI is an independent risk factor for mortality of COPD patients.

The mean reduction of the BODE index of COPD patients was significantly greater in the RAG than that in the PAG. Our study clearly demonstrated that BMI, %FEV_1, MRC criteria and 6MWD, within the BODE index, were improved in COPD patients after 12 weeks of acupuncture [9].

Celli et al. reported that the minimal difference which is clinically important for the BODE index is 1 U or more [40]. In the present study, therefore, the effect of acupuncture on the BODE index was satisfactory great.

It is conceivable that acupuncture may affect prognosis of COPD patients since the acupuncture treatment improved all factors included in the BODE index. This result suggests that acupuncture may have a considerable influence on the prognosis of COPD patients, especially for those with advanced disease.

Study limitation

Patients recruited in the present study did not have any supplement or vitamin newly prescribed by medical facilities for 6 months prior to the study. However, two patients in the PAG had been continually prescribed and used a supplement for at least 2 years prior to the study and five patients in the PAG and two patients in the RAG had personally purchased from drugstores and used multivitamins for at least 3 years prior to the study. We considered this would cause no effects on our study since all of them had been taking those supplements or vitamins for over the years and did not change their habits.

This study was performed in 4 different facilities. At one of these facilities, nutritional evaluation (Transferin, RBP) could not be obtained, and at two of them, inflammatory evaluation could not be assessed. Also, the number of blood sample was not large enough. In addition, since we did not record the amount of food intake and meal content of all patients, the details about changes in calorie intake and diet were unknown.

Conclusion

We demonstrated clinically relevant improvements in nutritional states (body composition, and nutritional hematological examination), prognosis (BODE index), muscle strength and inflammation biomarkers in COPD patients after 3 months of acupuncture treatment in our RCT. In order to clearly confirm the usefulness of acupuncture as an adjunctive therapy in COPD treatment, randomized trials with larger sample sizes and longer-term interventions with follow up evaluations are necessary.

Additional files

Additional file 1: Correlation between COHb and Prealbumin is shown. Prealbumin was negatively correlated with COHb ($r = -0.13$, $P = 0.318$), (Spearman's rank correlation coefficient). COHb; carboxyhemoglobin. Cross:Placebo Acupuncture Group, Open circle; Real Acupuncture Group.

Additional file 2: Prealbumin was negatively correlated with Hs-CRP ($r = -0.41$, $P = 0.049$). (Spearman's rank correlation coefficient). Hs-CRP; High sensitivity C-reactive protein. Cross:Placebo Acupuncture Group, Open circle; Real Acupuncture Group.

Additional file 3: Prealbumin was negatively correlated with TNF-α ($r = -0.44$, $P = 0.042$). (Spearman's rank correlation coefficient). TNF-α; Tumor Necrosis Factor-alpha. Cross:Placebo Acupuncture Group, Open circle; Real Acupuncture Group.

Additional file 4: Prealbumin was negatively correlated with IL-6 ($r = -0.54$, $P = 0.010$). (Spearman's rank correlation coefficient). IL-6; Interleukin

6. Cross:Placebo Acupuncture Group, Open circle; Real Acupuncture Group.

Additional file 5: Prealbumin was negatively correlated with SAA ($r = -0.44$, $P = 0.042$). (Spearman's rank correlation coefficient). SAA; Serum Amyloid A. Cross:Placebo Acupuncture Group, Open circle; Real Acupuncture Group.

Abbreviations

%IBW: Percent ideal body weight; 6MWD: 6-min walking distance; ANCOVA: analysis of covariance; BMI: Body mass index; CAT: COPD acupuncture trial; CI: confidence intervals; COHb: Carboxyhemoglobin; COPD: Chronic obstructive pulmonary disease; COX: Cyclooxygenase; CRP: C-reactive protein; FEV_1: Forced expiratory volume in one second; GOLD: Global initiative for chronic obstructive lung disease; Hb: Hemoglobin; HPA: Hypothalamus-pituitary-adrenal; H-s-CRP: High sensitivity C-reactive protein; IL-1β: Interleukin 1beta; IL-6: Interleukin 6; INF-γ: Interferon-gamma; iNOS: inducible-Nitric oxide synthase; MAC: Midupper arm circumference; MEP: maximum expiratory mouth pressure; MIP: Maximum inspiratory mouth pressure; MRC: Medical research council; PA: Pre-albumin; PAG: Placebo acupuncture group; QOL: Quality of Life; RAG: Real acupuncture group; RBP: Retinol-binding protein; REE: Rest energy expenditure; SAA: Serum amyloid A; SSF: Scapula skin folds (SSF); STF: Subscapular skinfold thickness; Tf: Transferrin; TNF-α: Tumor necrosis factor-alpha

Acknowledgements

The authors thank research assistant Rika Ishizuka (Office for Gender Equality Support in Fukushima medical university) for her assistance in manuscript preparation.

Trial registration

UMIN Clinical Trials Registry (UMIN000001277). Registration date July 30 2008.

Funding

This trial was funded by the Grants-in-Aid for scientific research from the Japan Society of Acupuncture and Moxibustion (JSAM). The Japan Society of Acupuncture and Moxibustion (JSAM) had no role in the design and conduct of the study; collection, management, analysis, and interpretation of the data; and preparation, review, or approval of the manuscript.

Authors' contributions

MS, SM, SS and MF developed the concept and designed study. MS, SS, TeS, KE, MM and TM did the acquisition of data. TeS, KE, MM, TM and TH supervised the investigation. NI developed analytical program and processed. MS, SM, ToS, MF and TH wrote the paper. All authors participated in the interpretation of the results and review of the manuscript for important intellectual content. All authors have read and approved the final version of the manuscript.

Competing interests

The authors declare that they have no competing interests.

¹
Author details

Department of Kampo Medicine, Aizu Medical Center, Fukushima Medical University School of Medicine, 21-2 Maeda, Tanisawa, Kawahigashi,

Aizuwakamatsu, Fukushima 969-3492, Japan. [2]Department of Respiratory Medicine, Nara Medical University, 840 Shijo-Cho, Kashihara, Nara 634-8521, Japan. [3]Respiratory Disease Center, Kitano Hospital, Tazuke Kofukai Medical Research Institute, 2-4-20 Ohgimachi, Kita-ku, Osaka 530-8480, Japan. [4]Course of Acupuncture and Moxibustion, Faculty of Health Sciences, Tsukuba University of Technology, 4-12-7 Kasuga, Tsukuba, Ibaraki 305-8521, Japan. [5]Department of Respiratory Medicine, Graduate School of Medicine, Kyoto University, Yoshida, Konoe-cho, Sakyo-ku, Kyoto 606-8501, Japan. [6]Department of Respiratory Medicine, Shiga General Hospital, 4-30 Moriyama-cho, Moriyama, Shiga 524-8524, Japan. [7]Department of Respiratory Medicine, Hyogo Prefectural Amagasaki General Medical Center, 2-17-77 Higashinanba-cho, Amagasaki, Hyogo 660-8550, Japan. [8]Noe Hospital, 1-3-25 Joto-ku, Osaka 536-001, Japan.

References

1. Landbo C, Prescott E, Lange P, Vestbo J, Almdal TP. Prognostic value of nutritional status in chronic obstructive pulmonary disease. Am J Respir Crit Care Med. 1999;160:1856–61.
2. Congleton J. The pulmonary cachexia syndrome: aspects of energy balance. Proc Nutr Soc. 1999;58:321–8.
3. Moore JA, Angelillo VA. Equations for the prediction of resting energy expenditure in chronic obstructive lung disease. Chest. 1988;94:1260–3.
4. Rabinovich RA, Bastos R, Ardite E, Llinàs L, Orozco-Levi M, Gea J, et al. Mitochondrial dysfunction in COPD patients with low body mass index. Eur Respir J. 2007;29:643–50.
5. Eid AA, Ionescu AA, Nixon LS, Lewis-Jenkins V, Matthews SB, Griffiths TL, et al. Inflammatory response and body composition in chronic obstructive pulmonary disease. Am J Respir Crit Care Med. 2001;164:1414–8.
6. Ogawa E, Nakano Y, Ohara T, Muro S, Hirai T, Sato S, et al. Body mass index in male patients with COPD: correlation with low attenuation areas on CT. Thorax. 2009;64(1):20–5.
7. Agustí AG, Noguera A, Sauleda J, Sala E, Pons J, Busquets X. Systemic effects of chronic obstructive pulmonary disease. Eur Respir J. 2003;21:347–60.
8. Gan WQ1, Man SF, Senthilselvan A, Sin DD. Association between chronic obstructive pulmonary disease and systemic inflammation: a systematic review and a metaanalysis. Thorax. 2004;59:574–80.
9. Suzuki M, Muro S, Ando Y, Omori T, Shiota T, Endo K, et al. A randomized, placebo-controlled trial of acupuncture in patients with chronic obstructive pulmonary disease (COPD): the COPD-acupuncture trial (CAT). Arch Intern Med. 2012;172:878–86.
10. Global Initiative for Chronic Obstructive Lung Disease. Global strategy for the diagnosis, management, And prevention of chronic obstructive pulmonary disease updated 2009. Available online at: https://goldcopd.org/
11. Jobst KA. A critical analysis of acupuncture in pulmonary disease: efficacy and safety of the acupuncture needle. J Altern Complement Med. 1995;1:57–85.
12. Suzuki M, Namura K, Ohno Y, et al. The effect of acupuncture in the treatment of chronic obstructive pulmonary disease. J Altern Complement Med. 2008;14:1097–105.
13. Park J, White A, Stevinson C, Ernst E, James M. Validating a new non-penetrating acupuncture device: two randomised controlled trials. Acupunct Med. 2002;20:168–74.
14. DeHoog S. Identifying patients at nutritional risk and determining clinical productivity: essentials for an effective nutrition care program. J Am Diet Assoc. 1985 Dec;85(12):1620–2.
15. Japanese Society of Nutritional Assessment. Japanese anthropometric reference data: (JARD2001). Osaka. In: Japan: medical review co; 2002.
16. Celli BR, Cote CG, Marin JM, Casanova C, Montes de Oca M, Mendez RA, et al. The body-mass index, airflow obstruction, dyspnea, and exercise capacity index in chronic obstructive pulmonary disease. N Engl J Med. 2004;350(10):1005–12.
17. ATS/ERS Statement on respiratory muscle testing. Am J Respir Crit Care Med 2002; 15: 116(4): 518–624.
18. Cohen J. Statistical power analysis. Curr Direct Psychol Sci. 1992;1(3):98–101.
19. Suzuki M, Namura K, Ohno Y, Egawa M, Sugimoto T, Ishizaki N, et al. Combined standard medication and acupuncture for COPD: a case series. Acupunct Med. 2012;30:96–102.
20. Nishimura Y, Tsutsumi M, Nakata H, Tsunenari T, Maeda H, Yokoyama M. Relationship between respiratory muscle strength and leanbody mass in men with COPD. Chest. 1995;107:1232–6.
21. Sahebjami H, Doers JT, Render ML, Bond TL. Anthropometric and pulmonary function test profiles of outpatients with stable chronic obstructive pulmonary disease. Am J Med. 1993;94:469–74.
22. Kawakita K, Itoh K, Okada K. Experimental model of trigger points using eccentric exercise. J Musculoskelet Pain. 2008;16:29–35.
23. Takaoka Y, Ohta M, Ito A, Takamatsu K, Sugano A, Funakoshi K, et al. Electroacupuncture suppresses myostatin gene expression: cell proliferative reaction in mouse skeletal muscle. Physiol Genomics 2007;18;30(2):102–110.
24. Gilson H, Schakman O, Kalista S, Lause P, Tsuchida K, Thissen JP. Follistatin induces muscle hypertrophy through satellite cell proliferation and inhibition of both myostatin and activin. Am J Physiol Endocrinol Metab. 2009;297(1):E157–64.
25. Donahoe M, Rogers RM, Wilson DO, Pennock BE. Oxygen consumption of the respiratory muscles in normal and in malnourished patients with chronic obstructive pulmonary diseases. Am Rev Respir Dis. 1989;140:385–91.
26. Yoshikawa M, Yoneda T, Fu A, Yamamoto C, Takenaka H, et al. Analysis of body composition by dual energy X-ray absorptiometry and its relation to pulmonary function in patients with pulmonary emphysema. Jap J Thor Dis. 1996;34(9):953–8.
27. Takahashi T. Acupuncture for functional gastrointestinal disorders. J Gastroenterol. 2006;41:408–17.
28. Hui KK, Liu J, Marina O, Napadow V, Haselgrove C, Kwong KK, et al. The integrated response of the human cerebro-cerebellar and limbic systems to acupuncture stimulation at ST 36 as evidenced by fMRI. Neuroimage. 2005; 27:479–96.
29. Ferreira IM, Brooks D, White J, Goldstein R. Nutritional supplementation for stable chronic obstructive pulmonary disease. Cochrane Database Syst Rev. 2012;12:CD000998.
30. Collins PF, Elia M, Stratton RJ. Nutritional support and functional capacity in chronic obstructive pulmonary disease: a systematic review and meta-analysis. Respirology. 2013;18:616–29.
31. Miki K, Maekura R, Nagaya N, Nakazato M, Kimura H, Murakami S, et al. Ghrelin treatment of cachectic patients with chronic obstructive pulmonary disease: a multicenter, randomized, double-blind, placebo-controlled trial. PLoS One. 2012;7(5):e35708.
32. Yende S, Waterer GW, Tolley EA, Newman AB, Bauer DC, Taaffe DR, et al. Inflammatory markers are associated with ventilatory limitation and muscle dysfunction in obstructive lung disease in well functioning elderly subjects. Thorax. 2006;61:10–6.
33. Broekhuizen R, Wouters EF, Creutzberg EC, Schols AM. Raised CRP levels mark metabolic and functional impairment in advanced COPD. Thorax. 2006;61:17–22.
34. McDonald JL, Cripps AW, Smith PK, Smith CA, Xue CC, Golianu B. The anti-inflammatory effects of acupuncture and their relevance to allergic rhinitis: a narrative review and proposed model. Evid Based Complement Alternat Med 2013; 2013: 591796.
35. Kavoussi B, Ross BE. The neuroimmune basis of anti-inflammatory acupuncture. Integr Cancer Ther. 2007;6:251–7.
36. Torres-Rosas R, Yehia G, Peña G, Mishra P, del Rocio Thompson-Bonilla M, Moreno-Eutimio MA, et al. Dopamine mediates vagal modulation of the immune system by electroacupuncture. Nat Med. 2014;20:291–5.
37. Tian L, Huang YX, Tian M, Gao W, Chang Q. Downregulation of electroacupuncture at ST36 on TNF-α in rats with ulcerative colitis. World J Gastroenterol. 2003;9:1028–33.
38. John M, Hoernig S, Doehner W, Okonko DD, Witt C, Anker SD. Anemia and inflammation in COPD. Chest. 2005;127:825–9.
39. Chung KF. Cytokines in chronic obstructive pulmonary disease. Eur Respir J. 2001;18(Suppl 34):50s–9s.
40. Celli BR, MacNee W. Standards for the diagnosis and treatment of patients with COPD: a summary of the ATS/ERS position paper. Eur Respir J. 2004;23: 932–46.

19

Effects of acupoint-stimulation for the treatment of primary dysmenorrhoea compared with NSAIDs: a systematic review and meta-analysis of 19 RCTs

Yang Xu[1,2†], Wenli Zhao[1,3†], Te Li[4], Huaien Bu[5], Zhimei Zhao[6], Ye Zhao[7,8*] and Shilin Song[9*]

Abstract

Background: Primary dysmenorrhoea (PD), defined as painful menses in women with normal pelvic anatomy, is one of the most common gynaecological syndromes. Acupoint-stimulation could potentially be an effective intervention for PD. Our aim was to determine the effectiveness of acupoint-stimulation compared with Non-Steroidal Anti-Inflammatory Drugs (NASIDs) in the treatment of PD.

Methods: Six databases were searched to December 2014. Sixteen studies involving 1679 PD patients were included. We included randomized controlled trials that compared acupoint-stimulation with NASIDs for the treatment of PD. The main outcomes assessed were clinical effectiveness rate, symptom score, visual analogue score, variation in peripheral blood prostaglandin F2α (PGF2α) and side effects. All analyses were performed using Comprehensive Meta-Analysis statistical software.

Results: (1) The total efficacy was better than control group: odds ratio = 5.57; 95% confidence interval (95% CI) = 3.96, 7.83; $P < 0.00001$; (2) The effect of intervention was positive in relieving the severity of PD symptoms: mean difference (MD) = 2.99; 95%CI = 2.49, 3.49; $P < 0.00001$; (3) No statistical difference existed between two groups in terms of a reduction in the VAS: MD = 1.24; 95%CI = −3.37, 5.85; $P = 0.60$; (4) The effect of intervention on the variation in peripheral blood PGF2α between two groups was positive: MD = 7.55; 95%CI = 4.29,10.82; $P < 0.00001$; (5) The side effects of control groups was more than the acupoint-stimulation group: OR = 0.03; 95%CI =0.00,0.22; $P = 0.0005$.

Conclusions: According to this article, acupoint-stimulation can relieve pain effectively in the treatment of PD and offers advantages in increasing the overall effectiveness.

Keywords: Acupoint-stimulation, Primary dysmenorrhoea, Meta-analysis, Systematic review, Non-steroidal anti-inflammatory drugs

Background

Dysmenorrhea is the most common gynecologic complaint among adolescent and young adult females. The prevalence of dysmenorrhoea appears to differ across the world, ranging from 80% in Western Australia [1], to 60% in Canada [2], 48.4% in Mexico [3], and 79.9% in Iran [4]. Over 50% of females of reproductive age have painful menstruation; among them, 10% have severe dysmenorrhoea, whereby their monthly lives' quality is impaired from 1 to 3 days differently [5]. It starts some hours before menstruation and continues for up to 48–72 h, and takes the form of pains and cramps in the lower abdomen radiating towards the inner side of the thighs [6]. Half of such cases experience systemic symptoms, such as nausea, vomiting, diarrhoea, fatigue, irritability and dizziness [7, 8], which reduce the quality of life. The patients with mild-to-moderate pain can manage their pain without

* Correspondence: zaky@ufl.edu; haiguagua@163.com
†Equal contributors
[7]Department of Chemical Engineering, University of Florida, 1006 Center Drive, Gainesville, FL 32611, USA
[9]Laboratory of Anatomy, School of Integrative Medicine, Tianjin University of Traditional Chinese Medicine, No. 88 Yu Quan Road, Nankai District, Tianjin 300193, China
Full list of author information is available at the end of the article

drugs or with a small amount of non-prescription drugs. However, approximately 15% of all women experience severe dysmenorrhoea to a level that affects work or study; such women need drugs to relieve their pain [9]. Dysmenorrhea in adolescents and young adults is usually primary, and is defined as painful menses in women with normal pelvic anatomy [10]. In ~ 10% of females with severe dysmenorrhea symptoms, pelvic abnormalities such as endometriosis or uterine anomalies may be found (secondary dysmenorrhea) [11]. This article mainly discusses primary dysmenorrhoea (PD).

In recent years, there are more and more researches about the pathogenesis of PD. In addition to factors relating to the body's nerve, genetic and immune systems, and psychological/social factors, the pathogenesis is generally considered to be mainly related to two factors: (1) abnormal uterine contraction, and (2) endocrine and metabolic factors. The state of uterine ischemia and hypoxia causes the uterine muscle to contract, increasing intrauterine tension, and so leading to abdominal pain. Patients with abnormal uterine contractions and the subjective feeling of abdominal colic have been consistently reported over time. Many types of molecular endocrine factors play an important role in the pathogenesis of PD, such as prostaglandins (PGs), oxytocin (OT) and vasopressin (VP), β-EPs, nitric oxide (NO), noradrenaline (NE), endothelins, and magnesium and calcium ions. In particular, prostaglandin F2α (PGF2α), cyclooxygenase (COX) metabolite of arachidonic acid, causes potent vasoconstriction and myometrial contractions, leading to uterine ischemia and pain [12].

Treatment for PD includes a variety of pharmacological and non-pharmacological methods. Common pharmacological interventions include Non-Steroidal Anti-Inflammatory Drugs (NASIDs) and oral contraceptives. NSAIDs are widely used as the first-line therapy for females with dysmenorrhoea [13, 14]. However, there are often adverse events associated with the use of NSAIDs, including stomach ache, diarrhoea, nausea, and liver or kidney damage after discontinuing medication [13]. Therefore, many patients with PD are seeking complementary and alternative techniques such as acupoint-stimulation to treat the symptoms of PD [15], which emphasizes stimulating the acupoint(s) to strengthen the body's endogenetic regulated function, so as to preventing and treating diseases by regulating the meridian system.

Although previously publications have reported that acupuncture-related treatments are effective for primary dysmenorrhea, the evidence is low convincing due to insufficient methodological quality and small sample size. Given the safety of acupoint-stimulation [16], therefore, the purpose of this systematic review and meta-analysis study is to determine the effectiveness of acupoint-stimulation in treating PD.

Methods
Search strategy
We searched six electronic databases that included PubMed, the Cochrane Library, Embase, the Chinese Academic Journals Full-text Database, the Chinese Science and Technology Journal Full-text Database (CNKI), Wanfang Data, and the Chinese Biomedical Literature Database (VIP). The index terms were the following: dysmenorrhoea, menorrhagia, painful menstruation, menstrual, pain, painful menstruation, menstrual pain, menstrual pains, acupuncture, moxibustion, auricular point, ear acupoint (administering persistent/temporary pressure with Cowherb seed/finger force to stimulate pressure points), electroacupuncture, acusector, acupoint application, randomized controlled trials, controlled clinical trials, and random. The above terms in Chinese were adapted and searched in Chinese databases. The studies were published between the first year they were available and December 2014, which of the language is Chinese and English.

Selection criteria and exclusion criteria
Selection criteria

- Research Type
- Research Subjects
- Interventions
- Outcomes (*Clinical effectiveness rate, Symptom score, Visual analogue score, Peripheral blood PGF2α, Side effects*)

Research type
Randomized controlled trials (RCTs).

Research subjects
Patients with a definite PD diagnosis: PD is defined as painful menses in women with normal pelvic anatomy. An eligible patient is diagnosed based on the PD Clinical Guideline of the Society of Obstetricians and Gynaecologists of Canada.

Interventions
Intervention groups – acupoint-stimulation, including acupuncture, moxibustion, ear acupressure, electroacupuncture, acupoint application; Control groups – NSAIDs.

Outcomes
(1) Clinical effectiveness rate

It was a dichotomous outcome and the overall effectiveness of acupoint-stimulation therapy as a subjective assessment, which was defined as the proportion of participants who got relieved pain and was based on response evaluation criteria used in the treatment of insomnia with acupoint-stimulation. What's more, it was

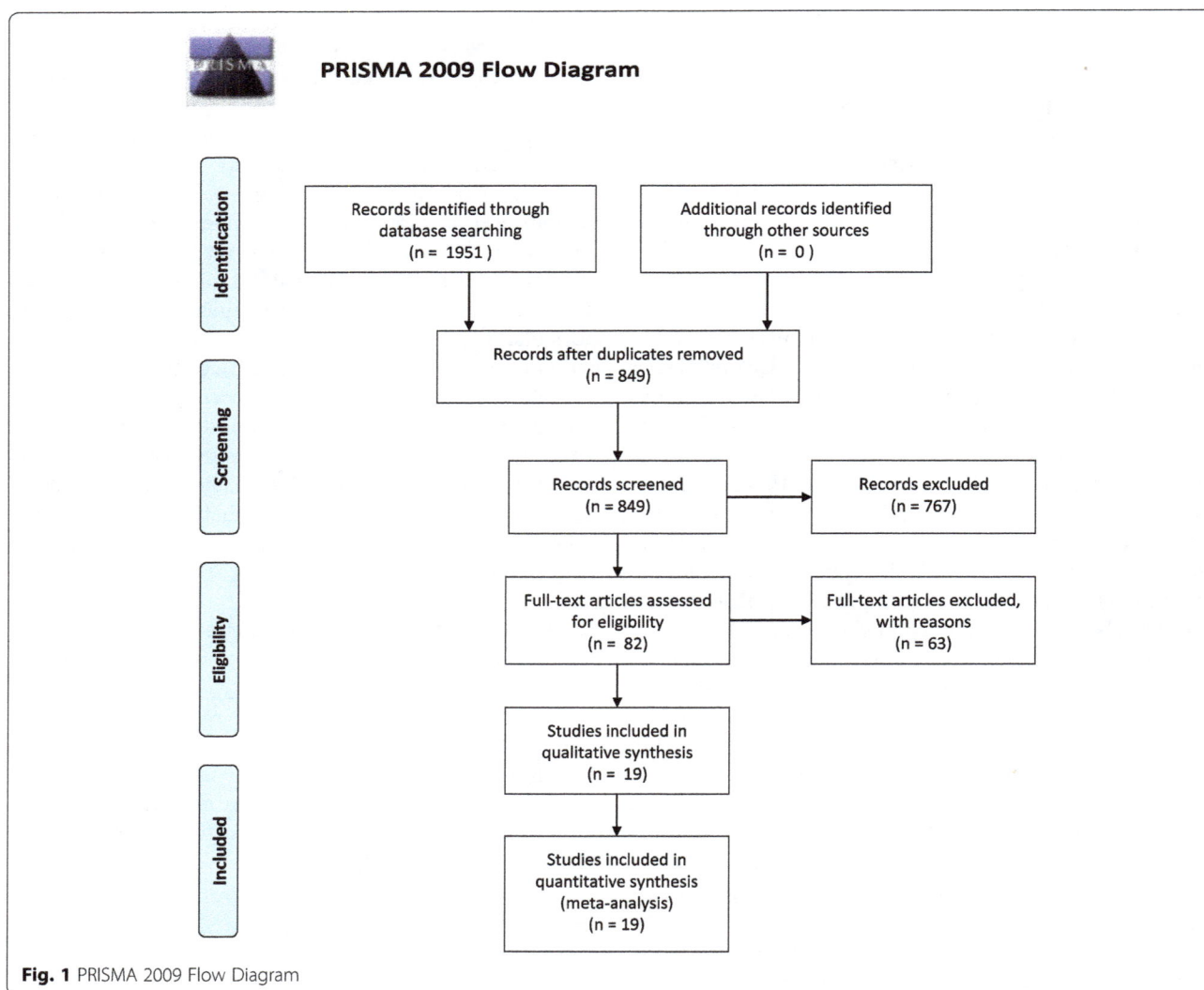

Fig. 1 PRISMA 2009 Flow Diagram

reported by trial participants themselves. For example, clinical therapeutic effect criteria were categorized as cure, markedly effective, effective, or ineffective. According to the Guideline for Clinical Trials of New Patent Chinese medicines (GCTNPCM) [17] evaluation standards, which define: Cured: after treatment, the score of symptoms was;restored to 0, abdominal pain and other symptoms disappeared and the dysmenorrhea did not recurred 3 menstrual cycles after treatment; Markedly effective: after treatment, the score of symptoms was decreased to less than 1/2 of the score before treatment, abdominal pain obviously relieved and other symptoms improved and the patient without taking analgesics could insist in work; Effective: after treatment,the score of symptoms decreased to 1/2–3/4 of the score before treatment, abdominal pain relieved and other symptoms improved, and the patient could work after taking analgesics; Ineffective: abdominal pain and other symptoms did not

change. The total number of "cure, markedly effective, effective" were used to calculate effective rate.

(2) Symptom score

In accordance with the GCTNPCM, the patients' symptom scores were recorded before and after treatment [18].

(3) Visual analogue score (VAS)

In the paper, we draw a 10 cm above the horizontal line and horizontal line of the end of 0, indicating no pain; on the other side of 10, said the pain; middle part of said varying degrees of pain. Feel the patient according to uniform mark on the horizontal line, indicating the degree of pain [19].

(4) Peripheral blood PGF2α.

The blood was taken from cubital vein within 24 h in the last menstrual period before treatment and within 24 h in the next menstrual period after treatment for one course, and the plasma PGF2α levels in the two groups were determined with radioimmunoassay.

(5) Side effects

Table 1 Characteristics of the 19 Trials Identified in the Literature Search

Studies	Randomization Method	Sample Size Intervention/Control	Age(I/C)	Intervention group	Control group	Outcomes Primary	Outcomes Secondary	Time of initiation of acupoint-stimulation and Course of Treatment	Follow-up Visit
Zhang LM et al. (2012) [22]	Random number table	45/45	13–27/11–25	Acupuncture at SP 10 SP 6 CV 6 LI 4	Indometacin	Clinical efficacy	N/A	The treatment started 3 days before menstrual onset, once every day and was given for 3 days for 3 menstrual cycles	3 months
Lin Q et al. (2012) [23]	Random number table	80/60	15–30/15–30	Eye acupuncture at the lower-*jiao* area; liver area; kidney area; the liver area; the heart area; the spleen area	Ibuprofen	Clinical efficacy	Uterine artery blood flow signals	The treatment started 5 days before menstrual onset, once every day and was given for 4–5 days for 3 menstrual cycles	3 months
Hu YL et al. (2012) [18]	Random number table	60/50	15–30/15–29	Eye acupuncture at the lower-*jiao* area; liver area; kidney area; the liver area; the heart area; the spleen area	Ibuprofen	Clinical efficacy	$PGF_{2\alpha}$ + recurrence rate	The treatment started 2 days before menstrual onset, once every day and was given for 4–5 days for 3 menstrual cycles	6 months
Cao Y et al. (2011) [24]	Random number table	29/30	15–29/20–28	Acupuncture at EX-B8 SP 8 BL 32	Ibuprofen	Clinical efficacy	symptom score+ VAS + side effects	The treatment started during the menstrual period, once every day and was given for 3 menstrual cycles	3 months
Zhi LX et al. (2007) [25]	SPSS Random number	60/60	19.60 ± 3.20/18.93 ± 2.60	Superficial needling at SP 6	Indometacin	Clinical efficacy	symptom score+ analgesic time	The treatment started 3 days before menstrual onset, once every day and was given for 5 days for 3 menstrual cycles	3 months
Bo LN et al. (2013) [26]	Random number table	69/64	13–35	Moxibustion at CV 4 CV 8 SP 6	Fenbid	N/A	$VAS + COX + PGF_{2\alpha} + OT$ + side effects	The treatment started 7 days before menstrual onset, once every day and was given for 7 days for 3 menstrual cycles	3 months
Ren XL et al. (2013) [27]	Registration order	40/40	16–28/18–27	Moxibustion at CV 4 SP 6	Ibuprofen	Clinical efficacy	$PGF_{2\alpha}$	The treatment started 3 days before menstrual onset, once every day and was given for 6 days for 3 menstrual cycles	3 months
Zhu Y et al. (2010) [28]	Random number table	51/51	18–26/19–25	Sandwiched moxibustion at CV 8	Indometacin	Clinical efficacy	symptom score +side effects	The treatment started 3 days before menstrual onset, once every day and was given for 5 days for 3 menstrual cycles	3 months
Li JM et al. (2012) [29]	Random number table	30/30	19–30	Electroacupuncture at BL 32	Fenbid	Clinical efficacy	symptom score	The treatment started during the menstrual period, once every day and was given for 3 menstrual cycles	3 months
Wang K et al. (2005) [30]	Random number table	30/28	16–28/15–24	Ear acupoint at TF 2 CO 18 CO 10 CO 12	Indometacin	Clinical efficacy	N/A	The treatment started 3 days before menstrual onset, once every day and was given for 6 days for 3 menstrual cycles	3 months
		36/36	14–28/13–27		Indometacin	Clinical efficacy	N/A		6 months

Table 1 Characteristics of the 19 Trials Identified in the Literature Search (Continued)

Study	Randomization	Sample size	Age	Intervention	Control	Outcome		Treatment schedule	Follow-up
Yang M et al. (2009) [31]	Random number table			Acupoint application at CV 4	Indometacin	Clinical efficacy	N/A	The treatment started 2 days before menstrual onset, once every day and was given for 4 days for 6 menstrual cycles	N/A
Chen LW et al. (2006) [32]	Random number table	30/28	16–28/15–24	Acupoint application at CV 4 CV 3 CV 6	Indometacin	Clinical efficacy	N/A	The treatment started 7 days before menstrual onset, once every day and was given for 10 days for 3 menstrual cycles	3 months
Liu C et al. (2011) [33]	Random number table	40/40	$21.22 \pm 5.86/20.96 \pm 6.12$	Moxibustion at CV 4 EX-B8	Fenbid	Clinical efficacy	symptom score	The treatment started 7 days before menstrual onset, once every day and was given for 10 days for 3 menstrual cycles	3 months
Zhu C et al. (2011) [34]	Random number table	20/20	17–28/18–27	Acupuncture at CV 4 CV 3 SP 10 SP 8 LI 4 LI 11	Indometacin	Clinical efficacy	N/A	The treatment started 7 days before menstrual onset, once every day and was given for 7 days for 3 menstrual cycles	3 months
Li ZL et al. (2012) [35]	Random number table	100/100	13–30/14–35	Acupoint application at CV 3 CV 8 BL 32 SP 6	Ibuprofen	Clinical efficacy	symptom score	The treatment started 7 days before menstrual onset, once every day and was given for 9 days for 6 menstrual cycles	6 months
Gurkan K et al. (2013) [19]	Registration order	11/24	$13.1 \pm 1.0/12.8 \pm 0.9$	Acupuncture at HT 7 PC 6 LI 4 LI 10 SP 6 LR 3 ST 36 GB 26 SP 15	Naproxen sodium	N/A	VAS	The treatment was given three times on the 5th and 2nd days prior to the expected menstruation date and on the third day of menstruation for 1 month	N/A
Jiang LY (2007) [36]	Registration order	34/34	$19.35 \pm 4.33/20.55 \pm 4.51$	Acupuncture at BL31 BL32 BL33 LI 3 SP 6 SP 8 CV 4 ST 36	Indometacin	Clinical efficacy	N/A	The treatment started 4 days before menstrual onset, once every day and was given for 7 days for 3 menstrual cycles	N/A
Xing QX (2011) [37]	Registration order	60/54	15–27/16–32	Pricking bloodletting at the liver area&kidney area; the liver area&the uterus area; HT 7	Indometacin	Clinical efficacy	N/A	The treatment started during the menstrual period, once every day and was given for 3 menstrual cycles	3 months
Ji L et al. (2012) [38]	Random number table	30/30	$22 \pm 3/22 \pm 2$	Sandwiched moxibustion at CV 8	Indometacin	Clinical efficacy	symptom score+ $PGF_{2\alpha} + PGE_2$	The treatment started 3 days before menstrual onset, once every day and was given for 6 days for 3 menstrual cycles	3 months

The above literatures didn't mention intention-to-treat or per-protocol analysis

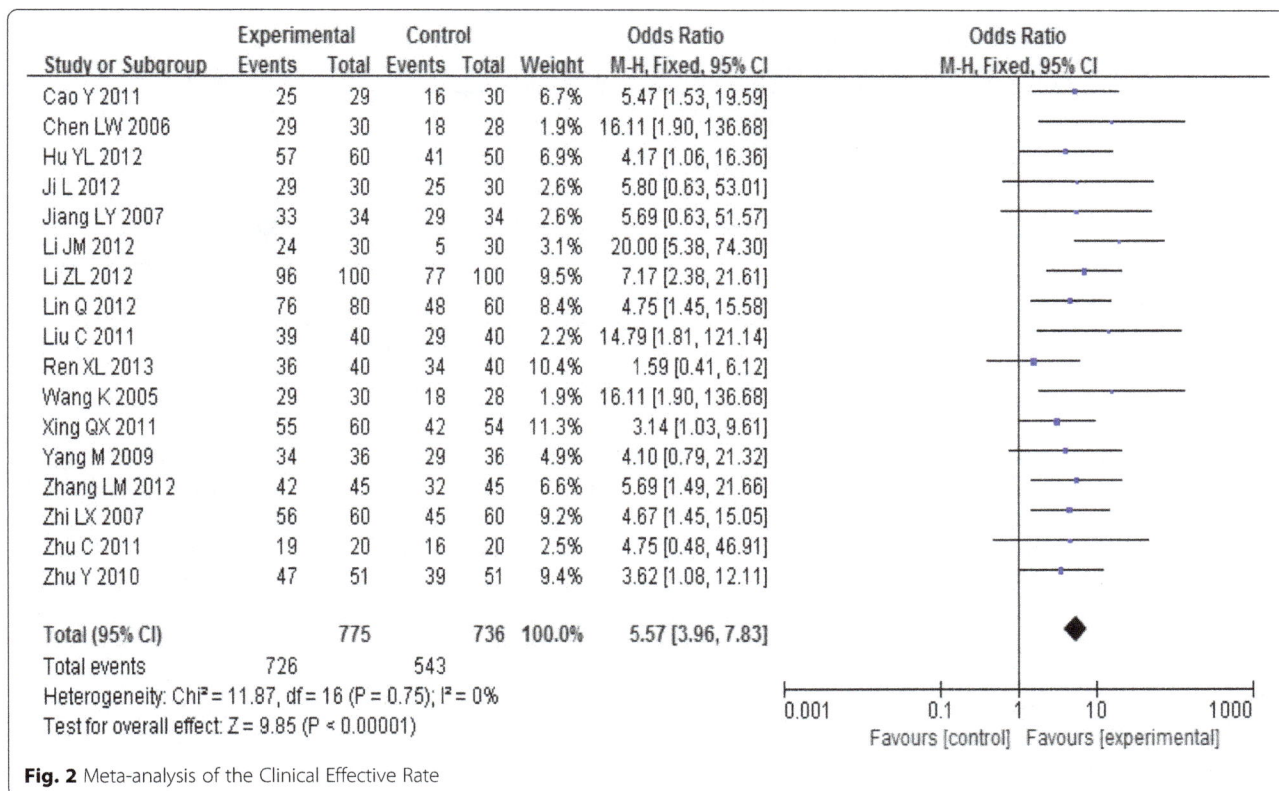

Fig. 2 Meta-analysis of the Clinical Effective Rate

To observe the vital signs before and after treatment and whether there were fainting, stomach ache, diarrhoea, nausea, and liver or kidney damage during the treatment and other adverse events occurred, and recorded.

Exclusion criteria

(1) Trials where it was unclear whether a randomized trial was being conducted;

(2) Trials conducted using combinations of treatments and many medical interventions;

(3) Trials in which the data were inadequate and difficult to extract.

Data extraction and quality assessment

Searches were conducted and the data extracted by two independent researchers. Each trial identified in the search was evaluated for design, eligibility criteria for participants, and outcome measures. Any disagreement

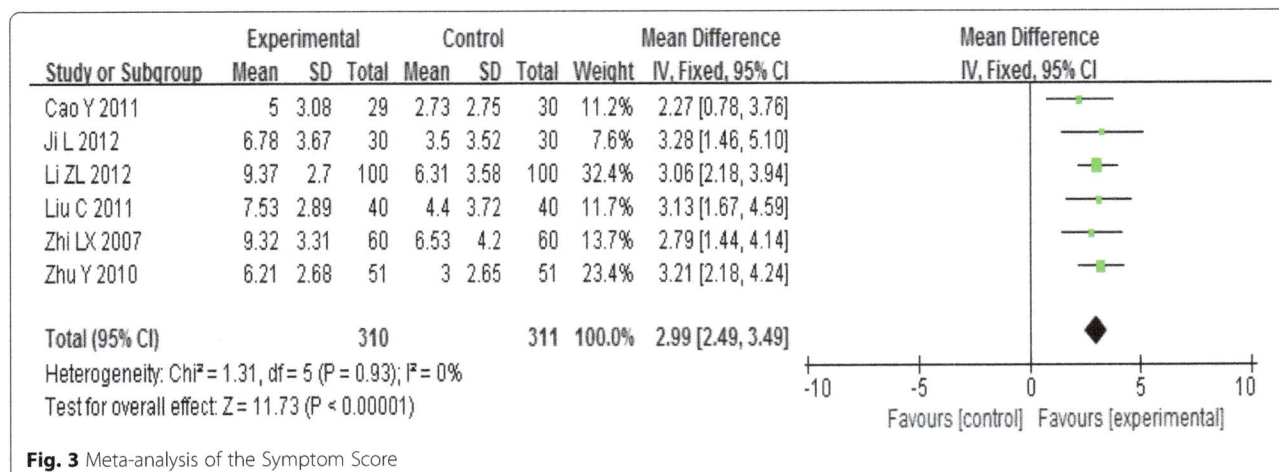

Fig. 3 Meta-analysis of the Symptom Score

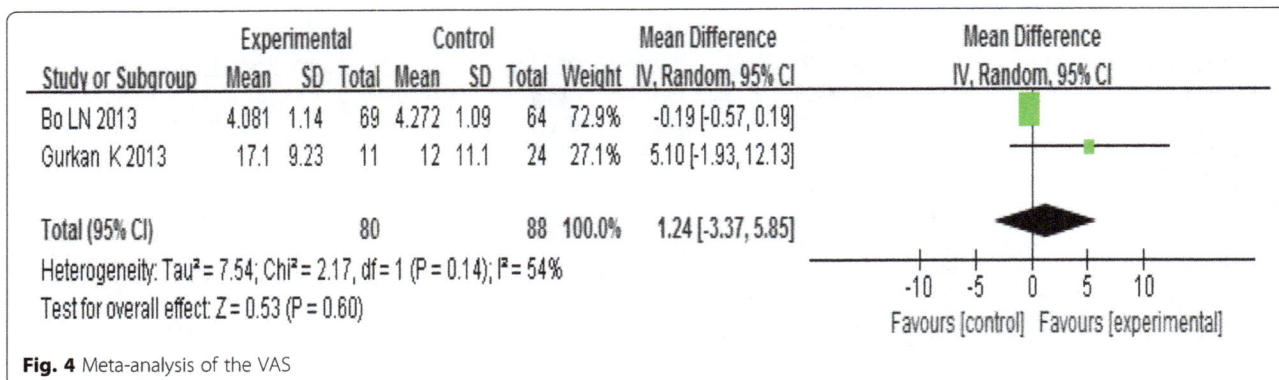

Fig. 4 Meta-analysis of the VAS

between researchers with regard to the eligibility of a trial was resolved by consulting a third researcher. We created a form for data extraction which included: (1) basic information about each trial, including the topic, first author, dateline and journal; (2) basic information about the patients, including the number of cases in each group and the mean age; (3) the study design and intervention; and (4) the outcomes.

The quality of the trials included in this study was assessed by other two researchers according to the Cochrane Handbook for Systematic Reviews of Interventions, Version 5.1.0.

Statistical analyses

All analyses were performed using Comprehensive Meta-Analysis statistical software, RevMan 5.1.0 (Cochrane Collaboration, Copenhagen, Denmark). Continuous outcome variables were analyzed using a standardized measure; dichotomous variables were compared and the results presented as odds ratios/risk ratios (OR/RR).

To obtain a standard deviation of the change from baseline for the experimental intervention, use (R_1 = 0.5) [20]:

$$SD(C) = \sqrt{SD(B)^2 + SD(F)^2 - (2 \times R_1 \times SD(B) \times SD \times (F))}$$

$SD(B)$ represents the standard deviation before intervention; $SD(F)$ represents the standard deviation after intervention.

The research team evaluated homogeneity among the trials via I^2. If I^2 was ≥50%, the trials were considered to be heterogeneous, and a random-effect model based on a Mantel-Haenszel (MH) or inverse variance (IV) statistical approach was selected. If I^2 was <50%, the studies were considered to be homogeneous, and a fixed-effects model based on an MH or IV statistical approach was used. Pooled summary statistics of the differences in the ratio or mean of the individual studies were developed. Pooled differences in ratios or means, and two-sided P-values were calculated and used as criteria for determining the level of statistical significance. $P < 0.05$ was considered to indicate statistical significance. Moreover, a sensitivity analysis was conducted based on the leave-one-out cross-validation procedure [21].

Results

Study selection

A flow chart of the included/excluded studies is shown in Fig. 1. Database searches yielded 70 studies from PubMed, 28 from the Cochrane Central Register of Clinical Trials, 215 from Embase, 552 from CNKI, 328 from Wanfang Data, 279 from VIP, and 479 from CBM. After removal of duplicate records, 849 records remained. Following the first review based on the title, 149 records were remained, and the abstracts were reviewed based on the pre-defined eligibility criteria. A total of 82 records were selected for full text review and data processing. During this

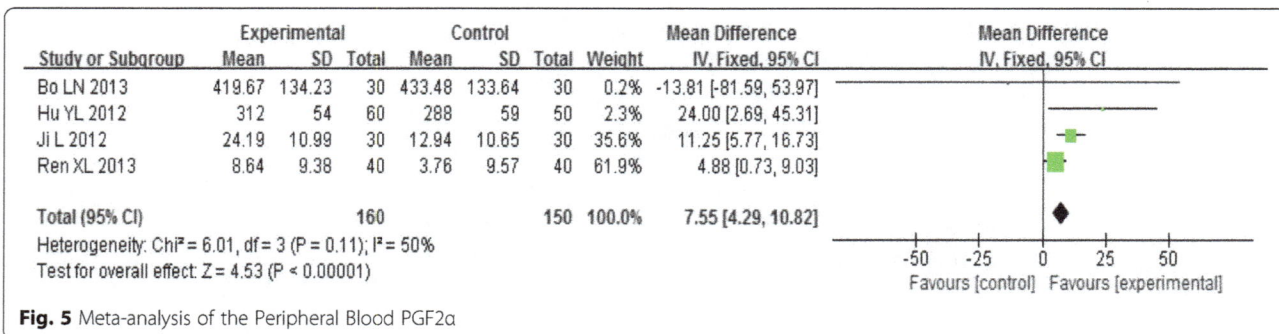

Fig. 5 Meta-analysis of the Peripheral Blood PGF2α

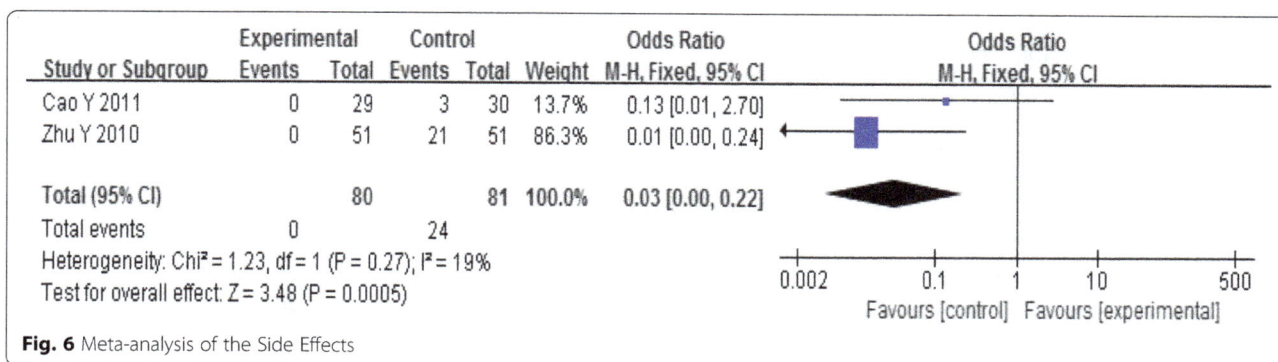

Fig. 6 Meta-analysis of the Side Effects

phase, 63 papers were excluded, so 19 studies were included in the final meta-analysis, comprising 1679 participants.

Characteristics of the included studies

Table 1 shows the main characteristics of the 19 RCTs [18, 19, 22–38].

Clinical outcomes

Clinical effectiveness rate

Seventeen trials examined the effects of acupoint-stimulation and reported the clinical effectiveness rate of treatment for participants with PD who used those therapies versus the rate for a control group. Analysis of pooled data using a fixed-effect model showed that the effect of intervention on the clinical effectiveness rate was positive [OR = 5.57, 95%CI (3.96, 7.83), $P < 0.00001$] (Fig. 2). That is to say, the clinical effectiveness rate, the acupoint-stimulation group being superior to the NSAIDs.

Symptom score

Six trials reported the symptom score. Analysis of pooled data using a fixed-effect model showed that the effect of intervention on the symptom score was positive [MD = 2.99, 95%CI (2.49, 3.49), $P < 0.00001$] (Fig. 3). The curative effect of acupoint-stimulation on PD is significant.

visual analogue score

Three trials reported the VAS; analysis of pooled data using a random-effect model showed that $I^2 = 98\%$, indicating heterogeneity. So, the trial by Cao (2011) was excluded from analysis, then analysis of the pooled data using a random-effect model showed that there was no statistical difference in variation of VAS between the groups receiving acupoint-stimulation and the control groups [MD = 1.24, 95%CI (−3.37,5.85), $P = 0.60$] (Fig. 4).

Peripheral blood PGF2α

Four trials examined the effects of acupoint-stimulation and reported peripheral blood PGF2α of participants with PD who used those therapies versus the rate for a control group. Analysis of the pooled data using a fixed-effect model showed that the effect of intervention on the variation in peripheral blood PGF2α between the groups receiving acupoint-stimulation and the control groups was positive [MD = 7.55, 95%CI (4.29, 10.82), $P < 0.00001$] (Fig. 5). In the study, it is indicated that acupoint-stimulation can effectively decrease peripheral blood PGF2α level in the patient of PD, so as to inhibit PGF2α-induced spastic contraction of uterine muscle, improve the decrease of blood flow, and relieve the symptoms of the patient of dysmenorrhea.

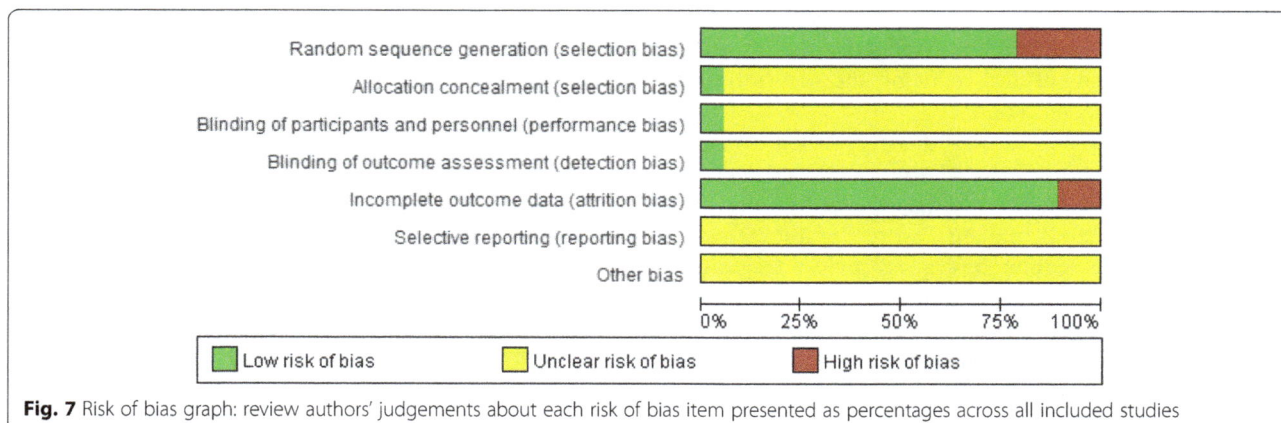

Fig. 7 Risk of bias graph: review authors' judgements about each risk of bias item presented as percentages across all included studies

Side effects

Three trials reported the side effects between acupoint-stimulation and control group. Analysis of pooled data using a random-effect model showed that $I^2 = 83\%$, indicating heterogeneity. So the trial by Bo (2013) was excluded from analysis, then analysis of the pooled data using a fixed-effect model showed that the side effects of control groups were more than the acupoint-stimulation group. [OR = 0.03, 95%CI (0.00, 0.22), $P = 0.0005$] (Fig. 6).

Quality assessment

The risks of seven biases among the 19 trials were evaluated, including random sequence generation, allocation concealment, blinding of participants and personnel, blinding of outcome assessment, incomplete outcome data, selective reporting, and other biases according to the criteria in the Cochrane Handbook for Systematic Reviews. Fifteen of the studies described correct randomization methods. There was only one trial with allocation concealment and blinding of participants and personnel and blinding of outcome assessment, and nearly all of the trials failed to mention allocation concealment, the blinding of the participants and personnel, and the blinding of outcome assessments. The methodological qualities of the included trials are summarized in Figs. 7 and 8.

Funnel plot of publication bias

The research team performed an analysis of all the included studies, using a funnel plot to determine publication bias in all of the literature. The outcome from the funnel plot analysis is summarized in Fig. 9. The outcome suggests that there was little publication bias.

Discussion

Meta-analysis of clinical effect

In the 19 RCTs included, 17 reported a clinical effectiveness rate and 6 reported symptom scores and 4 reported variation in the level of PGF2α in the peripheral blood of women with PD. The meta-analysis revealed that acupoint-stimulation is superior to NSAIDs in the treatment of PD in terms of clinical effectiveness rate and symptom improvement and reducing the concentration of PGF2α in peripheral blood.

Only one RCT reported uterine artery blood flow signals. The results showed that the uterine arterial pulsation index (PI) and uterine arterial resistance index (RI) of the dysmenorrheal patients were significantly increased in the eye acupuncture group before treatment. Moreover, most studies used a subjective, self-reported index of treatment effects as the outcome measure. Because participants self-reported without additional objective outcomes, their pain status could not be assessed accurately [39]. Furthermore, the included studies used

	Random sequence generation (selection bias)	Allocation concealment (selection bias)	Blinding of participants and personnel (performance bias)	Blinding of outcome assessment (detection bias)	Incomplete outcome data (attrition bias)	Selective reporting (reporting bias)	Other bias
Bo LN 2013	+	+	+	+	−	?	?
Cao Y 2011	+	?	?	?	−	?	?
Chen LW 2006	+	?	?	?	+	?	?
Gurkan K 2013	−	?	?	?	+	?	?
Hu YL 2012	+	?	?	?	+	?	?
Jiang LY 2007	−	?	?	?	+	?	?
Ji L 2012	+	?	?	?	+	?	?
Li JM 2012	+	?	?	?	+	?	?
Lin Q 2012	+	?	?	?	+	?	?
Liu C 2011	+	?	?	?	+	?	?
Li ZL 2012	+	?	?	?	+	?	?
Ren XL 2013	−	?	?	?	+	?	?
Wang K 2005	+	?	?	?	+	?	?
Xing QX 2011	−	?	?	?	+	?	?
Yang M 2009	+	?	?	?	+	?	?
Zhang LM 2012	+	?	?	?	+	?	?
Zhi LX 2007	+	?	?	?	+	?	?
Zhu C 2011	+	?	?	?	+	?	?
Zhu Y 2010	+	?	?	?	+	?	?

Fig. 8 Risk of bias summary: review authors' judgements about each risk of bias item for each included study

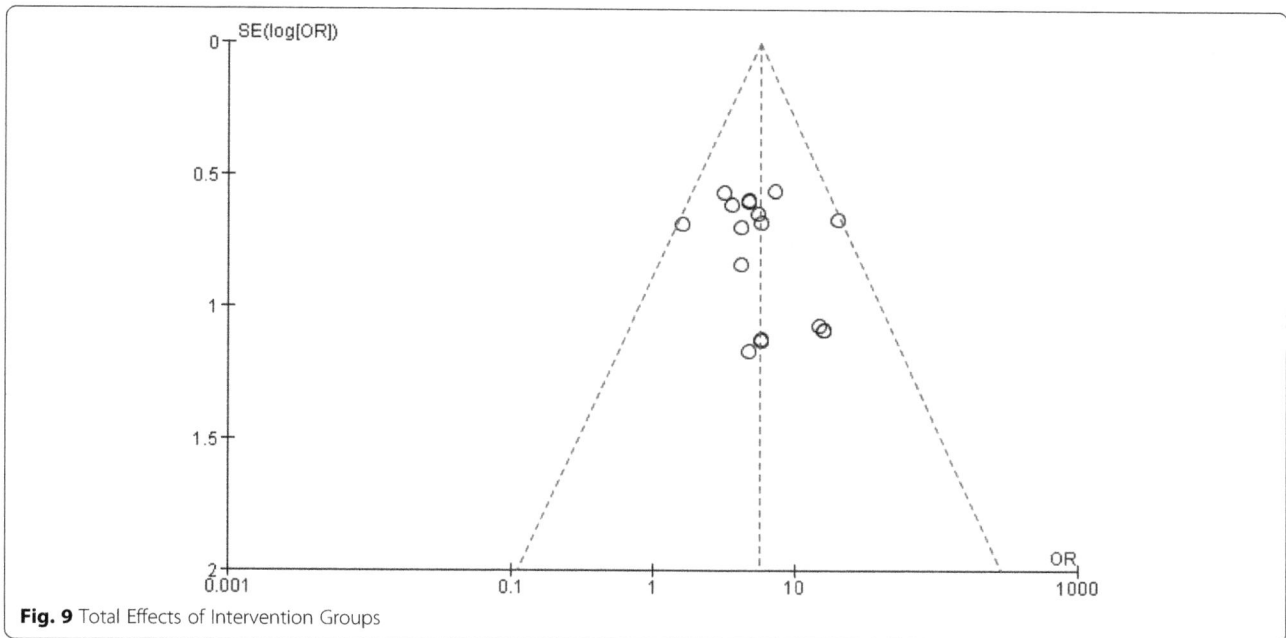

Fig. 9 Total Effects of Intervention Groups

different treatments for the intervention group, such as acupuncture, moxibustion, ear acupressure, electroacupuncture and acupoint application, which of the purpose is to highlight the specificity of acupoints.

The reason for NSAIDs being a drug of positive control

NSAIDs act by inhibiting the enzyme that catalyzes the conversion of arachidonic acid to cyclic endoperoxides, namely COX, which in turn inhibits the production of PGs [40, 41]. The resulting lower levels of PGs lead to less vigorous contractions of the uterus, and therefore to less discomfort. Thus, NSAIDs alleviate primary dysmenorrheic pain predominantly through the suppression of endometrial PGs synthesis [42]. Although NSAIDs is the first-line treatment for PD, it also has shortcomings, which can inhibit the synthesis of COX-1, as well as COX-2, finally it is easy to cause adverse reactions of gastrointestinal and central nervous system. Vane [43] indicated in 1994 that the effective treatment effect of NSAIDs was due to inhibition of COX-2, however, the adverse reactions imputed the suppression of COX-1. Therefore, we consider that NSAIDs may be used as a drug of positive control.

Although the results are encouraging, the conclusions from the current study should be carefully considered before being applied to clinical practice specific patients especially individuals with NSADIs contraindication. This study aims to collect all RCTs relating to acupoint-stimulation treatment of PD and use systematic review to gauge the effectiveness of acupoint-stimulation in the treatment of PD in order to use this treatment more widely in clinical practice.

Different conclusions of the published literature

Some evidence indicates that acupoint-stimulation is effective in treating primary dysmenorrhea [44–49], but that evidence was largely based on one small, randomized, controlled trial. However, two more recent sham acupuncture randomized controlled trials failed to show evidence of pain reduction [50, 51]. One of the major challenges may be the subjective nature of the symptoms' presentations and acupoints utilized. Although a few reviews [15, 21, 52, 53] of acupuncture for the treatment of PD are currently available, none of those reviews analyze the potential mechanism of acupuncture for the treatment of PD, which is the key research content in future. Therefore, a systematic review with a meta-analysis is necessary so that quality evidence can be put forward for the use (or not) of acupoint-stimulation for the treatment in individuals with PD.

Limitations and strengths

The limitations of this evaluation system are as follows: (1) most of the researches did not mention how the sample size was estimated, and most sample sizes were small, leading to a low inspection efficiency; (2) in some of the studies there was inadequate reporting of allocation concealment; implementing or not fully implementing allocation concealment will lead to an exaggerated curative effect; (3) the results were heterogeneous on account of their use of subjective indicators to evaluate the curative effect (symptom scores, VAS), so that implementation of the blinding method is important, but the included studies did not describe the implementation of the blinding method; (4) the study was limited to Chinese and

English research, leading to the possibility of selection bias, and the terminology or the guidelines used in clinical managements might not be in the same language.

The strengths of this evaluation system are as follows: this is the first report that comparing the effect of acupoint-stimulation and NSADIs in the treatment of PD, and it provides new evidence and open new horizons that acupoint-stimulation can relieve pain effectively in the treatment of PD and offers advantages in increasing the overall effectiveness.

Perspectives

In our future research, we will conduct some trials relating to acupoint-stimulation for the treatment of PD, which will focus on the following aspects to prevent bias: (1) an estimation of sample size, (2) a fully random design incorporating allocation concealment, and (3) a blind design for the proposer, performer and measurer.

Conclusion

The current evidence reveals that acupoint-stimulation in the treatment of PD has some obvious advantages compared with treatment by NSADIs. The advantages are that acupoint-stimulation can alleviate the symptoms of dysmenorrhoea, reduce the level of peripheral blood $PGF2\alpha$ and has fewer side effect, so it can be used to treat PD patients, especially individuals with NSADIs contraindication.

Abbreviations
CI: Confidence interval; CNKI: Chinese Science and Technology Journal Full-text Database; COX: Cyclooxygenase; COX-2: Cyclooxygenase 2; GCTNPCM: The Guideline for Clinical Trials of New Patent Chinese Medicines; IV: Inverse variance; MD: Mean difference; MH: Mantel-Haenszel; NE: Noradrenaline; NSAIDs: Non-Steroidal Anti-Inflammatory Drugs; OR: Odds ratios; OT: Oxytocin; PD: Primary dysmenorrhoea; $PGF2\alpha$: Prostaglandin $F2\alpha$; PGs: Prostaglandins; PI: Pulsation index; PRC: People's Republic of China; RCTs: Randomized controlled trials; RI: Resistance index; RR: Risk ratios; TCM: Traditional Chinese Medicine; VAS: Visual analogue score; VIP: Chinese Biomedical Literature Database; VP: Vasopressin.

Acknowledgments
Medical writing services were provided by YiHeAn Biotechnology Co. Ltd.. Authors retained full control of manuscript content.

Funding
This project was supported by the Science Foundation on Traditional Chinese Medicine/Integrative Medicine of the Tianjin Health and Family Planning Commission (2015036).

Authors' contributions
W.L.Z, Y.Z. And S.L.S conceived and designed the review; Y.X. And W.L.Z analyzed the data; H.E.B. Contributed reagents/materials/analysis tools; Z.M.Z., W.L.Z. And T.L. wrote the paper. All authors read and approved the final manuscript.

Authors' information
All authors contributed to the design and concept, performed the searches required for their assigned sections, wrote a section, read, revised and critiqued the successive versions, and approved the final manuscript. YZ coordinated the effort and integrated the sections and comments.

Competing interests
The authors declare that they have no competing interests.

Author details
Graduate School, Tianjin University of Traditional Chinese Medicine, Tianjin 300193, China. [2]Department of Gynecology and Obstetrics, Nankai Hospital, Tianjin Academy of Integrative Medicine, Tianjin 300100, China. [3]Department of Neurology, Nankai Hospital, Tianjin Academy of Integrative Medicine, Tianjin 300100, China. [4]Department of Chinese Medicine, Tianjin Hearing Impairment Specialist Hospital, Tianjin 300150, China. [5]Department of Public Health, School of Chinese Medicine, Tianjin University of Traditional Chinese Medicine, Tianjin 300193, China. [6]Department of Gynecology and Obstetrics of Chinese Medicine, First Teaching Hospital of Tianjin University of Traditional Chinese Medicine, Tianjin 300193, China. [7]Department of Chemical Engineering, University of Florida, 1006 Center Drive, Gainesville, FL 32611, USA. [8]Institute for Cell & Tissue Science and Engineering, University of Florida, Gainesville, FL 32611, USA. [9]Laboratory of Anatomy, School of Integrative Medicine, Tianjin University of Traditional Chinese Medicine, No. 88 Yu Quan Road, Nankai District, Tianjin 300193, China.

References
1. Hillen TIJ, Grbavac SL, Johnston PJ, Straton JAY, Keogh JMF. Primary dysmenorrhea in young western Australian women: prevalence, impact, and knowledge of treatment. J Adolesc Health. 1999;25(1):40–5.
2. Burnett MA, Antao V, Black A, Feldman K, Grenville A, Lea R, Lefebvre G, Pinsonneault O, Robert M. Prevalence of primary dysmenorrhea in Canada. J Obstet Gynaecol Can. 2005;27(8):765–70.
3. Ortiz MI, Rangel-Flores E, Carrillo-Alarcón LC, Veras-Godoy HA. Prevalence and impact of primary dysmenorrhea among Mexican high school students. Int J Gynecol Obstet. 2009;107(3):240–3.
4. Jalili Z, Safizadeh H, Shamsipoor N. Prevalence of primary dysmenorrhea in college students in Sirjan. Kerman Payesh. 2005;4(1):61–7.
5. Dawood MY. Dysmenorrhea. Clin Obstet Gynecol. 1983;26(3):719–27.
6. Jun EM, Chang S, Kang DH, Kim S. Effects of acupressure on dysmenorrhea and skin temperature changes in college students: a non-randomized controlled trial. Int J Nurs Stud. 2007;44(6):973–81.
7. Speroff L, Fritz MA. Clinical Gynecologic Endocrinology and Infertility (7th edition). Philadelphia: Lippincott Williams and Wilkins, 2005, Menstrual disorders; pp. 401–464.
8. Balbi C, Musone R, Menditto A, Prisco LD, Cassese E, D'Ajello M, et al. Influence of menstrual factors and dietary habits on menstrual pain in adolescence age. Eur J Obstet Gynecol Reprod Biol. 2000;91(2):143–8.
9. Ylikorkala O, Dawood MY. New concepts in dysmenorrhea. Am J Obstet Gynecol. 1978;130(7):833–47.
10. Pu BC, Fang L, Gao LN, Liu R, Li AZ. Animal study on primary dysmenorrhoea treatment at different administration times. Evid Based Complement Alternat Med. 2015;2015:367379.
11. Harel Z. Dysmenorrhea in adolescents and young adults: from pathophysiology to pharmacological treatments and management strategies. Expert Opin Pharmacother. 2008;9(15):2661–72.
12. Alvin PE, Litt IF. Current status of etiology and management of dysmenorrhea in adolescents. Pediatrics. 1982;70(4):516–25.
13. Dawood MY. Nonsteroidal anti-inflammatory drugs and changing attitudes toward dysmenorrhea. Am J Med. 1988;84(5):23–9.
14. Kaplan Ö, Nazıroğlu M, Güney M, Aykur M. Non-steroidal anti-inflammatory drug modulates oxidative stress and calcium ion levels in the neutrophils of patients with primary dysmenorrhea. J Reprod Immunol. 2013;100(2):87–92.
15. Yang H, Liu CZ, Chen X, Ma LX, Xie JP, Guo NN, Ma ZB, Zheng YY, Zhu J, Liu JP. Systematic review of clinical trials of acupuncture-related therapies for primary dysmenorrhea. Acta Obstet Gynecol Scand. 2008;87(11):1114–22.
16. Lin JG, Chen YH, Gao XY, Lao L, Lee H, Litscher G. Clinical efficacy, mechanisms, and safety of acupuncture and moxibustion. Evid Based Complement Alternat Med. 2014;2014:356258.
17. Zheng X-Y. Guideline for clinical trials of new patent Chinese medicines. 1st ed. Beijing: Ministry of Health of the People's Republic of China; 1993. p. 263–5.
18. Hu YL, Lin Q, Li Y, Zheng XM. Effect of eye acupuncture on plasma PGF 2α in patients of primary dysmenorrhea. World J Acupuncture-Moxibustion. 2012; 22(1):17–22.

19. Kiran G, Gumusalan Y, Ekerbicer HC, Kiran H, Coskun A, Arikan DC. A randomized pilot study of acupuncture treatment for primary dysmenorrhea. Eur J Obstet Gynecol Reprod Biol. 2013;169(2):292–5.

20. Higgins JP, Green S. Cochrane Handbook for Systematic Reviews of Interventions (Version 5.1.0). The Cochrane Collaboration, 2011, Available from: http://www.cochrane.org/handbook. Accessed 17 July 2015.

21. Xu T, Hui L, Juan YL, Min SG, Hua WT. Effects of moxibustion or acupoint therapy for the treatment of primary dysmenorrhea: a meta-analysis. Altern Ther Health Med. 2014;20(4):33–42.

22. Zhang LM, Yang HY. The 45 cases on single acupuncture treatment for primary dysmenorrhea. Fujian J TCM. 2012;43(2):25–6.

23. Lin Q, Chen WZ, Li Y, Hu YL. Effect of eye acupuncture on uterine artery blood flow in patients with primary dysmenorrhea. Shanghai J Acupunct Moxibustion. 2012;31(12):885–7.

24. Cao Y. Acupuncture clinical analysis of primary dysmenorrhea. Master Thesis Heilongjiang Chin Med College 2011: 26-29.

25. Zhi LX. Randomized controlled study on superficial needling for treatment of primary dysmenorrhea. Zhongguo Zhen Jiu. 2007;27(1):18–21.

26. Bo LN. A literature mining and randomized controlled trial of moxibustion in treating primary dysmenorrhea. Doctor Thesis Chengdu Chin Med College 2013: 43-60, 67-70.

27. Ren XL. Clinical study on the treatment of primary Dysmenorrhea with moxibustion. Global Traditional Chin Med. 2013;6(6):431–2.

28. Zhu Y, Chen RL, Le JI, Miao FR. Efficacy observation of primary dysmenorrhea treated with isolated-herbal moxibustion on Shenque (CV8). Zhongguo Zhen Jiu. 2010;30(6):453–5.

29. Li JM. Clinical study of electro—acupuncture treatment of primary dysmenorrhea Ci Liao acupoints. Master Thesis. Guangzhou Chin Med College. 2012: 15-17.

30. Wang K, Pan WY, Duan YH. Clinical study on the treatment of primary dysmenorrhea with auricular acupuncture. Guangdong Med J. 2005;26(12):1728–30.

31. Yang M. The clinical observation of 36 cases on dysmenorrhea moxibustion treatment of primary dysmenorrhea. Hainan Med J. 2009;20(7):226–7.

32. Chen LW. The clinical observation of primary dysmenorrhea treated with the Chinese native médicine sticks on the acupuncture point. Master Thesis Guangzhou Chin Med College 2006: 20-22.

33. Liu C, Zhang HY. Therapeutic effect of moxibustion on primary dysmenorrhea due to damp-cold retention. World J Acupuncture-Moxibustion. 2011;21(3):1–4.

34. Zhu C. Clinical study on the treatment of haemorrheological nature blood stasis type of primary dysmenorrhea with moxibustion. Hubei J TCM. 2011;33(1):65–6.

35. Li ZL, Li YQ, Pan FQ, Bian WH, Chu JZ, Zhu PQ. Clinical observation on Chinese herbs acupoint of Yugui wenjing decoction stick to treat haemorrheological nature blood stasis type of primary dysmenorrhea. Modern J Integrated Traditional Chinese Western Med. 2012;21(5):483–4.

36. Jiang LY. Clinical experience of acupuncture for treatment of 34 cases in primary dysmenorrhea. J Emerg Tradit Chin Med. 2007;16:620–1.

37. Xing QX. Observation on the therapeutic effect of pricking bloodletting at ear points on primary dysmenorrhea. Shanghai Zhenjiu Zazhi. 2011;30:235–6.

38. Ji L, Chen RL, Deng PY, Zhou LJ, Do SC, Zhu Y. Treatment effect of herb-partitioned moxibustion for dysmenorrhea of cold stagnation type and its effect on PGF2α and PGE2. Shanghai J Acupunct Moxibustion. 2012;31:882–4.

39. Sale H, Hedman L, Isberg A. Accuracy of patients' recall of temporomandibular joint pain and dysfunction after experiencing whiplash: a prospective study. J Am Dent Assoc. 2010;141(7):879–86.

40. Warner TD, Giuliano F, Vojnovic I, Bukasa A, Mitchell JA, Vane JR. Nonsteroid drug selectivities for cyclo-oxygenase-1 rather than cyclo-oxygenase-2 are associated with human gastrointestinal toxicity: a full in vitro analysis. Proc Natl Acad Sci U S A. 1999;96(13):7563–8.

41. Ruoff G, Lema M. Strategies in pain management: new and potential indications for COX-2 specific inhibitors. J Pain Symptom Manag. 2003;25(2):S21–31.

42. Dawood MY. Dysmenorrhea. J Reprod Med. 1990;33(1):168–78.

43. Vane JR. Towards a better aspirin. Nature. 1994;36(2):215–6.

44. Dawood MY. Primary dysmenorrhea: advances in pathogenesis and management. Obstet Gynecol. 2006;108(2):428–41.

45. Doty E, Attaran M. Managing primary dysmenorrhea. J Pediatr Adolesc Gynecol. 2006;19(5):341–4.

46. Proctor M, Farquhar C. Diagnosis and management of dysmenorrhea. BMJ. 2006;332(7550):1134–8.

47. Sanfilippo J, Erb T. Evaluation and management of dysmenorrhea in adolescents. Clin Obstet Gynecol. 2008;51(2):257–67.

48. French L. Dysmenorrhea. Am Fam Physician. 2005;71(2):285–91.

49. Durain D. Primary dysmenorrhea: assessment and management update. J Midwifery Women's Health. 2004;49(6):520–8.

50. Smith CA, Crowther CA, Petrucco O, Beilby J, Dent H. Acupuncture to treat primary dysmenorrhea in women: a randomized controlled trial. Evid Based Complement Alternat Med. 2011;2011:612464.

51. Kempf D, Berger D, Ausfeld-Hafter B. Laser needle acupuncture in women with dysmenorrhoea: a randomised controlled double blind pilot trial. Forsch Komplementmed. 2009;16(1):6–12.

52. Chung YC, Chen HH, Yeh ML. Acupoint stimulation intervention for people with primary dysmenorrhea: systematic review and meta-analysis of randomized trials. Complement Ther Med. 2012;20(5):353–63.

53. Abaraogu UO, Tabansi-Ochuogu CS. As acupressure decreases pain, acupuncture may improve some aspects of quality of life for women with primary Dysmenorrhea: a systematic review with meta-analysis. J Acupunct Meridian Stud. 2015;8(5):220–8.

20

Effect of acupuncture on Lipopolysaccharide-induced anxiety-like behavioral changes: involvement of serotonin system in dorsal Raphe nucleus

Tae Young Yang[1†], Eun Young Jang[1†], Yeonhee Ryu[2†], Gyu Won Lee[1], Eun Byeol Lee[1], Suchan Chang[1], Jong Han Lee[1], Jin Suk Koo[3], Chae Ha Yang[1] and Hee Young Kim[1,4*]

Abstract

Background: Acupuncture has been used as a common therapeutic tool in many disorders including anxiety and depression. Serotonin transporter (SERT) plays an important role in the pathology of anxiety and other mood disorders. The aim of this study was to evaluate the effects of acupuncture on lipopolysaccharide (LPS)-induced anxiety-like behaviors and SERT in the dorsal raphe nuclei (DRN).

Methods: Rats were given acupuncture at ST41 (*Jiexi*), LI11 (*Quchi*) or SI3 (*Houxi*) acupoint in LPS-treated rats. Anxiety-like behaviors of elevated plus maze (EPM) and open field test (OFT) were measured and expressions of SERT and/or c-Fos were also examined in the DRN using immunohistochemistry.

Results: The results showed that 1) acupuncture at ST41 acupoint, but neither LI11 nor SI3, significantly attenuated LPS-induced anxiety-like behaviors in EPM and OFT, 2) acupuncture at ST41 decreased SERT expression increased by LPS in the DRN.

Conclusions: Our results suggest that acupuncture can ameliorate anxiety-like behaviors, possibly through regulation of SERT in the DRN.

Keywords: Acupuncture, Anxiety, Dorsal raphe nucleus, LPS, Serotonin transporter

Background

Anxiety disorders, also called as generalized, social anxiety and panic disorder, are the most common mental health disorders which are characterized by irritability, fatigue, presence of restlessness, muscle tension, sleep problems, an intense and persistent fear of social, recurrent and unexpected panic attacks [1–3]. Anxiety disorders are also significantly related to other physiological dysfunctions such as migraine headaches, respiratory diseases, gastrointestinal diseases, and arthritis

---

* Correspondence: hykim@dhu.ac.kr

†Equal contributors

[1]College of Korean Medicine, Daegu Haany University, Daegu 42158, South Korea

[4]Department of Physiology, College of Korean Medicine, Daegu Haany University, Daegu 42158, South Korea

Full list of author information is available at the end of the article

and can negatively affect mobility, social function, and health care [4].

Among neurotransmitters, serotonin (5-hydroxytryptamine or 5-HT) is critically involved in the pathophysiology of mood and anxiety disorders [5]. Several lines of evidence indicate that serotonin transporter (SERT or 5-HTT), responsible for high-affinity serotonin uptake from extracellular fluid at the synaptic cleft, plays important roles in the pathology of depression and other mood disorders [6–8]. A previous study showed that reduction of tryptophan hydroxylase (enzyme for serotonin synthesis) and SERT in ventromedial prefrontal cortex (vmPFC) and increased SERT in dorsal raphe nucleus (DRN) are associated with mood- and anxiety-like behavior in animal model [9]. In addition, the patients with anxiety disorder reveal enhanced serotonin synthesis [10] and reduced serotonin 1A receptor levels [11] in the amygdala and prescribe selective serotonin reuptake inhibitors (SSRIs) targeting SERT [12, 13].

Lipopolysaccharide (LPS), a bacterial endotoxin, causes physiological or psychiatric changes such as anhedonia, anorexia, depressed mood, apathy [14, 15] and inflammation linked to anxiety and depression [16]. LPS can trigger depressive symptoms in humans [14] and anxiety- and depressive-like behaviors in experimental animals [16, 17]. The underlying mechanism includes increased serotonin turnover rates [18] and changes of SERT activity [19] by LPS.

Acupuncture has been increasingly used as an alternative therapy for mental disorders such as addiction, Parkinson's diseases, insomnia, and anxiety [20–23]. Especially, it was reported that acupuncture decreases tension, anxiety, and anger/aggression in anxiety disorder patients [23]. In addition, experimentally electroacupuncture regulates levels of T lymphocyte subsets in plasma and thymus in stress-induced anxiety rats [24]. Based on these studies, acupuncture may be effective in reducing anxiety, although the underlying mechanism is unclear.

To explore whether acupuncture can suppress anxiety-like behaviors by modulating SERT in the DRN, the present study examined the effects of acupuncture on LPS-induced anxiety-like behaviors and expressions of SERT in the DRN in rats.

Methods

Animals

Male Sprague-Dawley rats weighing 270–300 g (Daehan Animal, Seoul, Korea) were housed in groups of 2–3 rats per cage in controlled temperature (23 ± 2 °C) and humidity ($50 \pm 10\%$) on a 12 h light-dark cycle (lights on at 8:00 am) with ad libitum food and water. All experimental procedures were approved by the Institutional Animal Care and Use Committees of Daegu Haany University and conducted in accordance with National Institutes of Health guidelines for the care and use of laboratory animals.

Drug and chemicals

Lipopolysaccharide (LPS) and other chemicals were purchased from Sigma (Sigma, St. Louis, MO, USA). Primary antibodies for c-Fos (sc-52, Santa Cruz, CA, USA) and serotonin transporter (SERT; AB9726, Millipore, MA, USA) and donkey anti-rabbit Alexa Fluor 488 (A21206, Life Technologies, CA, USA) and 594 (A21207) were used for immunohistochemistry. LPS was dissolved in physiological saline and intraperitoneally (i.p.) administered at dose of 0.2 mg/kg.

Acupuncture treatment

Rats were given acupuncture at SI3, LI11, or ST41 acupoint for each 30 s before and after LPS administration (0.2 mg/kg, i.p.) and 2 h after LPS administration (Fig. 1a-c). The animals were then subjected to behavioral tests of elevated plus maze (EPM) and open field test (OPT) (Fig. 1c). For acupuncture treatment, stainless-steel needles (0.10 mm diameter and 7 mm length; Dongbang Medical Co., Korea) were inserted vertically to a depth of 3 mm from surface of skin, and manually performed twisted at a frequency of twice per second for 30 s, and the needles were then withdrawn. LI11 (*Qu Chi*) is located at the lateral of the transverse cubital crease midway, which is clinically prescribed for mental disorders in combination. SI3 (*Houxi*) is located on the dorsum of the hand, in the depression proximal to the ulnar side of the fifth metacarpophalangeal joint, at the border between the red and white flesh. ST41 (*Jiexi*) is located between two tendons on the dorsum of the foot which are more distinct when the ankle is dorsiflexion. In the present study, LI11 and SI3 acupoints were used as control points. The control groups were lightly grabbed without acupuncture needle insertion for 1 min.

Elevated Plus Maze (EPM)

Anxiety-like behavior produced by LPS was measured by using a modified EPM method [25]. Briefly, the maze was constructed of black acrylic and consisted of two open arms (50 cm × 10 cm) and two closed arms (50 cm × 10 cm × 40 cm) extending from a central platform (5 cm × 5 cm). Rats were placed at the center of EPM and time spent in the open arms was recorded for 5 min by a video tracking system (Ethovision, Nodus Information Technology BV, Wageningen, Netherlands).

Open field test (OFT)

A black rectangular box with a square floor (45 cm × 45 cm × 45 cm) was divided into nine equal sized zones (15 cm × 15 cm). Rats were placed at the central zone in an open field arena. Time spent was monitored and measured for 5 min in the central zone by a video tracking system (Ethovision, Nodus Information Technology BV, Wageningen, Netherlands).

Immunofluorescence for SERT or c-Fos

Rats were anesthetized with sodium pentobarbital (80 mg/kg, i.p.) and intracardially perfused with ice-cold saline followed by ice-cold 4% paraformaldehyde solution in 0.1 M phosphate buffered saline (PBS; pH 7.4). Brains were rapidly removed from the skull and then post-fixed with 10% sucrose/4% paraformaldehyde for 2 h and cryoprotected in 30% sucrose for at least

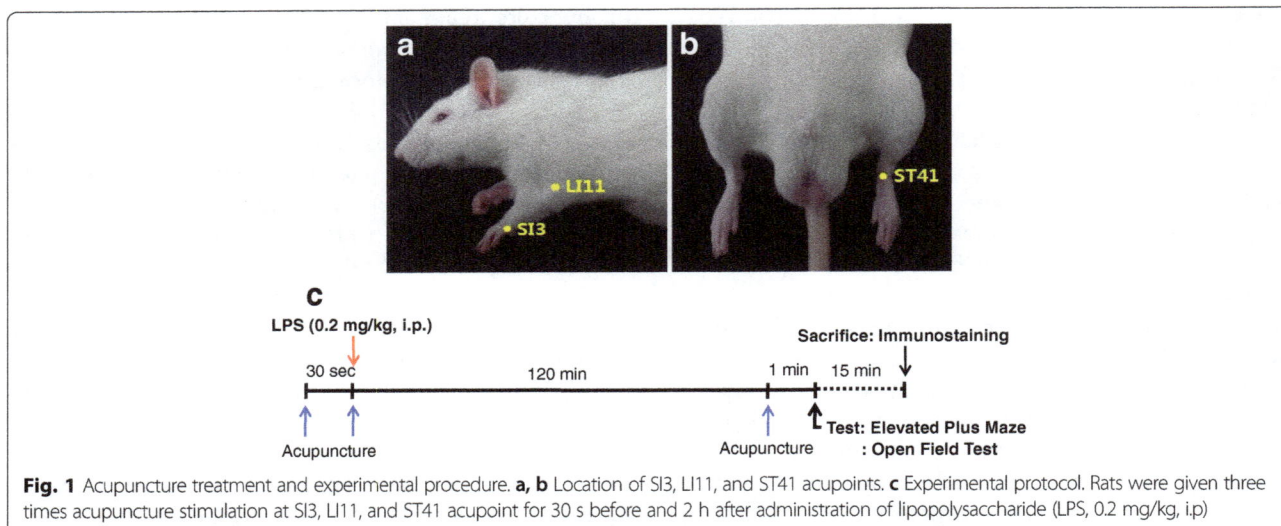

Fig. 1 Acupuncture treatment and experimental procedure. **a, b** Location of SI3, LI11, and ST41 acupoints. **c** Experimental protocol. Rats were given three times acupuncture stimulation at SI3, LI11, and ST41 acupoint for 30 s before and 2 h after administration of lipopolysaccharide (LPS, 0.2 mg/kg, i.p)

48 h. The brains were cryosectioned into 30 μm slices and incubated in blocking solutions containing 0.3% Triton X-100, 5% normal donkey serum in 0.01 M PBS at the room temperature for 1 h. After rinsing in PBS, the sections were incubated with primary antibody for c-Fos (red; 1:1000, Santa Cruz, CA, USA) and serotonin transporter (green; 1:500, Millipore, MA, USA) overnight at 4 °C. The sections were then processed with secondary antibody with donkey anti-rabbit Alexa Fluor 594 (red; 1:500, Life Technologies, CA, USA) and 488 (green; 1:500). All sections were cover-slipped with a mounting medium (Vector Laboratories, Burlingame, CA, USA) and were imaged under a 10 X objective using microscope (Zeiss Axioskop, Oberkochen, Germany). Fluorescence intensities (FI) of SERT in each section were estimated by computerized densitometry (i-solution, IMT, Daejeon, Korea).

Statistical analysis

Statistical analysis was carried out using SPSS 11.0 software. All data are presented as mean ± SEM (standard error of the mean) and were analyzed by one-way analysis of variance (ANOVA) followed by LSD post hoc test with statistical significance set at $^{\#}P < 0.05$, **, $^{\$\$}$ $P < 0.01$, and ***, $^{\#\#\#}$ $P < 0.001$.

Results
Effect of acupuncture on EPM parameter after LPS administration

LPS-treated group significantly spent less time in the open arms compared to normal group ($P < 0.001$). As shown in Fig. 2b, the LPS-treated rats displayed avoidance of the open arms while staying in closed arms. In acupuncture groups, rats received acupuncture treatment of 3 sessions:

before, immediately and 120 min after LPS administration (Fig. 1c). When time spent in the open arms was recorded for 5 min, acupuncture at ST41, but SI3, increased time spent in the open arms of EPM, compared to LPS-treated group (One-way ANOVA, $F_{(4,35)} = 22.775$, $P < 0.001$; post hoc, $P < 0.01$ vs. LPS). In contrast, acupuncture at LI11 (LPS + LI11) decreased time spent in the open arms of EPM compared to those of LPS or LPS + LI11 (Fig. 2; $P < 0.01$).

Effect of acupuncture on OFT parameter after LPS administration

Since rodents tend to avoid the center of the field under stress or depressive condition [26], the OFT was performed to further confirm the effects of acupuncture at ST41 on anxiety-like behaviors. When arena was subdivided into center and border zones, LPS-treated group spent lesser time in the central zone of the open field area than control group (Fig. 3a and b, $P < 0.001$), indicating anxiety-like behaviors by EPM. On the other hand, acupuncture at ST41, but neither LI11 nor SI3, group significantly elevated time spent in the central zone of open field area (Fig. 3c and d; One-way ANOVA, $F_{(4,29)} = 13.3707$, $P < 0.001$; post hoc $P < 0.05$ vs. LPS).

Effect of acupuncture on expression of SERT in the DRN

To see whether SERT expression is increased in activated neurons after LPS administration, c-Fos, a marker of neuronal activation, was double-stained with SERT in the DRN. Many red stained nuclei (c-Fos) surrounded by green cytoplasmic staining were observed in LPS group, indicating the expression of SERT in activated DRN neurons (Fig. 4b).

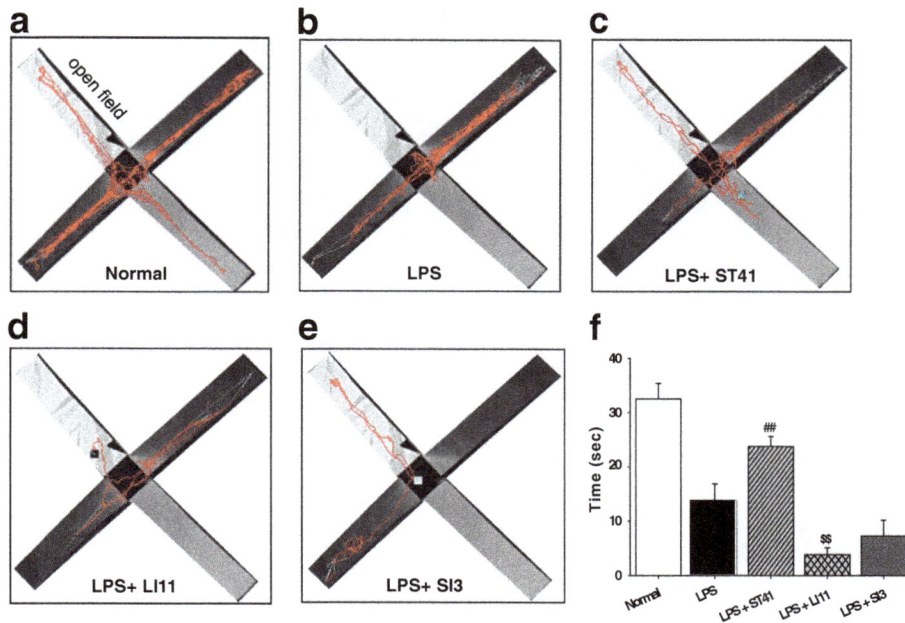

Fig. 2 Effect of acupuncture on LPS-induced anxiety-like behavior in the EPM. **a-e** Representative examples of traveling pattern for 5 min in the open arms. **f** Time spent in the open arms for 5 min presented as mean ± SEM. While LPS-administered rats spent less time in open arms compared to normal, acupuncture at ST41, but neither LI11 nor SI3, significantly spent more time in open arms compared to LPS-administered rats. *** $P < 0.001$ vs. normal, ## $P < 0.01$ vs. LPS, $$ $P < 0.01$ vs. LPS; $n = 6-7$ per group

Next, to explore the changes of SERT expression in the dorsal raphe nuclei (DRN) following acupuncture at ST41 in LPS-treated rats, the brains were taken out 15 min after last acupuncture treatment in one set of rats, according to experimental procedure shown in Fig. 1c. An enhanced expression in SERT fluorescence was observed in LPS-treated group compared to normal rats ($P < 0.01$). Acupuncture at ST41 significantly attenuated the SERT expression compared to LPS group (Fig. 5. One-way ANOVA, $F_{(2,12)} = 5.414$, $P = 0.021$, post hoc $P < 0.001$ vs. LPS).

Discussion

The present study demonstrated that acupuncture at ST41 results in 1) a decrease in LPS-induced anxiety-like behaviors in both EPM and OPF and 2) a reduction of SERT expression in the DRN enhanced by LPS.

LPS, a biologically active component of the outer membrane of gram negative bacteria, is widely used in experimental animal model in order to induce systemic inflammation [27], stimulate the release of pro-inflammatory cytokines in the brain areas [28] and produce sickness behaviors [29]. Peripheral LPS administration produces anxiety-like behaviors in EPM and OFT [30]. In accordance with others [31, 32], in the present study, LPS reduced time spent in open arms in EPM as well as in the center of zone in open filed area [33, 34], indicating induction of anxiety-like behaviors.

These behaviors were reversed by acupuncture at ST41, but neither SI3 nor LI11. These results suggest that anxiety-like behaviors were induced by acute treatment with LPS and acupuncture could suppress the development of the anxiety in rats in a point-specific manner. Acupuncture at ST41 has been used empirically in conjugation with other acupoints to treat neurological disorders in humans, but few experimental studies have been conducted to support the effects of single point ST41 on neurological symptoms. In one previous study, acupuncture at ST41, without combination with other points, can generate therapeutic effect on muscle fatigue by reducing glutathione levels in muscle tissues [35]. It is first time to show experimental evidence of anxiolytic effects of ST41 acupoint.

Behavioral alterations in anxiety or depression disorder are closely linked to abnormalities of serotonergic system [36, 37]. As a large number of serotonin cells is found in the DRN [38, 39], the DRN (synthesis or releasing of serotonin) is considered to be a critical region related to anxiety or depressive disorder. Serotonergic neurons project from the DRN to the extended amygdala, hippocampus, striatum, nucleus accumbens, and cortex [40]. Several lines of evidence have shown that transport capacity (Vmax) of cortical SERT, SERT activity and SERT protein level are enhanced in the frontal cortex of LPS-administered animal [19] and in the DRN of chronic social defect animal model [41]. In addition,

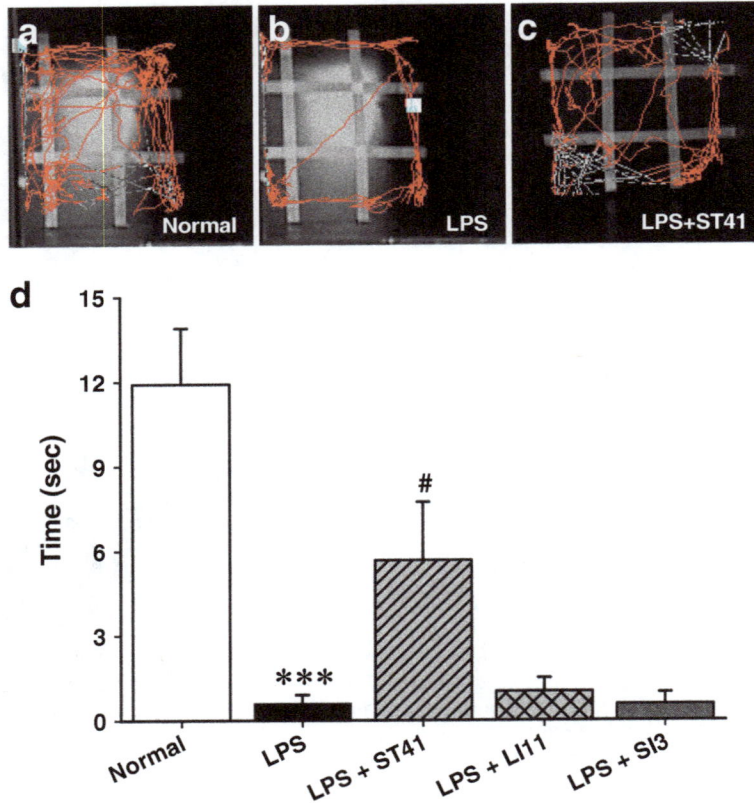

Fig. 3 Effect of acupuncture on LPS-induced anxiety-like behavior in the OFT. **a-c** Representative examples of traveling pattern for 5 min in the open field. **d** Time spent in the center of zone for 5 min presented as mean ± SEM. While LPS-treated rats spent less time in the center zone of open field arena compared to control, acupuncture at ST41, but neither LI11 nor SI3, spent more time in center zone of open field arena compared to LPS-treated rats. *** $P < 0.001$ vs. control, #$P < 0.05$ vs. LPS; $n = 6$–7 per group

serotonin level is decreased in the DRN in stress-depressed rats [42]. In the present study, to observe the relationship between anxiety-like behavior and SERT in the DRN, the changes of SERT expression following LPS treatment were evaluated by immunohistochemistry. Our results showing that SERT expression was increased in the DRN in LPS-induced group may suggest that

LPS-induced anxiety behaviors might be due to excessive reuptake of serotonin and in turn decreased level of serotonin in extrasynapse. Furthermore, in our present study, acupuncture at ST41, but not at control points (LI11 and SI3), significantly attenuated SERT expression in the DRN. These results indicate that acupuncture at ST41 could alleviate the anxiety-

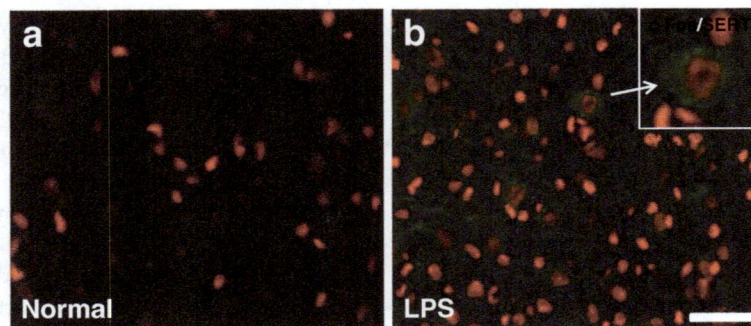

Fig. 4 Expression of SERT in activated neurons in the DRN. **a, b** Representative images of expression of SERT (green) and c-Fos (red) in the DRN of normal (**a**) and LPS-treated rats (**b**). Enlarged image in (**b**) shows a DRN neuron double-labelled with SERT/c-Fos. Scale bar = 50 μm

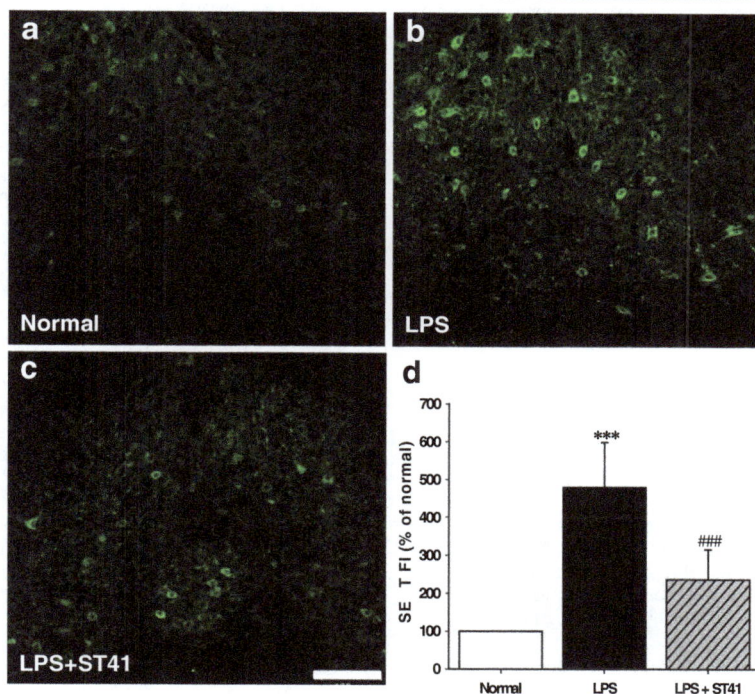

Fig. 5 Effect of acupuncture on SERT expression in the DRN. **a-c** Representative images of SERT expression in the DRN. **d** Summary of SERT *fluorescence intensity* (FI, D) in the DRN following LPS administration. Data are expressed as percentage of control (normal). Acupuncture at ST41 markedly decreased SERT expression produced by LPS in the DRN. **P* < 0.01 and ****P* < 0.001 vs. control, *###P* < 0.001 vs. LPS, *n* = 3–4 per group. Scale bar = 50 μm

like behavior by suppressing SERT expression. According to other studies, acupuncture increases the serotonin level in the DRN [43] and the nucleus accumbens [44] and serotonin/5-hydroxyphenlyacetic acid (5-HIAA) ratio in the DRN [43]. These studies support that acupuncture may regulate serotonin system in the DRN and thus attenuates anxiety-like behaviors.

As the other possible mechanism, acupuncture may regulate the level of inflammatory cytokines produced by LPS. Peripheral administration of LPS induces inflammatory cytokines such as tumor necrosis factor (TNF) α, interleukin (IL)-1β, IL-6 [45, 46] which may produce depressive or anxiety-like behavior [14, 17, 47, 48]. Several lines of evidence have shown that acupuncture significantly decreases the level of proinflammatory cytokines in the brain areas in stress-induced depression model [49, 50]. Therefore, acupuncture may have an anxiolytic effect by reducing the level of pro-inflammatory cytokines in LPS-induced anxiety model. Further studies should be performed to confirm the mechanisms underlying the anti-inflammatory effect of acupuncture on LPS-induced anxiety model.

Conclusions

In summary, acupuncture at ST41 acupuncture significantly can suppress LPS-induced anxiety-like behaviors in EPM and OFT and expression of SERT in the DRN produced by LPS. These results suggest that the anxiolytic-like effect of acupuncture may be achieved through regulation of SERT expression in the DRN.

Acknowledgements
Not applicable.

Funding
This study was supported by grants by Korea Institute of Oriental Medicine (Y15102 and K16070), NRF-2017R1E1A2A01079599 to HYK and National Research Foundation of Korea (NRF) funded by the Ministry of Education (2016R1D1A1B03935206) to EYJ.

Authors' contributions
HYK and YR designed the experiment, TYY, EYJ, GWL, EBL, SC, JHL and JSK performed the experiments and analyzed the data. EYJ, CHY and HYK drafted the manuscript. HYK were responsible for the overall direction of the project

and for edits to the manuscript. All authors have read and approved the final version of the manuscript.

Competing interests
The authors declare that they have no competing interests.

Author details
[1]College of Korean Medicine, Daegu Haany University, Daegu 42158, South Korea. [2]Korean Medicine Fundamental Research Division, Korea Institute of Oriental Medicine, Daejeon 34054, South Korea. [3]Department of Bioresource Science, Andong National University, Andong 36729, South Korea. [4]Department of Physiology, College of Korean Medicine, Daegu Haany University, Daegu 42158, South Korea.

References
1. Andrews G, Hobbs MJ, Borkovec TD, Beesdo K, Craske MG, Heimberg RG, Rapee RM, Ruscio AM, Stanley MA. Generalized worry disorder: a review of DSM-IV generalized anxiety disorder and options for DSM-V. Depress Anxiety. 2010;27(2):134–47.
2. Association AP. Diagnostic and statistical manual of mental disorders: DSM-I original edition. Arlington: editorial Benei Noaj; 2008.
3. Kessler RC, Chiu WT, Jin R, Ruscio AM, Shear K, Walters EE. The epidemiology of panic attacks, panic disorder, and agoraphobia in the National Comorbidity Survey Replication. Arch Gen Psychiatry. 2006; 63(4):415–24.
4. Sareen J, Jacobi F, Cox BJ, Belik SL, Clara I, Stein MB. Disability and poor quality of life associated with comorbid anxiety disorders and physical conditions. Arch Intern Med. 2006;166(19):2109–16.
5. Nemeroff CB, Owens MJ. Treatment of mood disorders. Nat Neurosci. 2002; 5(Suppl):1068–70.
6. Meyer JH. Imaging the serotonin transporter during major depressive disorder and antidepressant treatment. J Psychiatry Neurosci. 2007; 32(2):86–102.
7. Tafet GE, Idoyaga-Vargas VP, Abulafia DP, Calandria JM, Roffman SS, Chiovetta A, Shinitzky M. Correlation between cortisol level and serotonin uptake in patients with chronic stress and depression. Cogn Affect Behav Neurosci. 2001;1(4):388–93.
8. Won E, Ham BJ. Imaging genetics studies on monoaminergic genes in major depressive disorder. Prog Neuro-Psychopharmacol Biol Psychiatry. 2016;64:311–9.
9. Lim LW, Shrestha S, Or YZ, Tan SZ, Chung HH, Sun Y, Lim CL, Khairuddin S, Lufkin T, Lin VC. Tetratricopeptide repeat domain 9A modulates anxiety-like behavior in female mice. Sci Rep. 2016;6:37568.
10. Furmark T, Marteinsdottir I, Frick A, Heurling K, Tillfors M, Appel L, Antoni G, Hartvig P, Fischer H, Langstrom B, et al. Serotonin synthesis rate and the tryptophan hydroxylase-2: G-703T polymorphism in social anxiety disorder. J Psychopharmacol. 2016;30(10):1028–35.
11. Lanzenberger RR, Mitterhauser M, Spindelegger C, Wadsak W, Klein N, Mien LK, Holik A, Attarbaschi T, Mossaheb N, Sacher J, et al. Reduced serotonin-1A receptor binding in social anxiety disorder. Biol Psychiatry. 2007;61(9):1081–9.
12. Murrough JW, Yaqubi S, Sayed S, Charney DS. Emerging drugs for the treatment of anxiety. Expert Opin Emerg Drugs. 2015;20(3):393–406.
13. Dankoski EC, Carroll S, Wightman RM. Acute selective serotonin reuptake inhibitors regulate the dorsal raphe nucleus causing amplification of terminal serotonin release. J Neurochem. 2016. doi:10.1111/jnc.13528. (Epub ahead of print).
14. Dantzer R, O'Connor JC, Freund GG, Johnson RW, Kelley KW. From inflammation to sickness and depression: when the immune system subjugates the brain. Nat Rev Neurosci. 2008;9(1):46–56.
15. DellaGioia N, Hannestad J. A critical review of human endotoxin administration as an experimental paradigm of depression. Neurosci Biobehav Rev. 2010;34(1):130–43.
16. Salazar A, Gonzalez-Rivera BL, Redus L, Parrott JM, O'Connor JC. Indoleamine 2,3-dioxygenase mediates anhedonia and anxiety-like behaviors caused by peripheral lipopolysaccharide immune challenge. Horm Behav. 2012;62(3):202–9.
17. Jangra A, Lukhi MM, Sulakhiya K, Baruah CC, Lahkar M. Protective effect of mangiferin against lipopolysaccharide-induced depressive and anxiety-like behaviour in mice. Eur J Pharmacol. 2014;740:337–45.
18. van Heesch F, Prins J, Konsman JP, Korte-Bouws GA, Westphal KG, Rybka J, Olivier B, Kraneveld AD, Korte SM. Lipopolysaccharide increases degradation of central monoamines: an in vivo microdialysis study in the nucleus accumbens and medial prefrontal cortex of mice. Eur J Pharmacol. 2014;725:55–63.
19. Schwamborn R, Brown E, Haase J. Elevation of cortical serotonin transporter activity upon peripheral immune challenge is regulated independently of p38 mitogen-activated protein kinase activation and transporter phosphorylation. J Neurochem. 2016;137(3):423–35.
20. Cao Y, Yin X, Soto-Aguilar F, Liu Y, Yin P, Wu J, Zhu B, Li W, Lao L, Xu S. Effect of acupuncture on insomnia following stroke: study protocol for a randomized controlled trial. Trials. 2016;17(1):546.
21. Yoon SS, Yang EJ, Lee BH, Jang EY, Kim HY, Choi SM, Steffensen SC, Yang CH. Effects of acupuncture on stress-induced relapse to cocaine-seeking in rats. Psychopharmacology. 2012;222(2):303–11.
22. KW L, Yang J, Hsieh CL, Hsu YC, Lin YW. Electroacupuncture restores spatial learning and downregulates phosphorylated N-methyl-D-aspartate receptors in a mouse model of Parkinson's disease. Acupunct Med. 2017; 35(2):133-41.
23. de Lorent L, Agorastos A, Yassouridis A, Kellner M, Muhtz C. Auricular acupuncture versus progressive muscle relaxation in patients with anxiety disorders or major depressive disorder: a prospective parallel group clinical trial. J Acupunct Meridian Stud. 2016;9(4):191–9.
24. Huang WQ, Zhou QZ, Liu XG, Wei DN, He W, Zhang XD, Peng XH. Effects of acupuncture intervention on levels of T lymphocyte subsets in plasma and thymus in stress-induced anxiety rats. Zhen Ci Yan Jiu. 2015;40(4):265–9.
5. Valdez GR, Sabino V, Koob GF. Increased anxiety-like behavior and ethanol self-administration in dependent rats: reversal via corticotropin-releasing factor-2 receptor activation. Alcohol Clin Exp Res. 2004;28(6):865–72.
26. Walsh RN, Cummins RA. The open-field test: a critical review. Psychol Bull. 1976;83(3):482–504.
27. Szentirmai E, Krueger JM. Sickness behaviour after lipopolysaccharide treatment in ghrelin deficient mice. Brain Behav Immun. 2014;36:200–6.
28. Quan N, Sundar SK, Weiss JM. Induction of interleukin-1 in various brain regions after peripheral and central injections of lipopolysaccharide. J Neuroimmunol. 1994;49(1–2):125–34.
29. Orlandi L, Fonseca WF, Enes-Marques S, Paffaro VA Jr, Vilela FC, Giusti-Paiva A. Sickness behavior is accentuated in rats with metabolic disorders induced by a fructose diet. J Neuroimmunol. 2015;289:75–83.
30. Azizi-Malekabadi H, Hosseini M, Pourganji M, Zabihi H, Saeedjalali M, Anaeigoudari A. Deletion of ovarian hormones induces a sickness behavior in rats comparable to the effect of lipopolysaccharide. Neurol Res Int. 2015;2015:627642.
31. Bhatt S, Mahesh R, Devadoss T, Jindal A. Neuropharmacological evaluation of a novel 5-HT3 receptor antagonist (4-benzylpiperazin-1-yl)(3-methoxyquinoxalin-2-yl) methanone (6g) on lipopolysaccharide-induced anxiety models in mice. J Basic Clin Physiol Pharmacol. 2017;28(2):101-6.
32. Norouzi F, Abareshi A, Anaeigoudari A, Shafei MN, Gholamnezhad Z, Saeedjalali M, Mohebbati R, Hosseini M. The effects of Nigella Sativa on sickness behavior induced by lipopolysaccharide in male Wistar rats. Avicenna J Phytomed. 2016;6(1):104–16.
33. Claypoole LD, Zimmerberg B, Williamson LL. Neonatal lipopolysaccharide treatment alters hippocampal neuroinflammation, microglia morphology and anxiety-like behavior in rats selectively bred for an infantile trait. Brain Behav Immun. 2017;59:135-46.
34. Yang L, Wang M, Guo YY, Sun T, Li YJ, Yang Q, Zhang K, Liu SB, Zhao MG, YM W. Systemic inflammation induces anxiety disorder through CXCL12/CXCR4 pathway. Brain Behav Immun. 2016;56:352–62.
35. Toda S. Investigation of electroacupuncture and manual acupuncture on carnitine and glutathione in muscle. Evid Based Complement Alternative Med. 2011;2011:297130.
36. Anderson IM, Mortimore C. 5-HT and human anxiety. Evidence from studies using acute tryptophan depletion. Adv Exp Med Biol. 1999;467:43–55.
37. Soubrie P. Serotonergic neurons and behavior. J Pharmacol. 1986;17(2):107–12.
38. Waselus M, Galvez JP, Valentino RJ, Van Bockstaele EJ. Differential projections of dorsal raphe nucleus neurons to the lateral septum and striatum. J Chem Neuroanat. 2006;31(4):233–42.

39. Jacobs BL, Azmitia EC. Structure and function of the brain serotonin system. Physiol Rev. 1992;72(1):165–229.

40. Vertes RP. A PHA-L analysis of ascending projections of the dorsal raphe nucleus in the rat. J Comp Neurol. 1991;313(4):643–68.

41. Zhang J, Fan Y, Li Y, Zhu H, Wang L, Zhu MY. Chronic social defeat up-regulates expression of the serotonin transporter in rat dorsal raphe nucleus and projection regions in a glucocorticoid-dependent manner. J Neurochem. 2012;123(6):1054–68.

42. Yang LM, Hu B, Xia YH, Zhang BL, Zhao H. Lateral habenula lesions improve the behavioral response in depressed rats via increasing the serotonin level in dorsal raphe nucleus. Behav Brain Res. 2008;188(1):84–90.

43. Wei Q, Liu Z. Effects of acupuncture on monoamine neurotransmitters in raphe nuclei in obese rats. J Tradit Chin Med. 2003;23(2):147–50.

44. Yoshimoto K, Fukuda F, Hori M, Kato B, Kato H, Hattori H, Tokuda N, Kuriyama K, Yano T, Yasuhara M. Acupuncture stimulates the release of serotonin, but not dopamine, in the rat nucleus accumbens. Tohoku J Exp Med. 2006;208(4):321–6.

45. O'Connor JC, Lawson MA, Andre C, Moreau M, Lestage J, Castanon N, Kelley KW, Dantzer R. Lipopolysaccharide-induced depressive-like behavior is mediated by indoleamine 2,3-dioxygenase activation in mice. Mol Psychiatry. 2009;14(5):511–22.

46. Swiergiel AH, Dunn AJ. Effects of interleukin-1beta and lipopolysaccharide on behavior of mice in the elevated plus-maze and open field tests. Pharmacol Biochem Behav. 2007;86(4):651–9.

47. Yirmiya R. Endotoxin produces a depressive-like episode in rats. Brain Res. 1996;711(1–2):163–74.

48. Slavich GM, Irwin MR. From stress to inflammation and major depressive disorder: a social signal transduction theory of depression. Psychol Bull. 2014;140(3):774–815.

49. Lu J, Shao RH, Hu L, Tu Y, Guo JY. Potential antiinflammatory effects of acupuncture in a chronic stress model of depression in rats. Neurosci Lett. 2016;618:31–8.

50. Guo T, Guo Z, Yang X, Sun L, Wang S, Yingge A, He X, Ya T. The alterations of IL-1Beta, IL-6, and TGF-Beta levels in Hippocampal CA3 region of chronic restraint stress rats after Electroacupuncture (EA) pretreatment. Evid Based Complement Alternat Med. 2014;2014:369158.

21

Sinew acupuncture for knee osteoarthritis: study protocol for a randomized sham-controlled trial

Kwok Yin Au[1], Haiyong Chen[2,3]* (iD), Wing Chung Lam[4], Chiu On Chong[4], Andrew Lau[4], Varut Vardhanabhuti[5], Kin Cheung Mak[3,6], Fei Jiang[7], Wing Yi Lam[4], Fung Man Wu[4], Hiu Ngok Chan[4], Yan Wah Ng[4], Bacon Fung-Leung Ng[8], Eric Tat-Chi Ziea[8] and Lixing Lao[2,3]

Abstract

Background: Sinew acupuncture is a new modality of acupuncture in which needles are inserted into acupoints, ashi points or spasm points of sinew and muscles along the meridian sinew pathway. A previous observational study revealed that sinew acupuncture has immediate analgesic effects on various soft tissue injuries, including knee injuries. However, no rigorous trials have been conducted. This study aims to examine whether sinew acupuncture can safely relieve pain and symptoms of knee osteoarthritis (KOA) and improve patients' functional movement and quality of life.

Methods/design: A randomized, sham-controlled, patient- and assessor-blinded trial will be conducted to compare the efficacy of sinew acupuncture and sham acupuncture. Subjects will be assessed by the physician and acupuncturists. A sample of eighty-six eligible subjects will be randomized into either the sinew acupuncture group or the sham acupuncture group. The intervention will be performed in the Hong Kong Tuberculosis Association Chinese Medicine Clinic cum Training Centre of the University of Hong Kong by acupuncturists with over 3 years of acupuncture experience. Subjects will receive 10 sessions of interventions for 4 weeks, followed by a 6-week follow-up. The visual analogue scale (VAS) score at week 4 will be the primary outcome. The Western Ontario and McMasters University Osteoarthritis Index (WOMAC), Timed Up & Go Test (TUG), 8-step Stair Climb Test (SCT) and the 36-Item Short Form Survey (SF-36) will be secondary outcomes.

Discussion: Sinew acupuncture is a potential alternative non-pharmacological therapy for KOA. This rigorous trial will expand our knowledge of whether sinew acupuncture reduces pain intensity and improves symptoms, functional movements, and quality of life of KOA patients.

Trial registration: The study was registered at ClinicalTrials.gov (Identifier: NCT03099317) in March 2017.

Keywords: Sinew acupuncture, Sham acupuncture, Knee osteoarthritis, Pain, Randomized controlled trial, Protocol

Background

Osteoarthritis is one of the leading causes of disability in the elderly worldwide [1, 2]. The knee is the most commonly affected site [3]. Hip and knee osteoarthritis was ranked the 11th highest contributor to years lived with disability globally [4]. A US population-based survey

found that 30.8% of men above the age of 65 and 34.8% of elderly women have radiographic evidence of knee osteoarthritis (KOA) [5, 6]. A survey study with the same protocol conducted in China found that the prevalence of KOA in elderly men (27.6%) was similar, but the prevalence in elderly women (46.6%) was higher than that in the US study [6]. Furthermore, the two studies revealed that the prevalence of pain in KOA was 6.9% to 7.1% in elderly men and 11.6% to 15.4% in elderly women [6]. In 1997, the cost of osteoarthritis in the USA, Canada, UK, France, and Australia accounted for

* Correspondence: haiyong@hku.hk
[2]School of Chinese Medicine, The University of Hong Kong, 10 Sassoon Road, Pokfulam, Hong Kong, China
[3]Department of Chinese Medicine, The University of Hong Kong-Shenzhen Hospital, Shenzhen, China
Full list of author information is available at the end of the article

up to 1–2.5% of the gross national product in each of these countries [7]. Approximately one-third of direct osteoarthritis expenditures were from medications, mainly for pain-related agents [8]. The burden of osteoarthritis will continue to increase worldwide in the ageing population.

Knee pain largely affects KOA patients' quality of life and is the major reason patients seek medical help and advice [9]. Many modalities of non-pharmacological, pharmacological and surgical therapies have been implemented to reduce pain in KOA patients, including acupuncture, exercise, non-steroidal anti-inflammatory drugs (NSAIDs), COX – 2 selective agents, and joint replacement surgery [10]. NSAIDs and COX-2 inhibitors are commonly prescribed medications [10] but are associated with an increased risk of gastrointestinal bleeding and cardiovascular events [10].

Acupuncture has been widely used for KOA, although large-scale randomized controlled trials have shown contradictory results [11–14]. The discrepancies are caused by various factors such as the characteristics of controls [15, 16] and the dose of acupuncture treatment [16]. Systematic reviews have indicated that acupuncture is beneficial for patients with KOA [17, 18] and that the effects of acupuncture last for over 12 months [19].

Sinew acupuncture, a specific modality of acupuncture, was named by Professor Nongyu Liu. It was developed following the principles of *Huangdi Neijing*, a classic Chinese medical text, in conjunction with clinical experience [20–22]. *Huangdi Neijing* means "taking the [points of] tenderness as acupoints". Needles are inserted superficially at sinew points (spasm points, painful points, or acupoints close to or distal to the pain) along the meridian sinew pathway to achieve therapeutic effects [22, 23]. TCM treatments, based on the theory of meridian sinews, have recently been used for pain management [24–27]. Sinew acupuncture potentially reduces the risk of internal organ injuries. Sinew acupuncture generally causes less pain than traditional acupuncture, as it does not require deep insertion of needles or the Deqi sensation by manual manipulation of the needle, such as lifting, thrusting, twisting, and twirling [28].

Our previous observational studies have indicated that sinew acupuncture has immediate analgesic effects on soft tissue injuries at various locations (knee, elbow, back, neck and shoulders) [29]. As no controls were used in the previous observational studies, it is unclear whether the immediate analgesic effects are due to true effects or spontaneous remission of the tissue injury.

The proposed study aims to examine whether sinew acupuncture can relieve pain and symptoms of KOA and improve functional movement as measured by the visual analogue scale (VAS), the Western Ontario and McMasters University Osteoarthritis Index (WOMAC),

the Timed Up & Go Test (TUG) and the 8-Step Stair Climb Test (SCT). We will also evaluate whether sinew acupuncture can improve quality of life (QOL) as measured by the 36-Item Short Form Survey (SF-36). Furthermore, we will evaluate the safety of sinew acupuncture in treating KOA. We hypothesized that sinew acupuncture can safely relieve pain, enhance functional movement and improve QOL in KOA patients compared to sham acupuncture.

Methods/design
Study design
A randomized, sham-controlled, patient- and assessor-blinded trial will be conducted to compare the efficacy of sinew acupuncture and sham acupuncture. Subjects will receive 10 sessions of interventions, either sinew acupuncture or sham acupuncture, for 4 weeks followed by a 6-week follow-up period. The interventions will be performed by acupuncturists with more than 3 years of experience in acupuncture practice. Subjects will be blinded to the intervention and assessed by independent assessors using the primary outcome measure, VAS, and the secondary outcome measures, WOMAC, TUG and 8-step SCT. The details of the study design are shown in Fig. 1.

Study subjects
Subjects will be recruited from the Hong Kong Tuberculosis Association Chinese Medicine Clinic cum Training Centre of the University of Hong Kong, local nursing homes and community centres using advertisements in local newspapers. The eligibility of subjects will be assessed by the physician and acupuncturists using the criteria described below.

Inclusion criteria
Subjects are eligible to participate if they meet the following criteria: (i) are male or female Hong Kong permanent residents aged 50 years or above; (ii) meet the Clinical Classification Criteria for Osteoarthritis of the Knee as recommended by the American College of Rheumatology, have knee pain, have radiologic findings of osteoarthritis with Kellgren and Lawrence Grades 2–4, and have less than 30 min of morning stiffness or crepitus on active motion and osteophytes as determined by history and physical examination; (iii) have either unilateral knee pain or bilateral knee pain; (iv) have experienced pain for at least 6 months and knee pain > 40 mm on a visual analogue scale (VAS; 0 to 100 mm) within the past 7 days; and (v) are able to read and write Chinese and sign the informed consent form.

Exclusion criteria
Subjects will be excluded if they meet any of the following criteria: (i) are unable to walk; (ii) have a serious infection

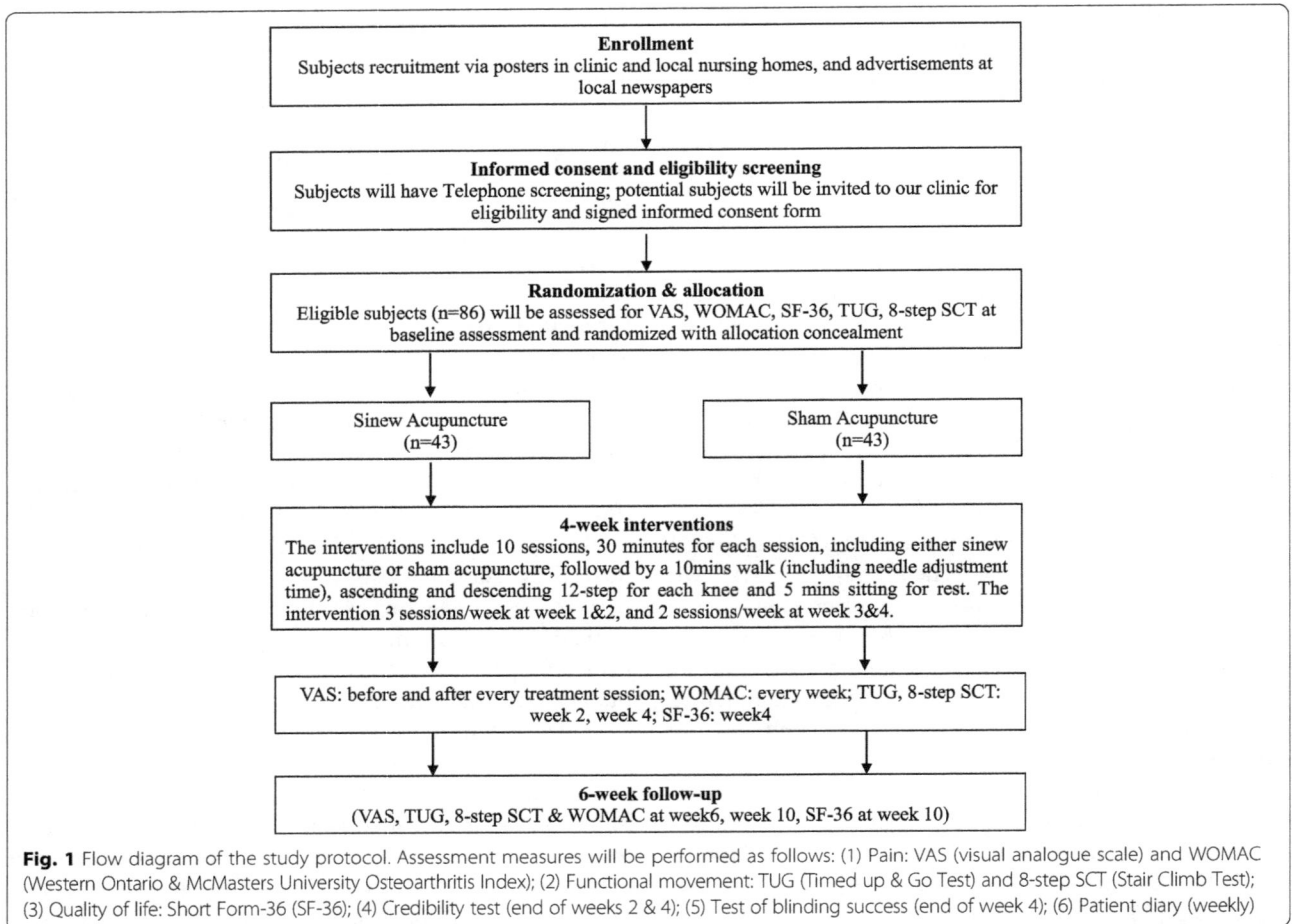

Enrollment
Subjects recruitment via posters in clinic and local nursing homes, and advertisements at local newspapers

Informed consent and eligibility screening
Subjects will have Telephone screening; potential subjects will be invited to our clinic for eligibility and signed informed consent form

Randomization & allocation
Eligible subjects (n=86) will be assessed for VAS, WOMAC, SF-36, TUG, 8-step SCT at baseline assessment and randomized with allocation concealment

Sinew Acupuncture
(n=43)

Sham Acupuncture
(n=43)

4-week interventions
The interventions include 10 sessions, 30 minutes for each session, including either sinew acupuncture or sham acupuncture, followed by a 10mins walk (including needle adjustment time), ascending and descending 12-step for each knee and 5 mins sitting for rest. The intervention 3 sessions/week at week 1&2, and 2 sessions/week at week 3&4.

VAS: before and after every treatment session; WOMAC: every week; TUG, 8-step SCT: week 2, week 4; SF-36: week4

6-week follow-up
(VAS, TUG, 8-step SCT & WOMAC at week6, week 10, SF-36 at week 10)

Fig. 1 Flow diagram of the study protocol. Assessment measures will be performed as follows: (1) Pain: VAS (visual analogue scale) and WOMAC (Western Ontario & McMasters University Osteoarthritis Index); (2) Functional movement: TUG (Timed up & Go Test) and 8-step SCT (Stair Climb Test); (3) Quality of life: Short Form-36 (SF-36); (4) Credibility test (end of weeks 2 & 4); (5) Test of blinding success (end of week 4); (6) Patient diary (weekly)

of the knee; (iii) have suspected tears in any ligaments or menisci or acute inflammation of the synovial capsule; (iv) have a history of trauma, ligament damage, fracture, or surgery on the knee(s) within 6 months, causing pain or functional problems (history of knee replacement will be excluded); (v) have a history of local tumour/malignancy at the knee; (vi) have physical or laboratory findings indicating infection, presence of autoimmune disease or inflammatory arthritis; (vii) have knee pain caused by radiculopathy/herniation of an intervertebral disc; (viii) have end-stage diseases or other suspected severe conditions such as deep vein thrombosis of the lower limb, oedema related to cancer or cancer treatment, severe blood coagulation disorders, uncontrolled systemic arterial hypertension and severe diabetes; (ix) have a history of prolotherapy, hyaluronic acid injections or corticosteroids injections within 3 months; (x) have received acupuncture, electro-acupuncture, Tui-na therapy, massage, or physiotherapy 8 weeks prior to enrolment in the trial; (xi) have severe pain in other regions; (xii) have severe mental disorder(s); (xiii) are oversensitive to needles; and (xiv) are insensitive to pain due to advanced diabetes, neuropathy or use of strong painkillers.

Eligible subjects will receive baseline assessments and will be randomly allocated to the sinew acupuncture group ($n = 43$) or the sham acupuncture group ($n = 43$) in a ratio of 1:1 by block randomization. The random digits and letters will be generated by SPSS, covered by aluminium foil, and sealed into opaque envelopes.

Subjects will be advised not to receive other acupuncture treatments, Tui-na, massage or physiotherapy. Subjects are not restricted from the use of painkillers (including herbs) or external ointments if they suffer intolerable pain. The use of rescue medications, the daily level of morning stiffness and exercise time will be recorded in patient diaries.

Interventions

Sinew acupuncture group

Subjects receiving sinew acupuncture will sit on a chair with the knee joint flexed at a most comfortable angle as close to 90 degrees as possible (if required, a block of A4 papers will be placed under the foot to adjust the angle). A hospital trolley table will be set up to block the vision of the subject to his/her knee (for blinding purposes). Routine disinfection will then be performed by the acupuncturist with a 75% alcohol pad. Acupoints (1–2 cm away from the point of tenderness, spasm or pain) along the meridian sinews near the knee(s) will be punctured through the skin by using sterile needles with a size of 0.30 mm × 40 mm (MOCM®) at an angle of 0–10 degrees pointing along the direction of the pain and the meridian sinew. The needles will be withdrawn immediately to a depth just under the skin and inserted forward smoothly 10 mm to 20 mm to avoid inducing pain. Five to eight points will be selected on each painful knee (while walking and climbing stairs) based on the theory of sinew acupuncture. Adjustments of the needles will be performed by extension and flexion of the knee joint to ensure that the needles do not cause pain during movement. Needles will be covered immediately by hypoallergenic bandages. The trolley table will be pulled away. Subjects will be advised to walk for 10 min (including the needle adjustment time). Needles will be adjusted at any time during walking if the subject has any pain induced by the acupuncture needle (for safety purposes) or primary pain of KOA (for the purpose of enhancing treatment effect). The trolley table will be used for blinding when the acupuncturist adjusts the needles. The acupuncturist will record the details of every adjustment procedure. After 10 min of walking, patients will be advised to step up and down from a step (~ 18 cm in height) for 12 rounds per knee. The pain points will be examined, and needle adjustments will be performed if necessary, followed by a period of rest by sitting for 5 min. After treatment, the needles will be removed while the subject is in a sitting position with the trolley table in place for blinding. Bandages will be applied in the same position for continuous blinding. The entire procedure will last 30 min

per session. Subjects will receive 10 sessions of interventions for 4 weeks, starting with thrice a week during the first 2 weeks and then twice a week during the last 2 weeks. The above procedures will be performed by the acupuncturist and blinded to subjects.

Sham acupuncture group

Subjects in the sham acupuncture group will undergo the same procedures as those in the sinew acupuncture group except that the non-insertion sham acupuncture will be applied. Briefly, subjects will sit in a chair and their vision of their knees will be blocked by the trolley table. After disinfection, sterile needles with a size of 0. 30 mm × 40 mm (MOCM ®) will be used to slightly puncture the acupoint without passing through the skin. The needles will immediately be covered with non-allergenic bandages to ensure sufficient blinding.

Outcome measures

The VAS at week 4 will be the primary outcome. The WOMAC, TUG, 8-step SCT, and SF-36 scores will be the secondary outcomes. The assessment schedule is shown in Table 1. Independent assessors who are not involved in acupuncture treatments will perform the VAS assessments (asking subjects to indicate the pain intensity at the most painful points during walking and ascending/descending a step and overall). Acupuncturists will complete a "Physical Examination and Treatment Form" including details of the medical history, diagnosis and treatment procedures. The acupuncturists will communicate with the subjects using neutral language. The administration of analgesics, external ointments and herbal medicines and the time of daily exercises will be collected weekly from patient diaries

Table 1 The schedule of enrollment, interventions, and assessments

Items	Enrollment	Allocation (baseline)	Interventions (± 2 days)										Follow-up	
Time points (week)	-2	0	1			2			3		4		6	10
Treatment sessions (n)	–	–	1	2	3	4	5	6	7	8	9	10	–	–
Eligibility screen	✓													
Informed consent	✓													
VAS		✓	✓	✓	✓	✓	✓	✓	✓	✓	✓	✓	✓	✓
WOMAC		✓				✓			✓		✓		✓	✓
SF-36		✓									✓			✓
TUG		✓							✓		✓		✓	✓
8-step SCT		✓							✓		✓		✓	✓
PE & Tx	✓		✓	✓	✓	✓	✓	✓	✓	✓	✓	✓	✓	✓
Patient Diary				✓		✓			✓		✓		✓	✓
Credibility Test											✓		✓	
Test of Blinding Success													✓	
Adverse events			✓	✓	✓	✓	✓	✓	✓	✓	✓	✓	✓	✓

PE & Tx, Physical Examination and Treatment Form; SCT, stair climb test; SF-36, 36-item short form; TUG, timed up & go test; VAS, visual analog scale; WOMAC, Western Ontario and McMasters University Osteoarthritis Index during the intervention period and at each visit during the follow-up period.

Measurement instruments

The 0–100 mm VAS is used to measure pain intensity. Subjects will indicate pain intensity on the VAS, with 0 mm representing no pain and 100 mm representing the most intolerable pain. Pain intensity will be measured at the most painful point during walking, the most painful point during ascending and descending a step, and the overall pain before and immediately after every treatment session and at follow-up at week 6 and week 10.

The WOMAC (Hong Kong Cantonese Version) [10] will be completed by subjects and will assess three domains: pain (5 items), stiffness (2 items) and physical function (17 items). The WOMAC will be measured at baseline, every week for the first 4 weeks, week 6 and week 10.

The SF-36 (Hong Kong Cantonese version) will be used to assess general QOL. The QOL will be collected by assessors at baseline, week 4 and week 10.

TUG and 8-step SCT will be evaluated by assessors at baseline, every 2 weeks after the last treatment session, and at week 6 and week 10.

Assessment of credibility

The Credibility of Treatment Rating Scale will be used to assess the credibility of the acupuncture treatments after the 6th treatment at week 2 and the last treatment at week 4. The 4-item scale is specifically designed to assess the credibility of acupuncture. The following questions will be asked to each subject by the assessors: (1) Do you believe this treatment will reduce the pain you are suffering? (2) Would you recommend this treatment to a friend or relative with the same problem? (3) Does the treatment seem to be a logical one? (4) Do you believe this treatment could be very effective in curing your knee osteoarthritis? [30].

Assessment of blinding success for acupuncture treatment

The blinding success of subjects will be evaluated by assessors after the last treatment session at week 4. Subjects in both groups will be asked the following question: "When you volunteered for the trial, you were informed that you had an equal chance of receiving sinew acupuncture or sham acupuncture treatment. Which acupuncture do you think you received?" Three options will be provided to the subjects, sinew acupuncture, sham acupuncture, and uncertain. Those who answered either sinew acupuncture or sham acupuncture will be asked to provide a reason for that assumption; the results will be recorded [12].

Adverse events/serious adverse events

Subjects will be encouraged to report adverse events at each treatment session using the TESS-adverse event form. For serious adverse events such as death, life threatening events, significant or persistent disability/incapacity, hospitalization or prolongation of existing hospitalization, the date, time, vital signs and reasons for treatment assignment disclosure should be noted in the Severe Adverse Event (SAE) Form, reported to the Institutional Review Board (IRB) and monitored within 48 h. If there are medical concerns such that the treatment protocol has to be revised due to safety, sudden serious adverse events or ethical reasons, the revision must be approved by the IRB before implementation. If a subject withdraws from the study, the reasons for withdrawal will be recorded.

Safety

Either sinew acupuncture or sham acupuncture will be performed by registered acupuncturists in Hong Kong who have at least 3 years of acupuncture experience. Throughout the trial, acupuncturists will follow the guideline from the Hong Kong Hospital Authority on Safety in Acupuncture for Chinese Medicine Practitioners (2nd amended version, 2016) including (1) prevention of fainting and syncope during acupuncture; (2) prevention of bleeding and bending or breaking of needles during acupuncture; and (3) prevention of performing acupuncture on the skin with local infections, ulcers, scars, or tumour. All acupuncture procedures adopted in our clinic (The Hong Kong Tuberculosis Association Chinese Medicine Clinic cum Training Centre of the University of Hong Kong) will follow (1) the introduction of the Notice for Patients Receiving Acupuncture and Tui-na Treatment at their first visit and (2) implementation of needle counting before and after each acupuncture session.

Adhesive bandages will consist of a flexible, nonwoven, low-adherence contact layer and a low-allergy, acrylic adhesive backing layer, which will be used to maintain the needle position during movement.

Potential risks and management

During the treatment, all acupoints will be located around the knee joint(s), and the needle insertion will be superficial/subcutaneous with standardized disinfection procedures. This method has very low risks of infection, pneumothorax or perforation of the viscera.

Small amounts of bleeding or bruising may occasionally occur. In clinical experience, a small amount of bleeding can be stopped by applying pressure with sterile cotton swabs/balls. Bruises usually disappear within 2–3 days.

A step test is used to evaluate the subjects' pain points while ascending/descending steps. To avoid falls, the step will be placed near a treatment bed, and a clinical assistant will accompany the subject at all times. The stairwell on the same floor of the hospital equipped with handles, bright lighting and anti-slip coating will be used for SCT assessment. Assessors will accompany the subjects during TUG and SCT assessments.

Ethics and dissemination

The ethical validity of the study has been assessed and approved by the Institutional Review Board of The University of Hong Kong/Hospital Authority Hong Kong West Cluster (HKU/HA HKW IRB, approved number UW 16–2007). The study was registered on Clinical-Trials.gov (Identifier: NCT03099317). The clinical study will be overseen by the HKU/HA HKW IRB. All subjects will receive sufficient information about the trial and must sign the informed consent form prior to enrolment. Case repot forms (CRFs) and study files will be archived for 3 years after completion of the final report and locked in a research cabinet. The Personal Data (Privacy) Ordinance (CAP 486) will be followed strictly.

Sample size estimation

G-power was used for sample size determination. The sample size was estimated by the VAS value with sinew acupuncture for knee pain using data from our pilot study [29]. The study observed 85 sessions of acupuncture treatments on the knee. After acupuncture treatments, the average VAS was reduced from 38.9 to 21.0 (change = − 17.9) with a standard deviation = 10.7. We estimated that the sham acupuncture (17.9*60% = 10.74) could reduce 60% of pain intensity compared to true acupuncture. The effect size was 0.673. With $\alpha = 0.05$ and power $(1-\beta)$ =0.8, the sample size was determined to be 37 per group. With the consideration of a 15% dropout rate, 86 subjects are required in each of the two groups.

Data analysis

All data will be doubly entered into a password-protected computer 1 week after data collection. The statistical analysis will be performed by SPSS 22.0 for Windows by a single statistician. The scores will be analysed by the intent-to-treat analysis. The last observation carried forward method will be used for missing data. Comparisons of continuous variables between the acupuncture and sham groups will be assessed using Student's t-test or analysis of covariance (ANCOVA) with baseline measures as covariates. Comparisons of categorical data between groups will be tested by the χ^2 test or the Mann–Whitney U-test. Changes in the scores from baseline within treatment groups will be assessed by the paired t-test or the Wilcoxon signed ranks test. Data from the patient diary will be assessed to analyse covariate balances in the two groups. If we find an imbalance, we will use the propensity score method [31] or the conditional inference method [32] to remove the confounding effect. All statistical tests will be two-sided at a 5% significance level.

Discussion

KOA is one of the most common diseases among the elderly. This study will evaluate the efficacy of sinew acupuncture for pain reduction, functional movement improvement, and QOL improvement in KOA patients. In our clinic, there are 8–10 new KOA patients each month. We estimate that recruitment will be completed in 10 months.

The study is conducted in collaboration with the School of Chinese Medicine, Department of Diagnostic Radiology and Department of Orthopaedics & Traumatology, Li Ka Shing Faculty of Medicine, HKU. The eligibility of KOA subjects will be assessed by clinical physicians. The intervention will be performed by experienced acupuncturists. The subjects and assessors will be blinded to subjects' allocations. The acupuncturist will not be involved in assessments or data entry. Data will be analysed by an independent statistician.

In acupuncture RCTs, it is critical to choose an appropriate control population. Vickers AJ et al. found that acupuncture was superior to both sham and no acupuncture controls for osteoarthritis pain with effect sizes of 0.16 and 0.57, respectively [18]. The small effect size in trials with sham acupuncture controls may be due to the following reasons: (1) the meta-analysis excluded outlying studies showing a very large effect size [18] and (2) according to Macpherson H, Vickers AJ, et al. in the same research group, acupuncture has a smaller effect size in trials with needle-insertion sham controls than in trials with needle non-insertion sham or non-sham controls [15]. Our previous study was consistent with their findings that acupuncture trials with needle non-insertion controls lead to more positive conclusions than those with needle-insertion sham controls [16]. In the present study, we will use needle non-insertion as the control, which may produce a smaller, nonspecific effect compared to needle-insertion sham controls. However, it should be noted that the effect size estimated from our pilot study [29] is larger than that of the previous study by Vickers AJ et al. [18]. If the power estimates prove to be high, the trail can be used to determine a more accurate effect size for future power calculations.

This trial will expand our knowledge of whether sinew acupuncture will reduce pain intensity, improve the symptoms and movements of KOA patients, and improve QOL. If this study is successful, the effectiveness of sinew acupuncture may be studied using a pragmatic trial design.

Acknowledgements

We are thankful to Chinese Medicine Department of Hospital Authority and The Hong Kong Tuberculosis Association Chinese Medicine Clinic cum

Training Centre of the University of Hong Kong for funding support. Acknowledgement is extended to colleagues in School of Chinese Medicine of The University of Hong Kong for their expert advice.

Funding
This study is funded by the Chinese Medicine Section, Hospital Authority, Hong Kong (The Train-the-Trainer Programme 2015/2016).

Authors' contributions
HYC conceived the study, designed the study protocol, sought ethical approval and wrote the manuscript. KYA designed the study protocol, sought funding and ethical approval, and wrote the manuscript. WCL, COC, AL, WYL, FMW, HNC and YWN contributed to development of the study protocol. VV and KCM designed the selection criteria of patients. FJ contributed to the sample size estimation and statistical analysis. BFN, ETZ and LL advised on the study design and protocol. All authors contributed to the research design and read, made critical revisions, wrote and approved the final manuscript.

Competing interests
The authors declare that they have no competing interests.

Author details
[1]Hong Kong Institute of Integrative Medicine, Faculty of Medicine, The Chinese University of Hong Kong, Hong Kong, China. [2]School of Chinese Medicine, The University of Hong Kong, 10 Sassoon Road, Pokfulam, Hong Kong, China. [3]Department of Chinese Medicine, The University of Hong Kong-Shenzhen Hospital, Shenzhen, China. [4]The Hong Kong Tuberculosis Association Chinese Medicine Clinic cum Training Centre of the University of Hong Kong, Hong Kong, China. [5]Department of Diagnostic Radiology, Li Ka Shing Faculty of Medicine, The University of Hong Kong, Hong Kong, China. [6]Department of Orthopaedics and Traumatology, Li Ka Shing Faculty of Medicine, The University of Hong Kong, Hong Kong, China. [7]Department of Statistics and Actuarial Science, The University of Hong Kong, Hong Kong, China. [8]The Chinese Medicine Department, Hospital Authority, Hong Kong, China.

References
1. Johnson VL, Hunter DJ. The epidemiology of osteoarthritis. Best Pract Res Clin Rheumatol. 2014;28(1):5–15.
2. Guccione AA, Felson DT, Anderson JJ, Anthony JM, Zhang Y, Wilson PW, Kelly-Hayes M, Wolf PA, Kreger BE, Kannel WB. The effects of specific medical conditions on the functional limitations of elders in the Framingham study. Am J Public Health. 1994;84(3):351–8.
3. Fransen M, Bridgett L, March L, Hoy D, Penserga E, Brooks P. The epidemiology of osteoarthritis in Asia. Int J Rheum Dis. 2011;14(2):113–21.
4. Cross M, Smith E, Hoy D, Nolte S, Ackerman I, Fransen M, Bridgett L, Williams S, Guillemin F, Hill CL, et al. The global burden of hip and knee osteoarthritis: estimates from the global burden of disease 2010 study. Ann Rheum Dis. 2014;73(7):1323–30.
5. Felson DT, Naimark A, Anderson J, Kazis L, Castelli W, Meenan RF. The prevalence of knee osteoarthritis in the elderly. The Framingham osteoarthritis study. Arthritis Rheum. 1987;30(8):914–8.
6. Zhang Y, Xu L, Nevitt MC, Aliabadi P, Yu W, Qin M, Lui LY, Felson DT. Comparison of the prevalence of knee osteoarthritis between the elderly Chinese population in Beijing and whites in the United States: the Beijing osteoarthritis study. Arthritis Rheum. 2001;44(9):2065–71.
7. March LM, Bachmeier CJ. Economics of osteoarthritis: a global perspective. Baillieres Clin Rheumatol. 1997;11(4):817–34.
8. Bitton R. The economic burden of osteoarthritis. Am J Manag Care. 2009; 15(8 Suppl):S230–5.
9. Neogi T. The epidemiology and impact of pain in osteoarthritis. Osteoarthr Cartil. 2013;21(9):1145–53.
10. Zhang W, Moskowitz RW, Nuki G, Abramson S, Altman RD, Arden N, Bierma-Zeinstra S, Brandt KD, Croft P, Doherty M, et al. OARSI recommendations for the management of hip and knee osteoarthritis, part II: OARSI evidence-based, expert consensus guidelines. Osteoarthr Cartil. 2008;16(2):137 62.

11. Witt C, Brinkhaus B, Jena S, Linde K, Streng A, Wagenpfeil S, Hummelsberger J, Walther HU, Melchart D, Willich SN. Acupuncture in patients with osteoarthritis of the knee: a randomised trial. Lancet. 2005;366(9480):136–43.
12. Berman BM, Lao LX, Langenberg P, Lee WL, Gilpin AMK, Hochberg MC. Effectiveness of acupuncture as adjunctive therapy in osteoarthritis of the knee - a randomized, controlled trial. Ann Intern Med. 2004;141(12): 901–10.
13. Hinman RS, McCrory P, Pirotta M, Relf I, Forbes A, Crossley KM, Williamson E, Kyriakides M, Novy K, Metcalf BR, et al. Acupuncture for chronic knee pain: a randomized clinical trial. JAMA. 2014;312(13):1313–22.
14. Scharf HP, Mansmann U, Streitberger K, Witte S, Kramer J, Maier C, Trampisch HJ, Victor N. Acupuncture and knee osteoarthritis: a three-armed randomized trial. Ann Intern Med. 2006;145(1):12–20.
15. MacPherson H, Vertosick E, Lewith G, Linde K, Sherman KJ, Witt CM, Vickers AJ, Acupuncture Trialists C. Influence of control group on effect size in trials of acupuncture for chronic pain: a secondary analysis of an individual patient data meta-analysis. PLoS One. 2014;9(4):e93739.
16. Chen HY, Ning ZP, Lam WL, Lam WY, Zhao YK, Yeung JWF, Ng BF-L, Ziea ETC, Lao LX. Types of control in acupuncture clinical trials might affect the conclusion of the trials: a review of acupuncture on pain management. J Acupunct Meridian. 2016;9(5):227–33.
17. Corbett MS, Rice SJC, Madurasinghe V, Slack R, Fayter DA, Harden M, Sutton AJ, MacPherson H, Woolacott NF. Acupuncture and other physical treatments for the relief of pain due to osteoarthritis of the knee: network meta-analysis. Osteoarthr Cartilage. 2013;21(9):1290–8.
18. Vickers AJ, Cronin AM, Maschino AC, Lewith G, MacPherson H, Foster NE, Sherman KJ, Witt CM, Linde K, Trialists' A. Acupuncture for chronic pain individual patient data meta-analysis. Arch Intern Med. 2012;172(19): 1444–53.
19. MacPherson H, Vertosick EA, Foster NE, Lewith G, Linde K, Sherman KJ, Witt CM, Vickers AJ. The persistence of the effects of acupuncture after a course of treatment: a meta-analysis of patients with chronic pain. Pain. 2017; 158(5):784–93.
20. Liu NY. Getting qi and arrival of qi. Zhongguo Zhen Jiu. 2014;34(8):828–30.
21. Liu N. Jingjin and weiqi. Zhongguo Zhen Jiu. 2015;35(2):185–8.
22. Liu N. Exploration and analysis on the mechanism of sinew acupuncture. Zhongguo Zhen Jiu. 2015;35(12):1293–6.
23. Ting H. Academic theory of sinew acupuncture by professor Liu Nongyu. Zhongguo Zhen Jiu. 2015;(s1):56–8.
24. Legge D. Acupuncture treatment of chronic low back pain by using the Jingjin (meridian sinews) model. J Acupunct Meridian. 2015;8(5):255–8.
25. Wei S, Chen ZH, Sun WF, Zhang GP, Li XH, Hou CF, Lu LD, Zhang L. Evaluating meridian-sinew release therapy for the treatment of knee osteoarthritis. Evid Based Complement Alternat Med. 2013;2013:182528.
26. Zhao H, Nie WB, Sun YX, Li S, Yang S, Meng FY, Zhang LP, Wang F, Huang SX. Warm needling therapy and acupuncture at meridian-sinew sites based on the meridian-sinew theory: hemiplegic shoulder pain. Evid Based Complement Alternat Med. 2015;2015:694973.
27. Chen YM, Zhao Y, Xue XL, Zhang QC, Wu XY, Li H, Zheng X, Zhao JN, He FD, Kong JH, et al. Distribution characteristics of meridian sinew (Jingjin) syndrome in 313 cases of whiplash-associated disorders. Chin J Integr Med. 2015;21(3):234–40.
28. Liu N, Liu H. Sinew Acupuncture. Beijing: Peoples's Medical Publishing House; 2016.
29. Liu N, Ren T, Xiang Y. Immediate analgesic effects of tendon acupuncture on soft tissue injury. Zhongguo Zhen Jiu. 2015;35(9):927–9.
30. Vas J, Rebollo A, Perea-Milla E, Mendez C, Font CR, Gomez-Rio M, Martin-Avila M, Carbrera-Iboleon J, Caballero MD, Olmos M, et al. Study protocol for a pragmatic randomised controlled trial in general practice investigating the effectiveness of acupuncture against migraine. BMC Complem Altern Med. 2008;8:12.
31. Rosenbaum PR, Rubin DB. The central role of the propensity score in observational studies for causal effects. Biometrika. 1983;70(1):41–55.
32. Jiang F, Tian L, Fu H, Hasegawa T, Pfeffer MA, Wei L: Robust alternatives to ANCOVA for estimating the treatment effect via a randomized comparative study. 2016.

22

Wrist-ankle acupuncture (WAA) for primary dysmenorrhea (PD) of young females: study protocol

Yingfan Chen[1], Sinan Tian[1], Jing Tian[2] and Shi Shu[1]*

Abstract

Background: Primary dysmenorrhea (PD) is one of the most common health complaints all over the world, specifically among young females. Acupuncture has been employed to relieve the pain-based symptoms and to avoid the side effects of conventional medication, and wrist-ankle acupuncture (WAA) has confirmed analgesic efficacy for various types of pain. The aim of this study is to evaluate the immediate analgesia effect of WAA on PD of young females.

Methods/design: This study will carry out a randomized parallel controlled single-blind trial to observe the immediate analgesia effect of WAA in PD of young females. Sixty participants who meet inclusion criteria will be recruited from September 2016 to September 2017 in Changhai hospital of China. They are randomly assigned to WAA therapy or sham acupuncture groups (30 patients for each group), and then receive real or sham acupuncture treatment, respectively. In this trial, the primary outcome measure is simple form of McGill pain questionnaire (SF-MPQ), while expectation and treatment credibility scale (ETCS), safety assessment, the COX menstrual symptom scale (CMSS), questionnaire about the feeling of being punctured are included in the secondary outcomes.

Discussion: This trial will be the first study protocol designed to evaluate the immediate analgesia effect of WAA in PD of young females. The strengths in methodology, including rigorous randomized, sham-controlled, participants-blinded and assessors-blinded, will guarantee the quality of this study. WAA doesn't require any needling sensation, so non-penetrating sham acupuncture can serve as an effective placebo intervention in this trial.

Trials registration: Chinese Clinical Trial Registry (identifier: ChiCTR-IOR-16008546; registration date: 27 May 2016).

Keywords: Wrist-ankle acupuncture (WAA), Primary dysmenorrheal (PD), Randomized controlled trial

Background

Dysmenorrhea is a common disease in females of reproductive age [1], leading to the activity limitation, efficiency impairment, and even life quality decrease. Moreover, the vast majority is primary dysmenorrhea (PD), defined as painful menses in women with normal pelvic anatomy. Due to the lack of standard methods for assessing the severity of dysmenorrhea, studies based on the different definitions of the condition have reported the prevalence of PD as between 45% and 95% of menstruating women [2]. PD has negative impact on physical and psychological aspects of health, and its harm to the health will in turn aggravate the symptoms of PD, which is a vicious cycle. It has become an important research field to alleviate the symptom of PD safely and to improve the quality of life and well-being rating of female.

Therapeutically, the conventional pharmacotherapy for the PD is the use of non-steroidal anti-inflammatory drugs (NSAIDs) and oral contraceptives [3, 4]. Although NSAIDs and other drugs can alleviate the pain of PD significantly, their application is limited, mostly because of their disability in curing the disease ultimately, along with their side effects and unaffordable high prices [5, 6].

Professor Zhang Xinshu and his colleagues from Changhai Hospital of Second Military Medical University, Shanghai, China invented and developed wrist-ankle acupuncture (WAA), a modern subcutaneous acupuncture technique, in the 1970s [7]. WAA which does not produce

* Correspondence: shushitcm@163.com
[1]Changhai Hospital of Traditional Chinese Medicine, Second Military Medical University, 168 Changhai Road, Yangpu District, Shanghai, China
Full list of author information is available at the end of the article

any pain or "needling sensation" is quite distinguished from the traditional acupuncture [8]. According to its unique theoretical system and the clinical evidence, WAA has demonstrated analgesic effects for both chronic and acute pain [9–11]. In addition, the active principle is considered to have correlation with the threshold of pain, or the regulation function of central nervous system, which is partly consistent with the analgesic mechanism of the traditional acupuncture [12–16]. There is a guaranteed guiding significance of WAA for PD's treatment. To date, there are few studies investigating the application of WAA in the alleviation of PD. The present study is aimed at investigating the immediate analgesia effects of WAA for young females with PD.

Methods/design
Objectives
The aims of this study are to:

1. observe the immediate analgesia effect of WAA in PD of young females;
2. provide high-quality evidence-based recommendations on further treatment.

Hypothesis
WAA therapy would relieve the pain of patients more effectively than sham acupuncture.

Study design
The randomized parallel controlled single-blind trial was designed to observe the immediate analgesia effect of wrist-ankle acupuncture in primary dysmenorrhea of young females (Fig. 1). The study will be conducted in Changhai hospital of China from September 2016 to September 2017.

Participants and recruitment
Posters of this trial will be put on notice boards to recruit potential participants in the hospital. And the trial information leaflets will be distributed to the patients. The protocol details are explained to the participants in the leaflets and posts. Participants will be included only if they meet the inclusion criteria and provide written informed consent.

Key inclusion and exclusion criteria
Inclusion criteria

1. patients conformed to the diagnostic criterion of PD according to the Primary Dysmenorrhea Consensus Guidelines [17];
2. nulliparous women of 18 to 30 years old;
3. instant pre-treatment VAS score of over 40 mm;
4. no experience with treatment of WAA;
5. signature of informed consent form.

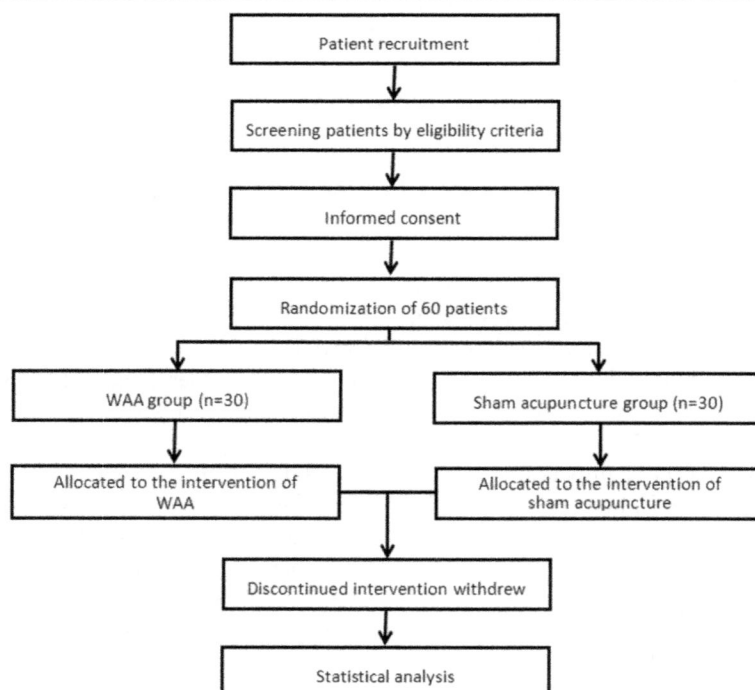

Fig. 1 Flowchart of the study design

Exclusion criteria

1. secondary dysmenorrhea caused by endometriosis, uterine myoma, endometrial polyps, pelvic inflammatory disease, or other gynecological problems confirmed by a gynecological abdominal ultrasound B examination;
2. females with irregular/infrequent menstrual cycles (outside of the typical range 21 to 35 days' cycle);
3. patients complicated with severe diseases (e.g. cerebral, liver, kidney, or hematopoietic system diseases), or mental defects;
4. take analgesic during the past 12 h;
5. received other alternative therapies such as massage, acupressure, herbal therapy in the previous three months;
6. poor treatment compliance (e.g. unstable working and living situation, difficult follow-up).

Data collection

Two identical scale questionnaires should be completed before and after the treatment for assessing the pain-based symptoms of PD in the current menstrual cycle. Participants will complete the first questionnaire 10 min before the treatment, while the second one will be collected immediately after the treatment. The researchers will be present when the questionnaires are completed to ensure the reliability and validity.

Interventions

According to the theory of WAA, each side of the body and each limb are longitudinally divided into six zones and one needling point is defined in each zone at the wrist or ankle. Needling the certain point will relieve the pain on the corresponding zone of the point. If the pain is on the upper (lower) part of the body (with the diaphragm as the demarcation), the needling point at the ipsilateral wrist (ankle) is selected [7, 18]. The pain sites of PD patients in the study are primarily located in the lower abdomen. To standardize the selection of the needling site and the treatment protocol, point 1 at both ankles will be needled (Fig. 2). Participants will be randomly assigned to the WAA group or the sham acupuncture group. The intervention will be applied during the first 24 h of the most intense dysmenorrhea's occurrence. A single registered acupuncturist, with at least one year of previous WAA experience, will administer the care to all subjects.

WAA group

WAA was administered on point 1 at both ankles on the first day when the pain occurs during the period. Retain the needle for 30 min. The subjects were asked to wear an eye mask. A disposable sterile WAA needle (0.25 mm in diameter and 25 mm in length, Suzhou Medical Appliance Factory, Jiangsu Province, China) was chosen in this trial. The target point was disinfected with an iodophordis infectant (Shanghai Likang Disinfectant Hi-tech Co. Ltd.). The processed needles were also held with thumb, index finger, and middle finger of the right hand. The skin near the target point was gently pressed with the left thumb to make it slightly taut. Then, the needle tip was swiftly inserted into the skin at the target point at an angle of 30°. The needle was lowered to the

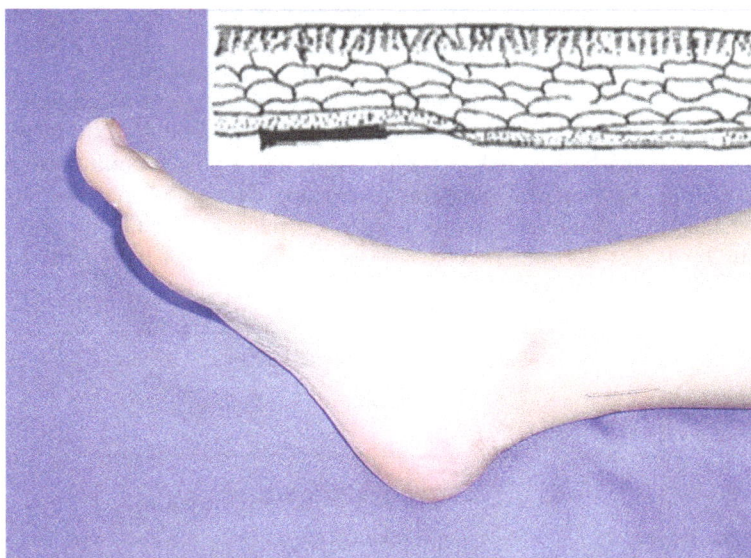

Fig. 2 WAA needling point 1 on the ankle zone (Point lower 1) after insertion. The location of Point lower 1 is close to the medial border of tendo calcaneus

horizontal position and slowly advanced until the entire needle (except the handle) entered the subcutaneous tissue. The handle was then fixed to the skin with an adhesive tape. The needles were retained in the subcutaneous tissue for 30 min. Upon withdrawal of the needle, dry sterilized cotton balls will be firmly applied to the insertion points. The patient will only feel a negligible stabbing pain when the tip of the needle pierces the skin.

Sham acupuncture group

Sham acupuncture was administered on point 1 at both ankles on the first day when the pain occurs during the period. Retain the needle for 30 min. The subjects were asked to wear an eye mask. The target site was also disinfected with an iodophordis infectant (Shanghai Likang Disinfectant Hi-tech Co. Ltd.). The tip and most body of the disposable sterile acupuncture needle will be cut off and blunted (0.25 mm in diameter and 25 mm in length, Suzhou Medical Appliance Factory, Jiangsu Province, China) (Fig. 3). This sham needle has been successfully used in the previous trail design [19]. Only 2-3 mm of the needle body in length was remained. The processed needles were also held with three right-hand fingers (thumb, index finger, and middle finger). The skin near the target site was gently pressed with the left thumb to make it slightly taut. The needle tip was swiftly punctured the skin at the target point at an angle of 30° (The tip actually was not inserted into the skin). Then, the needles remained in the point of skin horizontally for 30 min. The handle was also fixed to the skin with an adhesive tape. For a successful sham treatment, the patient will also only feel a little negligible stabbing pain when the tip of the needle pierces the skin, and no other needling sensation.

Randomization and blinding

An outside researcher who is not allowed to directly contact with the participants will perform computerized randomization. The assessor will also be blinded to the treatment allocation. The acupuncturist performing the WAA intervention and sham WAA intervention can't be completely blinded, but he is not allowed to reveal any information about treatment procedures and outcomes to the participants or the assessor. Thus, both the participants and the assessor won't distinguish clearly which intervention was given. A sealed envelope containing allocation sequence number for each participant will be opened after each participant is confirmed to meet the eligibility criteria and informed consent is made. If any error or disclosure with regard to randomization occurs, a new randomization sequence will be generated starting from the problematic serial number and applied to the participant from then on.

Outcome measures
The primary outcome
Simple form of McGill pain questionnaire (SF-MPQ):

The SF-MPQ consists of 3 parts, including the Visual Analogue Scales (VAS), Present Pain Intensity scale (PPI) and Pain Rate Index (PRI). The main component is composed of 15 descriptors, including 11 sensory and 4 affective, and the descriptors are rated on an intensity scale (0 = none, 1 = mild, 2 = moderate or 3 = severe).

Secondary outcomes
The COX menstrual symptom scale (CMSS) will be rated as the main secondary outcomes. The CMSS consists of 18 items and each item has 5 grades according to symptom severity, including the evaluation on general frequency of menstrual symptoms and average severity. 0 point for absence of discomfort; 1 point for mild discomfort; 2 points for moderate discomfort; 3 points for severe discomfort; and 4 points for extremely severe.

Expectation and treatment credibility scale (ETCS), safety assessment, participants' feeling of acupuncture questionnaire will also be included.

Sample size calculation
The sample size was determined according to the results of our previous pilot study, a two-arm design with WAA group and sham acupuncture group (the response rate was approximately 80% and 40%, respectively, showed by the pilot study). On the basis of the calculation performed by PASS11 with a two-sided significance level of

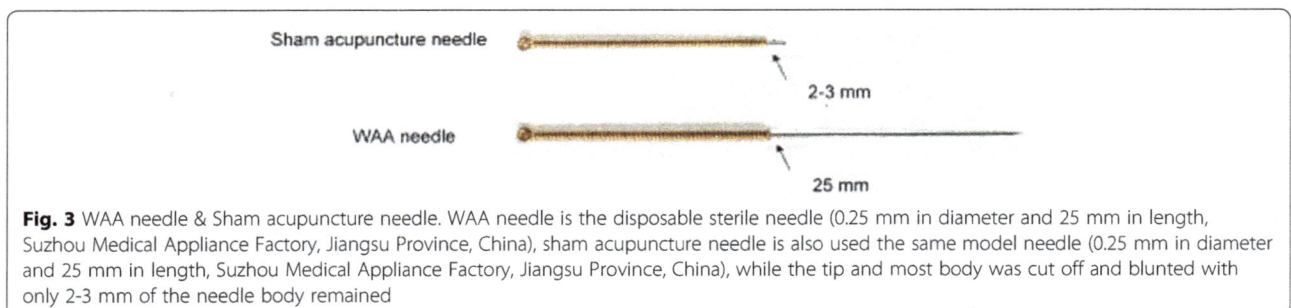

Fig. 3 WAA needle & Sham acupuncture needle. WAA needle is the disposable sterile needle (0.25 mm in diameter and 25 mm in length, Suzhou Medical Appliance Factory, Jiangsu Province, China), sham acupuncture needle is also used the same model needle (0.25 mm in diameter and 25 mm in length, Suzhou Medical Appliance Factory, Jiangsu Province, China), while the tip and most body was cut off and blunted with only 2-3 mm of the needle body remained

0.05 and power of 0.80, a total sample size of 52 would be required, with 26 for each group. Considering a maximum dropout tolerance of 15%, 30 initial participants in each group are required for this trial.

Statistical analysis

SPSS15.0 statistical software packages will be used to analyze the data. The statistician is blinded from the allocation of groups. For quantitative data, the distribution pattern and homogeneity of variance will be examined. If there is a symmetric distribution, the mean (M) ± standard deviation will be used for statistical description. Both paired samples t-test between the quantitative indices before and after treatment in one group and independent t-tests between the two groups will be used to determine and compare the effect of acupuncture. The entire statistical test will use bilateral examination, and the significance level sets at $P < 0.05$.

Discussion

The result of this trial is expected to provide high-quality clinical evidence that WAA is effective for young females with PD. Acupuncture has been used worldwide for various types of pain [20, 21], and the evidence from clinical studies also suggested that WAA has confirmed analgesic efficacy for many kinds of pain, like post-TACE pain or some cancer pain [15, 21–23]. Nowadays, the incidence of PD is increasing, especially among young females. At present, there are few attentions paid to the application of WAA for PD. Therefore, a trial about this direction deserves our devotion.

Based on TCM acupuncture theory, filiform needle therapy on the acupoints always needs participants to get the sensation of obtaining qi, which is usually experienced as sourness, numberness, distention and pain. Only the acupuncture trial design with request of obtaining qi can reflect the correct and obvious therapeutic effect of acupuncture [24]. Nevertheless, patients who experienced acupuncture treatment will perceive the difference between non-penetrating sham acupuncture and real acupuncture easily. For this reason, it is hard for common filiform needle in acupuncture intervention designed as a blind trial. However, Wrist-Ankle Acupuncture doesn't require any needling sensation. In the trial, the subjects were asked to wear an eye mask, so it is hard for them to distinguish the certain intervention in the following treatment. For this reason, we believe that non- penetrating sham acupuncture can serve as an effective placebo intervention in this trial. Meanwhile, participants' feeling of acupuncture questionnaire would arrange in the end of treatment in order to exclude breaking blind subjects. Therefore, a randomized controlled single-blind trial with a non- penetrating sham wrist-ankle acupuncture group was designed, and

it will be able to evaluate the immediate analgesia effect of WAA in PD of young females and provide useful advice of evidence-based medicine for further treatment.

Trial status
The trial is currently recruiting patients.

Acknowledgments
This work was supported by Incubation of Acupuncture and Tuina, Second Military Medical University.

Funding
This research received no specific grant from any funding agency in the public, commercial or not-for-profit sectors.

Authors' contributions
SS designed the methodology. CYF and TSN compiled the protocol. CYF was the project director. TSN registered the protocol in the Chinese Clinical Trial Registry and obtained the ethical approval. TJ were in charge of recruitment. All authors have read and approved the final manuscript.

Consent for publication
All authors signed and agreed to publish the paper according to the recommendations of Vancouver.
Written informed consent for publication of their clinical details and clinical images was obtained from the patient. A copy of the consent form is available for review by the Editor of this journal.

Competing interests
The authors declare that they have no competing interests.

Author details
[1]Changhai Hospital of Traditional Chinese Medicine, Second Military Medical University, 168 Changhai Road, Yangpu District, Shanghai, China. [2]Department of Nursing Science, Second Military Medical University, Shanghai, China.

References
1. Kennedy S. Primary dysmenorrhoea. Lancet. 1997;349(9059):1116.
2. Proctor M, Farquhar C. Diagnosis and management of dysmenorrhea. BMJ. 2006;332:1134–8.
3. French L. Dysmenorrhea. Am Fam Physician. 2005;12:85–291.
4. Dawood MY. Primary dysmenorrheal: advances in pathogenesis and management. Obstet Gynecol. 2006;108(2):428–41.
5. Nevatte T, O'Brien PM, Bäckström T, Brown C, Dennerstein L, Endicott J, Epperson CN, Eriksson E, Freeman EW, Halbreich U, Ismail K. ISPMD consensus on the management of pre-menstrual disorders. Arch Women's Ment Health. 2013;16(4):279–91.
6. Zhang WY, Li WPA. Efficacy of minor analgesics in primary dysmenorrhoea: a systematic review. BJOG Int J Obstet Gynaecol. 1998;105(7):780–9.
7. Zhang XS, Ling CQ, Zhou QH. Practical wrist-ankle acupuncture therapy. Beijing: People's Medical Publishing House; 2002.
8. Lao HH. Wrist-ankle acupuncture: methods and applications. 2nd ed. New York: Oriental Healthcare Center 1999: 1–43.
9. Zhu ZZ, Wang XP. Clinical observation on the therapeutic effects of wrist-ankle acupuncture in treatment of pain of various origins. J Tradit Chin Med. 1998;18:192–4.
10. Su JT, Zhou QH, Li R, et al. Immediate analgesic effect of wrist-ankle acupuncture for acute lumbago: a randomized controlled trial. Chinese Acupuncture & Moxibustion. 2010;30(8):617–22.
11. Marra C, Pozzi I, Ceppi L, et al. Wrist-ankle acupuncture as perineal pain relief after mediolateral episiotomy: a pilot study. Journal of Alternative & Complementary Medicine. 2011;17(3):239–41.
12. Yang J, Huang J. Electro-acupuncture analgesia can enhance the counteraction to pain via the p38 MAPK signal pathway. Nervous Diseases and Mental Health. 2007;7(5):371–3.

13. Wang ZF, Yu XM, Tao J. Study on the analgesic effect of wrist ankle acupuncture and its application in Fmri. Chinese Journal of Ethnomedicine and Ethnopharmacy. 2016;24:50–2.

14. Zhou YL, Liu YJ, Fu JN, Wei W. Effect of Huaisanzhen on central analgesic transmitters in the rat of the nerve root pain caused by protrusion of lumbar intervertebra disc. Chinese Acupuncture & Moxibustion. 2017;27(12):923–6.

15. Li BZ, Chan WC, Lo KC, et al. Wrist-ankle acupuncture for the treatment of pain symptoms: a systematic review and meta-analysis. Evidence-Based Complementray and Alternative Medicine. 2014;14(1):261709.

16. Xia HU, Wei GU, Zhou QH. Analgesic efficacy and mechanism of wrist-ankle acupuncture on pain caused by liver cancer. Chinese Journal of Integrated Traditional & Western Medicine on Liver Diseases. 2005;15(3):131–3.

17. Lefebvre G, Pinsonneault O, Antao V, Black A, Burnett M. Feldman K: Primary dysmenorrhea consensus guideline. J Obstet Gynaecol Can. 2005,27(12):1117–1146.

18. Zeng K, Dong HJ, Chen HY, et al. Wrist-ankle acupuncture for pain after transcatheter arterial chemoembolization in patients with liver cancer: a randomized controlled trial. Am J Chin Med. 2014;42(2):289–302.

19. Shu S, Zhan M, You YL, et al. Wrist-ankle acupuncture (WAA) for precompetition nervous syndrome: study protocol for a randomized controlled trial. Trials. 2015;16(1):1–6.

20. Gemma M, Nicelli E, Gioia L, et al. Acupuncture accelerates recovery after general anesthesia: a prospective randomized controlled trial. Journal of Integrative Medicine. 2015;13(2):99–104.

21. Lin JG, Chen YH. The role of acupuncture in cancer supportive care. Am J Chin Med. 2012;40(2):219–29.

22. Hu X, Ling CQ. Biomechnical mechanism of analgesic effect of wrist-ankle acupuncture. Chinese Acupuncture & Moxibustion. 2004;24(5):361–3.

23. Hu X, Ling CQ, Zhou QH. Clinical observation on wrist-ankle acupuncture for treatment of pain of middle-late liver cancer. Chinese Acupuncture & Moxibustion. 2004;24(3):149–51.

24. To M, Alexander C. The effects of park sham needles: a pilot study. Journal of Integrative Medicine. 2015;13(1):20–4.

23

Effects of acupuncture on vascular dementia (VD) animal models

Ze-Yu Zhang[1], Zhe Liu[2]* (ID), Hui-Hui Deng[1] and Qin Chen[3]

Abstract

Background: Vascular dementia is the second most common type of dementia that causes cognitive dysfunction. Acupuncture, an ancient therapy, has been mentioned for the treatment of vascular dementia in previous studies. This study aimed to evaluate the effects of acupuncture in animal models of vascular dementia.

Methods: Experimental animal studies of treating vascular dementia with acupuncture were gathered from Embase, PubMed and Ovid Medline (R) from the dates of the databases' creation to December 2016. We adopted the CAMARADES 10-item checklist to evaluate the quality of the included studies. The Morris water maze test was considered as an outcome measure. The software Stata12.0 was used for the meta-analysis. Heterogeneity was examined using I^2 statistics, and we conducted subgroup analyses to determine the causes of heterogeneity for escape latency and duration in original platform.

Results: Sixteen studies involving 363 animals met the inclusion criteria. The included studies scored between 4 and 8 points, and the mean was 5.44. The results of the meta-analysis indicated remarkable differences with acupuncture on increasing the duration in the former platform quadrant both in EO models (SMD = 1.56, 95% CI: 1.02 ~ 2.11; $p < 0.00001$) and 2-VO models (SMD 4.29, 95% CI 3.23 ~ 5.35; $p < 0.00001$) compared with the control groups.

Conclusions: Acupuncture may be effective in improving cognitive function in vascular dementia animal models. The mechanisms of acupuncture for vascular dementia are multiple such as anti-apoptosis, antioxidative stress reaction, and metabolism enhancing of glucose and oxygen.

Keywords: Acupuncture, Vascular dementia, Systematic review, Meta-analysis

Background

Vascular dementia (VD) is a heterogeneous group of brain disorders of which the cognitive impairment can be ascribed to cerebrovascular pathologies; more than 20% cases of dementia are vascular dementia, making it the second most prevalent form of dementia, second only to Alzheimer's disease (AD) [1]. Advanced age, diabetes, hypertension, smoking and atrial fibrillation are all risk factors for vascular dementia [2]. Level of education, which is considered to be an effective alternative indicator of cognitive reserves, has a significant association with the expression of VD in that higher education appears to be associated with

fewer cognitive deficits [3, 4]. As the populations of North America and European countries age, the risk of VD in these regions approximately doubles every 5.3 years. However, the current study suggests that effective therapy for vascular dementia has proven to be more difficult than for Alzheimer's disease. While memantine and cholinesterase inhibitor drugs have been proven to be significantly effective in treating Alzheimer's disease and are therefore labeled for this indication, they are not recommended for use in the treatment of vascular dementia by either regulatory bodies or guideline groups due to their overall low effectiveness and possible side effects [5–7].

Acupuncture, an economical type of traditional Chinese therapy with minimal side effects, has been used for many diseases in Asian countries for thousands of years and is widely used for rehabilitation after stroke [8]. Usually after a

---

* Correspondence: ssrsliu@163.com
[2]Department of of Neurobiology and Acupuncture Research, Third Clinical College of Zhejiang Chinese Medical University, Hangzhou, Zhejiang, China
Full list of author information is available at the end of the article

stroke, 15–30% of subjects will develop vascular dementia within three months, and delayed dementia will develop in the long term due to recurrent stroke in 20–25% of subjects [9]. In recent years, more and more studies, and especially animal experiment studies, have been published to illustrate the effectiveness of acupuncture for vascular dementia.

Until now, no systematic meta-analysis has been published to analyze the effects of acupuncture on enhancing cognitive function in vascular dementia animal models. A systematic review of animal experiments can be beneficial for future experimental designs and provide a basis for clinical studies. Additionally, it can provide valuable directions for further research. It is for these reasons that we conducted this systematic review and meta-analysis.

Methods

This systematic review and meta-analysis complied with standard guidelines (See Additional file 1).

Search strategy

The following electronic databases were searched from database inception to December 2016: Embase, PubMed and Ovid Medline (R), and the following keywords were used: acupuncture, electroacupuncture, acupoint, vascular dementia, multi-infarct dementia and multiinfarct dementia. The search language was limited to English, and we also tried to collect records from other sources. The detailed search strategies are shown in Additional file 2.

Inclusion criteria

(1) Subjects: Animal models of vascular dementia were included.
(2) Intervention: Only manual acupuncture and electroacupuncture (EA) were included.
(3) Outcome: The Morris water maze test was used to evaluate cognitive functions in animal models.
(4) Language: Only articles published in English were included.
(5) No publication date limit was set, and the search was conducted in December 2016.

Exclusion criteria

(1) Duplicate articles;
(2) Studies that have no control group;
(3) Auricular acupuncture, laser acupuncture and other acupuncture techniques;
(4) Acupuncture therapy combined with the use of traditional Chinese medicines or Western drugs;
(5) Studies aiming to compare different acupuncture techniques;
(6) Studies that only compared acupuncture with traditional Chinese medicines.

Study selection and data extraction

One reviewer (ZYZ) generated the search strategy, searched the databases, and made a list of all the records. Two evaluators (HHD, QC) independently evaluated the articles based on the inclusion and exclusion criteria. Disagreements were solved together through discussions (ZYZ, HHD, QC). Two reviewers (HHD, QC) independently extracted the data.

The following data were extracted: publication year, the last name of the first author, model of vascular dementia, weight range of the included animals, number of animals included, method of treatment with timing and duration in the acupuncture and control groups, the assessment of trials, and the results of each article (positive or negative). The final outcomes were extracted if several outcomes were presented. When the outcome data were only shown graphically, we attempted to contact the authors to obtain the detailed data; if we received no response to our request, we used GetData software to measure the data. Differences were solved together through discussions (HHD, QC, ZYZ).

Risk of bias assessment

We evaluated methodological quality against an ten-item checklist [10]: (1) peer-reviewed journal; (2) temperature control; (3) animals were randomly allocated; (4) blind established model; (5) blinded outcome assessment; (6) anesthetics used without marked intrinsic neuroprotective properties; (7) animal model (diabetic, advanced age or hypertensive); (8) calculation of sample size; (9) statement of compliance with animal welfare regulations; (10) possible conflicts of interest.

The quality of each study was evaluated by a score from zero to ten. Two evaluators (HHD, QC) independently extracted the data and assessed the quality of each study. Disagreements were resolved through discussion (HHD, QC, ZYZ).

Statistical analysis

For statistical analysis, we used the statistical software package Stata version 12.0. The data of the Morris water maze test, such as escape latency, time in the quadrant in which the former platform was located, and frequency of crossing through the former platform were considered continuous data, and we therefore calculated standard mean differences (SMD) with confidence intervals (CIs) established at 95%. Heterogeneity in the studies was examined using I^2 statistics. If the I^2 statistic was higher than 50%, we considered significant heterogeneity to be present, and we used a random effects model. Otherwise, we used a fixed effect model. When significant heterogeneity existed, the subgroup analysis would be conducted based on animal species, acupuncture methods and modeling methods. We used Egger's test and Begg's test to assess publication bias.

Results

We identified 194 possibly relevant studies in the initial search. After duplicates had been removed, we screened the titles and the abstracts of 105 remaining records, and 82 records were excluded. For further screening, 23 remaining articles were downloaded. Eventually, 16 studies met the inclusion criteria [11–26]. The selection process flow diagram is shown in Fig. 1 [27].

Study characteristics

The 16 studies included involved 363 rats, 174 of which were in an acupuncture group and 189 of which were in a control group. All the studies stated the weight range of the rats, which ranged from 180 to 490 g. A total of 7 of the 16 studies mentioned the age of the animals [11, 14, 16–18, 23, 25], which ranged from 2 months old to 12 months old. Sixteen of the included studies used different subtests of the Morris water maze test; all the studies met the inclusion criteria by using escape latency as outcome data, while two studies used swimming speed [24, 26], five studies used duration in the quadrant of the former platform position [12, 13, 21, 24, 26], one used swimming distance [19], and three used frequency of crossing former platform [12, 15, 16]. Two species of rats were used in the 16 studies: seven studies used Sprague–Dawley (SD) rats [11, 13, 15, 17–19, 25], and nine studies used Wistar rats [12, 14, 16, 20–24, 26]. The basic characteristics of the studies are listed in Table 1 [28].

Model preparation method

Various methods were used to establish a vascular dementia (VD) model in the different studies (Table 1) [29]. The 4-vessel occlusion (4-VO) method was used in two studies [11, 13]; 7 studies used bilateral common carotid artery occlusion (2-VO) [15, 17–20, 24, 26]; 6 studies used embolic occlusion (EO) [12, 14, 16, 21–24]; and the remaining trial used middle cerebral artery occlusion (MCAO) [25].

Description of acupuncture

A range of acupuncture techniques was employed with regard to the combinations of acupoints, the stimulation method (EA or manual acupuncture) and manipulation. Five studies used acupoints CV6 (Zhongji), CV12 (Zhongwan), CV17 (Danzhong), SP10 (Xiehai), ST36 (Zusanli) [12, 14, 16, 21, 24], which was the most commonly used technique. Three studies chose to apply acupuncture

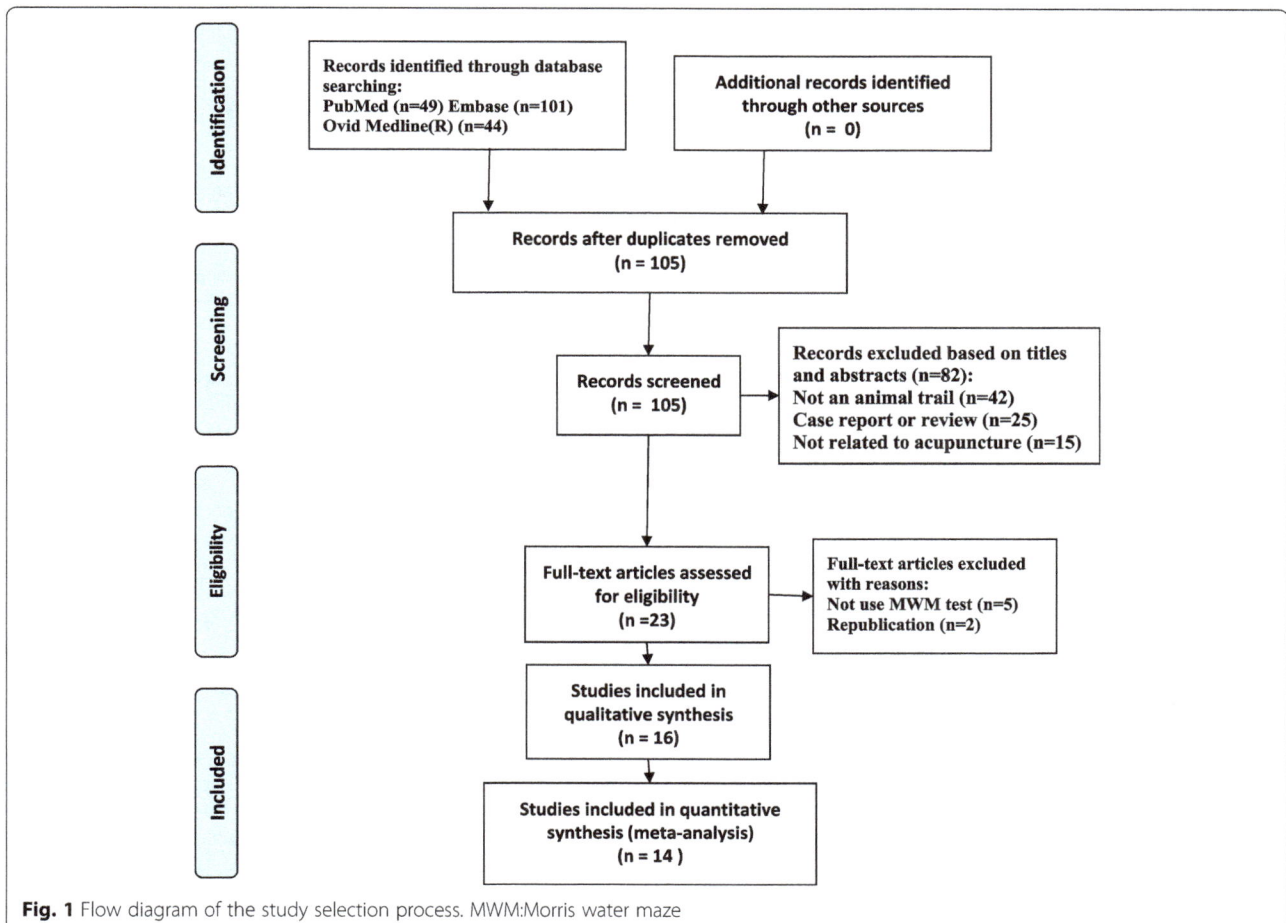

Fig. 1 Flow diagram of the study selection process. MWM:Morris water maze

Table 1 Data of 16 included studies

Trial	Species (Na/Nc)	Age(month)	Weigh(g)	Model	Acupuncture(acupoints)	Control intervention	Outcome assessment	Result
Wang 2004 [11]	SD rats (14/13) SD rats (14/13)	2~3	200–250	4-VO	EA,20 min/d for 15d, 150HZ, 2 mA, continuous Waveform (GV14, GV20)	No treatment Nimodipine	Escape latency Escape latency	$P < 0.01$ $P > 0.05$
Yu 2005 [12]	Wistar rats (15/14)	NR	340 ± 40	EO	manual acupuncture, 30 s/d for 21 d (CV6, CV12, CV17, SP10, ST36)	Placebo-acupuncture	Escape latency Duration in former platform position Frequency crossing former platform	$P < 0.05$ $P < 0.05$ $P < 0.05$
Shao 2008 [13]	SD rats (9/8) SD rats (9/8)	NR	180–220	4-VO	EA,20 min/d for 15 d, 150 HZ, 1–2 mA, Continuous Waveform (BL17, BL20, BL23, GV20)	No treatment Nimodipine	Escape latency Escape latency	$P < 0.01$ $P > 0.05$
Wang 2009 [14]	Wistar rats(11/11)	10	300 ± 40	EO	manual acupuncture, 30 s/d for 21 d (CV6, CV12, CV17, SP10, ST36)	Placebo-acupuncture	Escape latency Duration in former platform position	$P < 0.05$ $P < 0.01$
Wei 2011 [15]	SD rats (10/10)	NR	200–250	2-VO	EA, 20 min/d for 10 d, 50 HZ,1.0 mA, continuous Waveform (GV14, GV20)	No treatment Nimodipine	Escape latency Frequency crossing former platform Escape latency Frequency crossing former platform	$P < 0.01$ $P < 0.01$ $P > 0.01$ $P > 0.01$
Zhao 2011 [16]	Wistar rats(10/10)	4	240 ± 20	EO	manual acupuncture, 30 s/d for 21 d(CV6, CV12, CV17, SP10, ST36)	Placebo-acupuncture	Escape latency Swimming Speed	$P < 0.01$ $P > 0.05$
Zhu 2011 [17]	SD rats (11/12)	9	460 ± 30	2-VO	EA, 20 min/d for 30 d,4HZ, 2.0 mA, continuous waveform (BL23, GV14, GV20)	No treatment	Escape latency	$P < 0.01$
Zhu 2012 [18]	SD rats (12/10)	12	400 ± 30	2-VO	EA, 20 min/d for 30 d,4 HZ, 2.0 mA, continuous waveform (BL23, GV14, GV20)	No treatment	Escape latency	$P < 0.05$
Zhu 2013 [19]	SD rats (6/6)	NR	432 ± 30	2-VO	EA, 20 min/d for 30 d, 4HZ, continuous waveform (BL23, GV14, GV20)	No treatment	Escape latency	$P < 0.05$
Yang 2014 CG [20]	Wistar rats (12/12)	NR	200–250	2-VO	manual acupuncture, 360 min/d for 21 d (Frontal region, frontoparietal region and parietal region)	No treatment	Escape latency Swimming distance	$P < 0.05$ $P < 0.05$
Yang 2014 CG [20]	Wistar rats (12/12)	NR	200–250	2-VO	manual acupuncture, 360 min/d for 21 d (Frontal region, frontoparietal region and parietal region)	No treatment	Escape latency Swimming distance	$P < 0.05$ $P < 0.05$
Zhang 2014 [21]	Wistar rats (10/10)	NR	300–320	EO	manual acupuncture, 30 s/d for 21 d (CV6, CV12, CV17, SP10, ST36)	Placebo-acupuncture	Escape latency Frequency crossing former platform Duration in former platform position	$P < 0.01$ $P < 0.01$ $P < 0.01$
Li 2015 [22]	Wistar rats (11/11)	NR	320–360	EO	manual acupuncture,30 s/d for 14 d (ST36)	Placebo-acupuncture	Escape latency	$P < 0.05$
Li 2015 [23]	Wistar rats (10/10)	2	300–320	EO	manual acupuncture, 30 s/d for 14 d (ST36	Placebo-acupuncture	Escape latency	$P < 0.05$
Wang 2015 [24]	Wister rats(10/10)	NR	200–220	2-VO	manual acupuncture, 30 s/d for 21 d (CV6, CV12, CV17, SP10, ST36)	Placebo-acupuncture	Escape latency Swimming speed Duration in former platform position	$P < 0.05$ $P > 0.05$ $P < 0.05$

Table 1 Data of 16 included studies *(Continued)*

Trial	Species (Na/Nc)	Age(month)	Weigh(g)	Model	Acupuncture(acupoints)	Control intervention	Outcome assessment	Result
Fang 2016 [25]	SD rats (18/18)	9	300–450	MCAO	EA, 20 min/d for 30 d, 30HZ, 6-15 V, sparse wave (BL23, GV14, GV20)	No treatment	Escape latency	$P < 0.05$
Li 2016 [26]	Wister rats (14/14)	NR	270–320	2-VO	manual acupuncture, 30 s/d for 14 d (ST36)	Placebo-acupuncture	Escape latency Duration in former platform position Swimming speed	$P < 0.01$ $P < 0.01$ $P > 0.05$

Na number of animals in the acupuncture group, *EA* electroacupuncture, *Nc* number of animals in the control group, *SD* Sprague Dawley, *4-VO* 4-vessel occlusion, *EO* embolic occlusion, *2-VO* bilateral common carotid artery occlusion, *NR* no record, *PG* positive control group, *CG* cluster-needling group, *MCAO* middle cerebral artery occlusion

treatment to a single acupoint, ST36 (Zusanli) [22, 23, 26]. Four studies used BL23 (Shenshu), GV14 (Dazhui), and GV20 (Baihui) [17–19, 25]. Two studies used GV14 (Dazhui) and GV20 (Baihui) [11, 15]. One study used BL17 (Geshu), BL20 (Pishu), BL23 (Shenshu), and GV20 (Baihui) [13]. The final study had two acupuncture groups [20]: the group called the positive control group used GV14 (Dazhui) and GV20 (Baihui), and the other group, the cluster-needling group, used the frontal region, the frontoparietal region, and the parietal region. Nine studies chose manual acupuncture as the method of stimulation [12, 14, 16, 20–24, 26], while the other seven studies used electroacupuncture [11, 13, 17–19, 25]. Almost all of the studies that used manual acupuncture adopted 30s as their treatment duration; the exception was the study that had two acupuncture groups [20], the positive control group and the cluster-needling group, which used 60 min and 360 min. Of the 7 EA studies, six of the studies adopted continuous waves [11, 13, 15, 17–19], of which the frequency ranged from 4 Hz to 150 Hz, and the current density was from 1 to 2 mA. The remaining study adopted sparse wave [25], of which the frequency was 30 Hz. A summary of the acupuncture treatment protocols is shown in Table 1.

Control interventions

Ten studies adopted some interventions in the control groups. The Western medicine nimodipine was used as a control intervention in three studies [11, 13, 15], and the remaining seven studies adopted placebo-acupuncture as a control intervention [12, 14, 16, 22–24, 26].

Study quality assessment

The study quality scores ranged from 4 to 8. Four studies scored points in 4 items [13, 16, 21, 23]; four studies scored points in 5 items [11, 12, 14, 17]; six studies scored points in 6 items [15, 18, 19, 24–26]; one study scored 7 points [22]; and the remaining study scored 8 points [20]. All of the included studies were published in peer-reviewed journals. Eleven of the studies mentioned control of temperature [11–13, 15, 18–20, 22, 24–26], which included room temperature or the temperature of the water in the

maze. All of the studies adopted random allocation. Blinded building of the model was adopted in 13 studies [11, 12, 14–17, 19–22, 24–26]. Blinded outcome assessment was adopted in 2 studies [22, 23]. Twelve studies stated the use of anesthetics without marked intrinsic neuroprotective properties [11, 12, 14, 15, 17–20, 22–24, 26]. No study adopted a diabetic, hypertensive or aged animal model, and no study reported sample size calculations. Eight studies mentioned compliance with animal welfare regulations [14, 15, 18, 20, 21, 23–26]. Seven studies stated possible conflicts of interest [13, 16–18, 20, 22, 25]. The study quality assessment is shown in Table 2.

Morris water maze outcomes analyses

Escape latency

Twelve studies adopted escape latency as an outcome index. And all of these studies reported the positive effectiveness of acupuncture on reducing escape latency, except for the one study [20] that was designed with two acupuncture groups, the positive control group and cluster-needling group, which showed negative results and positive results, respectively. Of these 12 studies, six of them provided detailed data regarding the marked effect of acupuncture [11, 13, 15, 18–20], and we extracted the data from the other six studies that demonstrated the data in a graphical representation by using GetData software [16, 21–26]. To avoid double-counting [30], the effects of different acupuncture intervention arms included in a single study were averaged and entered once in the analysis [20] [$n = 280$, SMD = -3.06, 95%CI (-4.04~ -2.09), $p < 0.00001$; heterogeneity $I^2 = 87.1\%$, random effects model, Fig. 2a] [31–33]. Three studies compared the effect of acupuncture with nimodipine [11, 13, 15], and all three of these studies concluded that escape latency was not significantly different between the medication group and the acupuncture group [$n = 64$, SMD = -0.07, 95% CI (-0.56 ~ 0.42), $p = 0.775 > 0.05$; heterogeneity $I^2 = 0\%$, fixed effect model, Fig. 2b].

Duration in original platform

Five studies showed the effect of acupuncture on improving the duration in the quadrant of the former platform compared with the control group (VD group or

Table 2 Methodological quality assessment of the included studies

Study	1	2	3	4	5	6	7	8	9	10	Score
Wang 2004 [11]	Y	Y	Y	Y	N	Y	N	N	N	N	5
Yu 2005 [12]	Y	Y	Y	Y	N	Y	N	N	N	N	5
Shao 2008 [13]	Y	Y	Y	N	N	U	N	N	N	Y	4
Wang 2009 [14]	Y	N	Y	Y	N	Y	N	N	Y	N	5
Wei 2011 [15]	Y	Y	Y	Y	N	Y	N	N	Y	N	6
Zhao 2011 [16]	Y	N	Y	Y	N	U	N	N	N	Y	4
Zhu 2011 [17]	Y	N	Y	Y	N	Y	N	N	N	Y	5
Zhu 2012 [18]	Y	Y	Y	N	N	Y	N	N	Y	Y	6
Zhu 2013 [19]	Y	Y	Y	Y	N	Y	N	N	N	N	6
Yang 2014 [20]	Y	Y	Y	Y	N	Y	N	N	Y	Y	8
Zhang 2014 [21]	Y	N	Y	Y	N	U	N	N	Y	N	4
Li 2015 [22]	Y	Y	Y	Y	Y	Y	N	N	N	Y	7
Li 2015 [23]	Y	N	Y	N	Y	Y	N	N	N	N	4
Wang 2015 [24]	Y	Y	Y	Y	N	Y	N	N	Y	N	6
Fang 2016 [25]	Y	Y	Y	Y	N	U	N	N	Y	Y	6
Li 2016 [26]	Y	Y	Y	Y	N	Y	N	N	Y	N	6

(1) Peer-reviewed journal. (2) Temperature control. (3) Animals were randomly allocated. (4) Blind established model. (5) Blinded outcome assessment. (6) Anesthetics used without marked intrinsic neuroprotective properties. (7) Animal model (diabetic, advanced age or hypertensive). (8) Calculation of sample size. (9) Statement of compliance with animal welfare regulations. (10) Possible conflicts of interest
Y, Yes(low risk bias); N, No(high risk bias); U, Unclear

placebo-acupuncture group) [12, 14, 21, 24, 26]. All five of these studies reported positive results, but none of them provided detailed data [13]; we therefore extracted the data from the figures [$n = 119$, SMD = 2.52, 95%CI (1.34 ~ 3.69), $p < 0.00001$; heterogeneity $I^2 = 82.0\%$, random effects model, Fig. 2c].

Frequency of crossing former platform

Three studies reported the positive results of acupuncture on increasing the frequency of crossing the former platform location [12, 15, 21] [$n = 69$, SMD = 1.84, 95% CI (0.95 ~ 2.74), $p < 0.00001$; heterogeneity $I^2 = 56.3\%$, random effects model, Fig. 2d].

There was no significant difference observed in the animals' swimming speed in the water maze in the two studies that measured it, although the detailed data were unavailable [24, 26].

Subgroup analyses
Escape latency

Animal species Acupuncture was found to have a remarkable effect on reducing escape latency time in both Sprague-Dawley rats (SMD −3.33, 95% CI −5.18 ~ − 1.47; $p < 0.00001$) and Wister rats (SMD −2.85, 95% CI −3.79~ − 1.91; $p = 0.002$). The subgroup analysis observed that

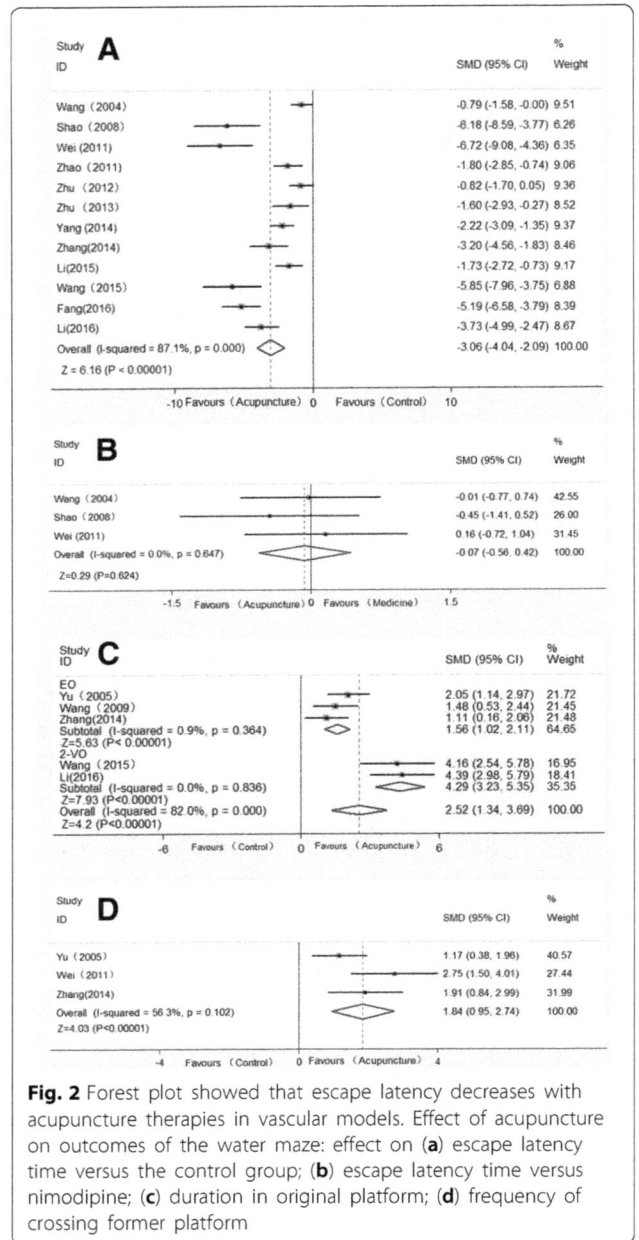

Fig. 2 Forest plot showed that escape latency decreases with acupuncture therapies in vascular models. Effect of acupuncture on outcomes of the water maze: effect on (**a**) escape latency time versus the control group; (**b**) escape latency time versus nimodipine; (**c**) duration in original platform; (**d**) frequency of crossing former platform

Wister rats had slightly reduced heterogeneity ($I^2 = 73.5\%$), while Sprague-Dawley rats did not ($I^2 = 92.1\%$).

Acupuncture methods We performed a subgroup analysis of the methods of acupuncture used (Table 3) and observed significant effects of manual acupuncture (SMD −3.11, 95% CI −4.23 ~ − 2.00; $p = 0.002$) and electro-acupuncture (SMD −3.05, 95% CI −4.56~ − 0.78; $p < 0.00001$) on reducing escape latency time. Subgroup analysis of the acupuncture methods indicated that manual acupuncture had reduced heterogeneity ($I^2 = 75.9\%$), while electroacupuncture did not ($I^2 = 90.5\%$).

Table 3 Subgroup analysis for the effect of acupuncture on reducing escape latency time

		SMD	LL	HL	Degrees of freedom	Heterogeneity I^2	Effect size Z	P
Species	SR	−3.33	−5.18	−1.47	5	92.10%	3.52	$P < 0.00001$
	WR	−2.85	−3.79	−1.91	5	73.50%	5.93	$P = 0.002$
Modeling	2-VO	−2.97	−4.21	−1.73	6	85.80%	4.69	$P < 0.00001$
	4-VO	−3.36	−8.63	1.92	1	94.30%	1.25	$P = 0.212$
	EO	−2.38	−3.82	−0.95	1	65.80%	3.26	$P = 0.001$
	MCAO	−5.19	−6.58	−3.79	0	−	7.29	$P < 0.00001$
Methods	EA	−3.05	−4.56	−1.53	6	90.50%	3.94	$P < 0.00001$
	MA	−3.11	−4.23	−2.00	4	75.90%	5.47	$P = 0.002$
OVERALL		−3.06	−4.04	−2.09	11	87.10%	6.04	$P < 0.00001$

SR Sprague–Dawley Rats, *WR* Wister Rats, *2-VO* bilateral common carotid artery occlusion, *VO* 4-vessel occlusion, *EO* embolic occlusion, *MCAO* middle cerebral artery occlusion, *EA* Electroacupuncture, *MA* Manual acupuncture

Modeling methods We also conducted a subgroup analysis of the modeling methods (Table 3) [31]. This subgroup analysis showed that acupuncture had a significant effect on 2-VO models (SMD −2.97, 95% CI −4.21~ − 1.73; $p < 0.00001$), EO models (SMD −2.38, 95% CI −3.82~ − 0.95; $p = 0.001$), and MCAO models (SMD −5.29, 95% CI −6.58~ − 3.79; $p < 0.00001$), but no remarkable difference was found in the 4-VO models (SMD −3.36, 95% CI −8.63 ~ 1.92; $p = 0.212 > 0.05$).

Duration in original platform

Modeling methods For all five of the studies that regarded duration in original platform as an outcome measure, adopted electroacupuncture, and used Wister rats, we only conducted a subgroup analysis of the modeling methods (Fig. 2c). Both the EO models (SMD 1.56, 95% CI 1.02 ~ 2.11; $p < 0.00001$) and the 2-VO models (SMD 4.92, 95% CI 3.23 ~ 5.35; $p < 0.00001$) found a remarkable effect with the use of electroacupuncture, and this subgroup analysis significantly reduced the heterogeneity (EO: $I^2 = 0.9\%$, 2-VO: $I^2 = 0\%$).

Publication bias test

We performed a publication bias test for the outcome of escape latency using Egger's test (Pr > |z| = 0.001 < 0.05, continuity corrected) and Begg's test (Pr > |z| = 0.005 < 0.05, continuity corrected, Fig. 3). The results of these two tests indicated the potential existence of publication bias across all of the included studies [34]. We did not conduct a publication bias test for the other outcome measures, because there were fewer than ten included studies for each measure [35].

Signaling pathways

Of the sixteen included studies, fifteen described possible mechanisms of acupuncture in ameliorating cognitive function. The main signaling pathways were summarized in three aspects, oxidative stress damage reduction, nerve apoptosis suppression and neurogenesis. See Table 4 [36, 37].

Discussion

To the best of our knowledge, this report describes the first systematic meta-analysis exploring the effect of acupuncture on vascular dementia in animal experiments with the results of the Morris water maze test as the outcome assessment.

Implications

This study indicates that electroacupuncture could increase the duration in the former platform quadrant both in EO models (SMD = 1.56, 95% CI: 1.02 ~ 2.11; $p < 0.00001$; heterogeneity: I-squared = 0.9%) and 2-VO models (SMD = 4.29, 95% CI: 3.23 ~ 5.35; $p < 0.00001$; heterogeneity: I-squared = 0%) compared with the control groups. This finding suggests that acupuncture may play a potential role in ameliorating cognitive dysfunction in animal models. A previous study indicates that the addition of acupuncture therapy to routine care may have beneficial effects on improvements in cognitive status but limited efficacy on health-related quality of life in vascular dementia patients [38].

The high heterogeneity between the studies based on escape latency time cannot be completely explained. We conducted subgroup analyses based on the method of stimulation, the modeling method and the animal species used, but no evident cause was found. Meanwhile, the subgroup analysis of the modeling methods that regarded the duration in former platform as an outcome measure obviously reduced the heterogeneity. We found all five of the studies in this analysis adopted the same method of stimulation, the same animal species, and similar acupoint combinations. Four of the five studies used CV6, CV12, CV17, SP10, and ST36, the other study used ST36. These

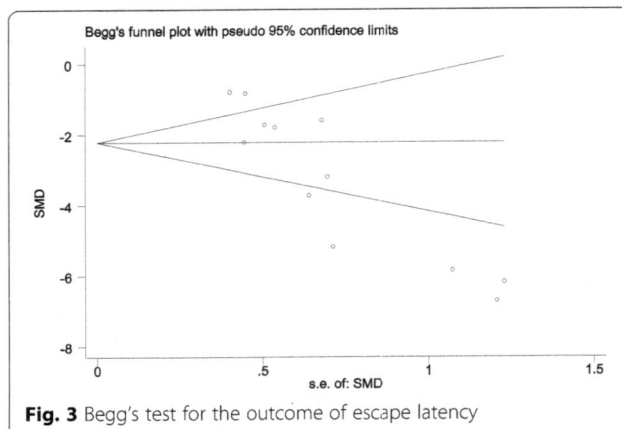

Fig. 3 Begg's test for the outcome of escape latency

findings indicate that, in addition to the differences in stimulation method, modeling methods and animal species used, acupoint combinations may be another source of heterogeneity among the studies.

Systematic reviews can help promote the methodological quality of preclinical animal studies. Systematic

Table 4 Proposed mechanisms

Study	Findings & Proposed mechanisms
Wang 2004 [11]	• Reduced NO, NOS and MDA • Increased SOD and GSH-Px
Shao 2008 [13]	Increased AVP and SS
Wang 2009 [14]	• Up-regulating the expression of Bcl-2 • Counter-regulated the pro-apoptotic Bax
Wei 2011 [15]	Promoting synaptic function and structure
Zhao 2011 [16]	Enhanced hexokinase, pyruvate kinase and glucose 6 phosphate dehydrogenase activities
Zhu 2011 [17]	Inhibiting expression of p53 and Noxa
Zhu 2012 [18]	Increased p70S6K and ribosomal protein S6
Zhu 2013 [19]	Increased mTOR and eIF4E
Yang 2014 [20]	Increased hippocampal ACh, DA, and 5-HT
Zhang 2014 [21]	Increased CBF
Li 2015 [22]	Increase pyramidal neuron number in hippocampal CA1 area
Li 2015 [23]	• Inhibited PDE activity • Activated ERK and cAMP/PKA/CREB
Wang 2015 [24]	Enhanced Nrf2
Fang 2016 [25]	Decreased TNF-α mRNA, IL-6 mRNA and IL-1β mRNA
Li 2016 [26]	• Increased complex I, II, IV and cox IV • Decreased ROS

NO nitric oxide, *NOS* nitric oxide synthase, *MDA* malondialdehyde, *GSH-Px* glutathione peroxidase, *AVP* arginine vasopressin, *SS* somatostatin, *Bcl-2* B-cell lymphoma-2, *Bax* Bcl-2 associated X protein, *P53* Tumor protein P53, *P70S6K* P70 ribosomal protein S6 kinase, *mTOR* mammalian target of rapamycin, *eIF4E* eukaryotic translation initiation factor, *Ach* acetylcholine, *DA* dopamine, *5-HT* 5-hydroxytryptamine, *CBF* cerebral blood flow, *PDE* phosphodiesterase, *ERK* extracellular signal-regulated kinase, *cAMP* 3',5'-cyclic AMP/protein kinaseA, *PKA* protein kinaseA, *CREB* cAMP/PKA/cAMP response element binding protein, *Nrf2* nuclear factor erythroid-related factor 2, *TNF* tumor necrosis factor, *IL* interleukin, *coxIV* cytochrome oxidase IV, *ROS* reactive oxygen species

reviews can help promote the methodological quality of preclinical animal studies. Essential methodological details are significant to measure the quality of a body of evidence and to assess the bias risk in animal trials. However, the insufficiency of the methodology is evident in many aspects of the present study. For instance, an adequate target animal model represents an important aspect to improve the quality of the experimental design. All included studies were performed on healthy and young animals. However, vascular dementia [39] generally occurs in aged, diabetic or hypertensive patients; therefore, experiments using young and healthy animals may overestimate the effectiveness of the intervention [10]. Hence, appropriate target animal models (hypertensive, advanced age and diabetic) should be used in future experimental research.

The included studies investigated several signaling pathways to gain a better understanding of the mechanism of improving cognitive function via acupuncture, including modulating the production and degradation of free radicals to reduce brain damage [11], exerting anti-apoptotic effects by up-regulating B-cell lymphoma-2 (Bcl-2) and counter-regulating Bcl-2-associated X protein (Bax) to protect neurons [14], enhancing glucose metabolism in the brain [16], reducing tumor protein P53 and Noxa expression to protect pyramidal cells from apoptosis [17], increasing cerebral blood flow for increased glucose and oxygen supply to neurons [21], exerting neuroprotective effects via an antioxidative pathway mediated by nuclear factor erythroid2-related factor 2 (Nrf2) [24], and increasing complex enzymes to protect neurons from oxidative stress [26]. The present study indicated that acupuncture protects neurons during vascular dementia mainly through enhancing oxygen and glucose metabolism and anti-apoptosis and antioxidant properties. However, the signaling pathways targeted by acupuncture were infrequently and incompletely reported. Therefore, this field should be further explored in future clinical studies.

Limitations

This systematic meta-analysis has several limitations, the first of which is language bias. We limited the language of our searches to English only, which may cause potential publication bias. The results may have differed if we had included studies reported in Chinese, Korean, Japanese or other languages. Second, the total sample size was still not big enough, although we made a concerted effort to search all of the studies that met the inclusion criteria. Third, the quality of the included studies was unsatisfactory, which had an important influence on the results of the systematic meta-analysis. Fourth, evident availability bias was caused by two included studies from which the data cannot be extracted [35]. We tried to contact the authors by e-mail, but we received no reply.

Fifth, we performed Begg's test and Egger's test for publication bias assessment, and the results indicated potential publication bias.

In view of the limitations above, we recommend that non-English language literature should be included in future systematic meta-analyses. Furthermore, blind outcome assessments, use of target animal models (hypertensive, advanced age and diabetic), calculation of sample size, statement of compliance with animal welfare regulations, possible conflicts of interest and detailed data publishing should be considered in future animal model studies.

Conclusions

From a methodological perspective, animal experiments should be standardly and appropriately designed and transparently reported. Acupuncture may play a potential role in ameliorating cognitive dysfunction in animal models. Furthermore, our findings indicates that acupuncture could protect neurons in animal models of vascular dementia through enhanced oxygen and glucose metabolism, as well as antioxidant and anti-apoptosis effects. Thus, this field should be further explored in vascular dementia clinical trials.

Acknowledgements
We would like to extend our gratitude to Professor Bo-Yi Liu, from Department of Acupuncture, Zhejiang Chinese Medical University, Hangzhou, Zhejiang, China, for revising the manuscript. And we thank American Journal Experts (AJE) for English language editing. This manuscript was edited for English language by American Journal Experts (AJE).

Funding
This work was supported by the Natural Science Foundation of Zhejiang Province of China (no.LY16H270004 and no.LY13H270012); the National Natural Science Foundation of China (no. 81273822 and no.81503645). The funders had no role in study design, data collection and analysis, decision to publish, or preparation of the manuscript.

Authors' contributions
Conceived and designed the experiments: ZL, ZYZ. Performed the experiments: QC, HHD, ZYZ. Analyzed the data: QC, HHD, ZYZ. Contributed reagents/materials/analysis tools: ZYZ. Wrote the paper: ZL, ZYZ. Revised the manuscript: QC, ZL. Agreed with the manuscript's results and conclusions: QC, HHD, ZL, ZYZ. All the authors read and approved the final manuscript.

Competing interests
The authors declare that they have no competing interests.

Author details
[1]Department of Traditional Chinese Medicine, Third Clinical Medical College of Zhejiang Chinese Medical University, Hangzhou, Zhejiang, China.
[2]Department of of Neurobiology and Acupuncture Research, Third Clinical College of Zhejiang Chinese Medical University, Hangzhou, Zhejiang, China.
[3]Department of Acupuncture, Zhejiang Chinese Medical University Affiliated Third Hospital, Hangzhou, Zhejiang, China.

References

1. Gorelick PB, Scuteri A, Black SE, DeCarli C, Greenberg SM, Iadecola C, Launer LJ, et al. Vascular contributions to cognitive impairment and dementia: a statement for healthcare professionals from the American Heart Association/American Stroke Association. Stroke. 2011;42(9):2672–713.
2. Sahathevan R, Brodtmann A, Donnan GA. Dementia, stroke, and vascular risk factors: a review. Stroke. 2012;7:61–73.
3. Stern Y. Cognitive reserve in ageing and Alzheimer's disease. Lancet Neurol. 2012;11:1006–12.
4. Zieren N, Duering M, Peters N, Reyes S, Jouvent E, Hervé D, Gschwendtner A, et al. Education modifies the relation of vascular pathology to cognitive function: cognitive reserve in cerebral autosomal dominant arteriopathy with subcortical infarcts and leukoencephalopathy. Neurobiol Aging. 2013; 34(2):400–7.
5. Román GC. Vascular dementia may be the most common form of dementia in the elderly. J Neurol Sci. 2002;s203–204(1):7–10.
6. O'Brien JT, Thomas A. Vascular dementia. Lancet. 2015;386(10004):1698–706.
7. Health, NCCFM. Dementia: supporting people with dementia and their carers in health and social care. Nhs National Institute for Health & Clinical Excellence; 2006.
8. Rabinstein AA, Shulman LM. Acupuncture in clinical neurology. Neurologist. 2003;9(9):137–48.
9. Pendlebury ST, Rothwell PM. Prevalence, incidence, and factors associated with pre-stroke and post-stroke dementia: a systematic review and meta-analysis. Lancet Neurol. 2009;8(11):1006–18.
10. Macleod MR, O'Collins T, Howells DW, Donnan GA. Pooling of animal experimental data reveals influence of study design and publication bias. Stroke. 2004;35(5):1203–8.
11. Wang L, Tang CZ, Lai XS. Effects of electroacupuncture on learning, memory and formation system of free radicals in brain tissues of vascular dementia model rats. J Tradit Chin Med. 2004;24(2):140–3.
12. Yu J, Liu C, Zhang X, Han J. Acupuncture improved cognitive impairment caused by multi-infarct dementia in rats. Physiol Behav. 2005;86(4):434–41.
13. Shao Y, Fu Y, Qiu L, Yan B, Lai XS, Tang CZ. Electropuncture influences on learning, memory, and neuropeptide expression in a rat model of vascular dementia. Neural Regen Res. 2008;3(3):267–71.
14. Wang T, Liu CZ, Yu JC, Jiang W, Han JX. Acupuncture protected cerebral multi-infarction rats from memory impairment by regulating the expression of apoptosis related genes bcl-2 and bax in hippocampus. Physiol Behav. 2008;96(1):155–61.
15. Wei D, Jia X, Yin X, Jiang W. Effects of electroacupuncture versus nimodipine on long-term potentiation and synaptophysin expression in a rat model of vascular dementia. Neural Regen Res. 2011;06(30):2357–61.
16. Zhao L, Shen P, Han Y, Zhang X, Nie K, Cheng H, et al. Effects of acupuncture on glycometabolic enzymes in multi-infarct dementia rats. Neurochem Res. 2011;36(5):693–700.
17. Zhu Y, Zeng Y. Electroacupuncture protected pyramidal cells in hippocampal ca1 region of vascular dementia rats by inhibiting the expression of p53 and noxa. CNS Neurosci Ther. 2011;17(6):599–604.
18. Zhu Y, Wang X, Ye X, Gao C, Wang W. Effects of electroacupuncture on the expression of p70 ribosomal protein S6 kinase and ribosomal protein S6 in the hippocampus of rats with vascular dementia. Neural Regen Res. 2012;7(3):207–11.
19. Zhu Y, Zeng Y, Wang X, Ye X. Effect of electroacupuncture on the expression of mTOR and eIF4E in hippocampus of rats with vascular dementia. Neurol Sci. 2013;34(7):1093–7.
20. Yang J, Litscher G, Li H, Guo W, Liang Z, Zhang T, et al. The effect of scalp point cluster-needling on learning and memory function and neurotransmitter levels in rats with vascular dementia. Evid Based Complement Alternat Med. 2014. https://doi.org/10.1155/2014/294103.
21. Zhang X, Wu B, Nie K, Jia Y, Yu J. Effects of acupuncture on declined cerebral blood flow, impaired mitochondrial respiratory function and oxidative stress in multi-infarct dementia rats. Neurochem Int. 2014;65(1):23–9.
22. Li F, Yan CQ, Lin LT, Li H, Zeng XH, Liu Y, et al. Acupuncture attenuates cognitive deficits and increases pyramidal neuron number in hippocampal ca1 area of vascular dementia rats. BMC Complement Altern Med. 2015. https://doi.org/10.1186/s12906-015-0656-x.
23. Li QQ, Shi GX, Yang JW, Li ZX, Zhang ZH, He T, et al. Hippocampal cAMP/PKA/CREB is required for neuroprotective effect of acupuncture. Physiol Behav. 2015. https://doi.org/10.1016/j.physbeh.
24. Wang XR, Shi GX, Yang JW, Yan CQ, Lin LT, Du SQ, et al. Acupuncture ameliorates cognitive impairment and hippocampus neuronal loss in

experimental vascular dementia through Nrf2-mediated antioxidant response. Free Radic Biol Med 2015. dio: https://doi.org/10.1016/j.freeradbiomed.2015.10.426

25. Fang Y, Sui R. Electroacupuncture at the WANGU acupoint suppresses expression of inflammatory cytokines in the Hippocampus of rats with vascular dementia. Afr J Tradit Complement Altern Med. 2016;13(5):17–24.

26. Li H, Liu Y, Lin LT, Wang XR, Du SQ, Yan CQ, et al. Acupuncture reversed hippocampal mitochondrial dysfunction in vascular dementia rats. Neurochem Int. 2015;92:35–42.

27. Moher D, Liberati A, Tetzlaff J, Altman DG, The PRISMA group. Preferred reporting items for systematic reviews and meta-analyses: the PRISMA statement. PLoS Med. 2009;6(7):e1000097. https://doi.org/10.1371/journal.pmed.1000097

28. Huang KY, Liang S, Yu ML, Fu SP, Chen X, Lu SF. A systematic review and meta-analysis of acupuncture for improving learning and memory ability in animals. BMC Complement Altern Med. 2016 Aug 19. https://doi.org/10.1186/s12906-016-1298-3.

29. Venkat P, Chopp M, Chen J. Models and mechanisms of vascular dementia. Exp Neurol. 2015;272:97–108.

30. Senn SJ. Overstating the evidence – double counting in meta-analysis and related problems. BMC Med Res Methodol. 2009;9(1):1–7.

31. Harris R, Bradburn M, Deeks J, Harbord R, Altman D, Steichen T, et al. Metan: stata module for fixed and random effects meta-analysis. Stat Softw Components. 2006;8(1):3–28.

32. Harris RJ, Bradburn MJ, Deeks JJ, Harbord RM, Altman DG, Sterne JAC. Metan: fixed- and random-effects meta-analysis. Stata J. 2008;8(1):3–28.

33. Palmer TM, Sterne JAC. Meta-analysis in Stata. Systematic reviews in health care: meta-analysis in context, second edition. BMJ publishing. Group. 2001:347–69.

34. Sterne J, Egger M, Smith G. Systematic reviews in health care: investigating and dealing with publication and other biases in meta-analysis. BMJ. 2001;323(7304):101–5.

35. Ahmed I, Sutton AJ, Riley RD. Assessment of publication bias, selection bias, and unavailable data in meta-analyses using individual participant data: a database survey. BMJ. 2011;344(7838):d7762.

36. Qi S, Mizuno M, Yonezawa K, Nawa H, Takei N. Activation of mammalian target of rapamycin signaling in spatial learning. Neurosci Res. 2010;68:88–93.

37. Leung MC, Yip KK, Ho YS, Siu FK, Li WC, Garner B. Mechanisms underlying the effect of acupuncture on cognitive improvement: a systematic review of animal studies. J NeuroImmune Pharmacol. 2014;9(4):492–507.

38. Bekinschtein P, Katche C, Slipczuk LN, Igaz LM, Cammarota M, Izquierdo I, et al. mTOR signaling in the hippocampus is necessary for memory formation. Neurobiol Learn Mem. 2007;87:303–7.

39. Shi GX, Li QQ, Yang BF, Liu Y, Guan LP, Wu MM, et al. Acupuncture for Vascular Dementia: A Pragmatic Randomized Clinical Trial. Sci World J. 2015;(4):161439.

Permissions

List of Contributors

Bongjun Sur, Bombi Lee, Mijung Yeom, Ju-Hee Hong and Sunoh Kwon
Acupuncture and Meridian Science Research Center, College of Korean Medicine, Kyung Hee University, Hoegi-ding, Dongdaemoon-gu, Seoul 130-701, Republic of Korea

Hyang Sook Lee, Hi-Joon Park, Hyejung Lee and Dae-Hyun Hahm
Acupuncture and Meridian Science Research Center, College of Korean Medicine, Kyung Hee University, Hoegi-ding, Dongdaemoon-gu, Seoul 130-701, Republic of Korea
The Graduate School of Basic Science of Korean Medicine, College of Korean Medicine, Kyung Hee University, Seoul 130-701, Republic of Korea

Seung-Tae Kim
Division of Meridian and Structural Medicine, School of Korean Medicine, Pusan National University, Yangsan 628-870, Republic of Korea

O sang Kwon, Kwang-Ho Choi, Junbeom Kim, Seong Jin Cho, Suk-Yun Kang, Ji-Young Moon and Yeon Hee Ryu
KM Fundamental Research Division, Korea Institute of Oriental Medicine, Daejeon, Korea

Sook-Hyun Lee
Department of Applied Korean Medicine, Graduate School, Kyung Hee University, Seoul, Republic of Korea

Sabina Lim
Department of Applied Korean Medicine, Graduate School, Kyung Hee University, Seoul, Republic of Korea
Research Group of Pain and Neuroscience, WHO Collaborating Center for Traditional Medicine, East–west Medical Research Institute, Kyung Hee University, Seoul, Republic of Korea
Department of Meridian & Acupoint, College of Korean Medicine, Kyung Hee University, 26 Kyungheedae-ro,Dongdaemun-gu, Seoul 130-70102447, Republic of Korea

Maurits van den Noort
Research Group of Pain and Neuroscience, WHO Collaborating Center for Traditional Medicine, East–west Medical Research Institute, Kyung Hee University, Seoul, Republic of Korea

Peggy Bosch
Donders Institute for Brain, Cognition and Behaviour, Radboud University, 6525 HR Nijmegen, The Netherlands

Jing-jing Wei, Wen-ting Yang, Su-bing Yin, Chen Wang, Yan Wang and Guo-qing Zheng
Department of Neurology, the Second Affiliated Hospital and Yuying Children's Hospital of Wenzhou Medical University, Wenzhou, China

Yangseok Lee, Hi-Joon Park and Dae-Hyun Hahm
Acupuncture and Meridian Science Research Center, College of Korean Medicine, Kyung Hee University, 26, Kyungheedae-ro, Dongdaemun-gu, Seoul 02447, Republic of Korea
Department of Basic Science of Korean Medicine, Graduate School, Kyung Hee University, 26, Kyungheedae-ro, Dongdaemun-gu, Seoul 02447, Republic of Korea

Sunoh Kwon
Acupuncture and Meridian Science Research Center, College of Korean Medicine, Kyung Hee University, 26, Kyungheedae-ro, Dongdaemun-gu, Seoul 02447, Republic of Korea
Department of Psychiatry and Behavioral Sciences, Northwestern University Feinberg School of Medicine, Chicago 60611, USA
KM Fundamental Research Division, Korea Institute of Oriental Medicine, Daejeon 34054, Republic of Korea

Sook-Hyun Lee and Sung Min Lim
Department of Clinical Research on Rehabilitation, Korea National Rehabilitation Research Institute, 58 Samgaksan-ro, Gangbuk-gu, Seoul 142-070, Republic of Korea

Kwang-Ho Choi, O Sang Kwon, Seong Jin Cho, Sanghun Lee, Seok-Yun Kang and Yeon Hee Ryu
KM Fundamental Research Division, Korea Institute of Oriental Medicine, 1672 Yuseong-daero, Yuseong-Gu, Daejeon 305-811, South Korea

Felicity L. Bishop and Lucy Yardley
Psychology, Faculty of Social and Human Sciences, University of Southampton, Building 44 Highfield Campus, Southampton SO17 1BJ, UK

Cyrus Cooper
MRC Lifecourse Epidemiology Unit, University of Southampton, Southampton General Hospital, Tremona Road, Southampton SO16 6YD, UK

Paul Little and George Lewith
Primary Care and Population Sciences, Aldermoor Health Centre, University of Southampton, Southampton SO16 5ST, UK

Xuanming Hu, Mengqian Yuan, Yin Yin, Yidan Wang, Yuqin Li, Na Zhang, Xueyi Sun, Zhi Yu and Bin Xu
Key Laboratory of Integrated Acupuncture and Drugs Constructed, Nanjing University of Chinese Medicine, Ministry of Education, Nanjing 210023, China

Yali Liu, Xiuxia Li and Dang Wei
Evidence-Based Medicine Center, School of Basic Medical Sciences, Lanzhou University, Lanzhou 730000, China
Key Laboratory of Evidence Based Medicine and Knowledge Translation of Gansu Province, Lanzhou 730000, China

Xiaoqin Wang and and Kehu Yang
Evidence-Based Medicine Center, School of Basic Medical Sciences, Lanzhou University, Lanzhou 730000, China
Key Laboratory of Evidence Based Medicine and Knowledge Translation of Gansu Province, Lanzhou 730000, China
Chinese GRADE Center, Lanzhou 730000, China

Xiue Shi
Evidence-Based Medicine Center, School of Basic Medical Sciences, Lanzhou University, Lanzhou 730000, China
Key Laboratory of Evidence Based Medicine and Knowledge Translation of Gansu Province, Lanzhou 730000, China

Chinese GRADE Center, Lanzhou 730000, China
Gansu Rehabilitation Center Hospital, Lanzhou 730000, China

Xu Zhao
Evidence-Based Medicine Center, School of Basic Medical Sciences, Lanzhou University, Lanzhou 730000, China
Department of Hypertension, Lanzhou University Second Hospital, Lanzhou 730000, China

Jing Gu
Gansu University of Chinese Medicine, Lanzhou 730000, China

Jungtae Leem
Korean Medicine Clinical Trial Center, College of Korean Medicine, Kyung Hee University, Seoul, South Korea
Department of Clinical Research of Korean Medicine, College of Korean Medicine, Kyung Hee University, Seoul, South Korea

Sanghoon Lee
Korean Medicine Clinical Trial Center, College of Korean Medicine, Kyung Hee University, Seoul, South Korea
Department of Acupuncture and Moxibustion, College of Korean Medicine, Kyung Hee University, Hoegi-dong 1, Dongdaemun-gu, Seoul 130-701, Republic of Korea

Gajin Han
Korean Medicine Clinical Trial Center, College of Korean Medicine, Kyung Hee University, Seoul, South Korea
Department of Gastroenterology, College of Korean Medicine, Kyung Hee University, Seoul, South Korea

Junhee Lee
Korean Medicine Clinical Trial Center, College of Korean Medicine, Kyung Hee University, Seoul, South Korea
Department of Sasang Constitutional Medicine, College of Korean Medicine, Kyung Hee University, Seoul, South Korea

Jimin Park
Department of Acupuncture and Moxibustion, College of Korean Medicine, Kyung Hee University, Hoegi-dong 1, Dongdaemun-gu, Seoul 130-701, Republic of Korea

Seulgi Eun and Kyungmo Park
Department of Biomedical Engineering, Kyung Hee University, Yongin, Gyeonggi, South Korea

Meena M. Makary
Department of Biomedical Engineering, Kyung Hee University, Yongin, Gyeonggi, South Korea
Systems and Biomedical Engineering Department, Faculty of Engineering, Cairo University, Giza, Egypt

Emery R. Eaves
Department of Anthropology, Northern Arizona University, 5 E. McConnell Drive, , Flagstaff, AZ 86011-5200, USA

Amy Howerter, Judith S. Gordon, Cheryl Ritenbaugh and Myra L. Muramoto
Department of Family and Community Medicine, College of Medicine, University of Arizona, 1450 N Cherry Ave, Tucson, AZ 85719, USA

Mark Nichter
School of Anthropology, College of Social and Behavioral Sciences, Department of Family and Community Medicine, College of Medicine, University of Arizona, , Tucson, AZ 85721-0030, USA

Lysbeth Floden
Department of Pharmacy Practice & Science, College of Pharmacy, University of Arizona, 1295 N. Martin, , Tucson, AZ 85721, USA

Wei-Chen Tang
Department of Chinese Medicine, Tainan Municipal An-Nan Hospital, Tainan, Taiwan

Yao-Chin Hsu
Department of Chinese Medicine, Chi-Mei Medical Center, Tainan, Taiwan

Che-Chuan Wang
Department of Neurosurgery, Chi-Mei Medical Center, Tainan, Taiwan
Department of Medical research, Chi-Mei Medical Center, Tainan, Taiwan
Department of Child Care, Southern Taiwan University of Science and Technology, Tainan, Taiwan

Chiao-Ya Hu and Chung-Ching Chio
Department of Medical research, Chi-Mei Medical Center, Tainan, Taiwan

Jinn-Rung Kuo
Department of Medical research, Chi-Mei Medical Center, Tainan, Taiwan
Department of Biotechnology, Southern Taiwan University of Science and Technology, Tainan, Taiwan
Traumatic,Brain Injury Center, Chi Mei Hospital, No. 901, Zhonghua Rd., Yongkang Dist.,Tainan City 710, Taiwan, ROC

Chao Liang, Bin Xu and Zhi Yu
Nanjing University of Chinese Medicine, Nanjing 210046, Jiangsu Province, China

Kaiyue Wang
Xi'an Traditional Chinese Medicine Brain Disease Hospital, Xi'an 710000, China

Alexandra Jocham, Antonius Schneider and Klaus Linde
Institute of General Practice, Klinikum rechts der Isar, Technical University of Munich, Orleansstrasse 47, 81667 Munich, Germany

Levente Kriston
Department of Medical Psychology, University Medical Center Hamburg-Eppendorf, Hamburg, Germany

Pascal O. Berberat
TUM Medical Education Center, TUM School of Medicine, Technical University of Munich, Munich, Germany

Xinrong Li, Yang Liu, Qinxiu Zhang and Xiaopei Wang
Department of Otorhinolaryngology, Head and Neck Surgery of the Teaching Hospital of Chengdu University of Traditional Chinese Medicine, Chengdu, Sichuan Province 610072, People's Republic of China

Nan Xiang, Miao He, Juan Zhong and Qing Chen
Chengdu University of Traditional Chinese Medicine, Chengdu, Sichuan Province 610072, People's Republic of China

To-Yi Lam and Li-Zhu Lin
Department of Oncology, Guangzhou University of Chinese Medicine, Guangzhou 510405, China

Li-Ming Lu
The Second Affiliated Hospital of Guangzhou University of Chinese Medicine, Guangdong Provincial Hospital of Chinese Medicine, Guangzhou 510120, China

Wai-Man Ling
Department of Clinical Oncology, Pamela Youde Nethersole Eastern Hospital, 3 Lok Man Road, Chai Wan, Hong Kong

Tomoko Suzuki and Tadamichi Mitsuma
Department of Kampo Medicine, Aizu Medical Center, Fukushima Medical University School of Medicine, 21-2 Maeda, Tanisawa, Kawahigashi, Aizuwakamatsu, Fukushima 969-3492, Japan

Masao Suzuki
Department of Kampo Medicine, Aizu Medical Center, Fukushima Medical University School of Medicine, 21-2 Maeda, Tanisawa, Kawahigashi, Aizuwakamatsu, Fukushima 969-3492, Japan
Respiratory Disease Center, Kitano Hospital, Tazuke Kofukai Medical Research Institute, 2-4-20 Ohgimachi, Kita-ku, Osaka 530-8480, Japan

Shigeo Muro
Department of Respiratory Medicine, Nara Medical University, 840 Shijo-Cho, Kashihara, Nara 634-8521, Japan

Motonari Fukui
Respiratory Disease Center, Kitano Hospital, Tazuke Kofukai Medical Research Institute, 2-4-20 Ohgimachi, Kita-ku, Osaka 530-8480, Japan

Naoto Ishizaki
Course of Acupuncture and Moxibustion, Faculty of Health Sciences, Tsukuba University of Technology, 4-12-7 Kasuga, Tsukuba, Ibaraki 305-8521, Japan

Susumu Sato and Toyohiro Hirai
Department of Respiratory Medicine, Graduate School of Medicine, Kyoto University, Yoshida, Konoe-cho, Sakyo-ku, Kyoto 606-8501, Japan

Tetsuhiro Shiota
Department of Respiratory Medicine, Shiga General Hospital, 4-30 Moriyama-cho, Moriyama, Shiga 524-8524, Japan

Kazuo Endo
Department of Respiratory Medicine, Hyogo Prefectural Amagasaki General Medical Center, 2-17-77 Higashinanba-cho, Amagasaki, Hyogo 660-8550, Japan

Michiaki Mishima
Noe Hospital, 1-3-25 Joto-ku, Osaka 536-001, Japan

Yang Xu
Graduate School, Tianjin University of Traditional Chinese Medicine, Tianjin 300193, China
Department of Gynecology and Obstetrics, Nankai Hospital, Tianjin Academy of Integrative Medicine, Tianjin 300100, China

Wenli Zhao
Graduate School, Tianjin University of Traditional Chinese Medicine, Tianjin 300193, China
Department of Neurology, Nankai Hospital, Tianjin Academy of Integrative Medicine, Tianjin 300100, China

Te Li
Department of Chinese Medicine, Tianjin Hearing Impairment Specialist Hospital, Tianjin 300150, China

Huaien Bu
Department of Public Health, School of Chinese Medicine, Tianjin University of Traditional Chinese Medicine, Tianjin 300193, China

Zhimei Zhao
Department of Gynecology and Obstetrics of Chinese Medicine, First Teaching Hospital of Tianjin University of Traditional Chinese Medicine, Tianjin 300193, China

Ye Zhao
Department of Chemical Engineering, University of Florida, 1006 Center Drive, Gainesville, FL 32611, USA
Institute for Cell & Tissue Science and Engineering, University of Florida, Gainesville, FL 32611, USA

Shilin Song
Laboratory of Anatomy, School of Integrative Medicine, Tianjin University of Traditional Chinese Medicine, No. 88 Yu Quan Road, Nankai District, Tianjin 300193, China

Tae Young Yang, Eun Young Jang, Gyu Won Lee, Eun Byeol Lee, Suchan Chang, Jong Han Lee and Chae Ha Yang
College of Korean Medicine, Daegu Haany University, Daegu 42158, South Korea

Hee Young Kim
College of Korean Medicine, Daegu Haany University, Daegu 42158, South Korea
Department of Physiology, College of Korean Medicine, Daegu Haany University, Daegu 42158, South Korea

Yeonhee Ryu
Korean Medicine Fundamental Research Division, Korea Institute of Oriental Medicine, Daejeon 34054, South Korea

Jin Suk Koo
Department of Bioresource Science, Andong National University, Andong 36729, South Korea

Kwok Yin Au
Hong Kong Institute of Integrative Medicine, Faculty of Medicine, The Chinese University of Hong Kong, Hong Kong, China

Haiyong Chen and Lixing Lao
School of Chinese Medicine, The University of Hong Kong, 10 Sassoon Road, Pokfulam, Hong Kong, China
Department of Chinese Medicine, The University of Hong Kong-Shenzhen Hospital, Shenzhen, China

Kin Cheung Mak
Department of Chinese Medicine, The University of Hong Kong-Shenzhen Hospital, Shenzhen, China
Department of Orthopaedics and Traumatology, Li Ka Shing Faculty of Medicine, The University of Hong Kong, Hong Kong, China

Wing Chung Lam, Chiu On Chong, Andrew Lau, Wing Yi Lam, Fung Man Wu, Hiu Ngok Chan and Yan Wah Ng
The Hong Kong Tuberculosis Association Chinese Medicine Clinic cum Training Centre of the University of Hong Kong, Hong Kong, China

Varut Vardhanabhuti
Department of Diagnostic Radiology, Li Ka Shing Faculty of Medicine, The University of Hong Kong, Hong Kong, China

Fei Jiang
Department of Statistics and Actuarial Science, The University of Hong Kong, Hong Kong, China.

Bacon Fung-Leung Ng and Eric Tat-Chi Ziea
The Chinese Medicine Department, Hospital Authority, Hong Kong, China

Yingfan Chen, Sinan Tian and Shi Shu
Changhai Hospital of Traditional Chinese Medicine, Second Military Medical University, 168 Changhai Road, Yangpu District, Shanghai, China

Jing Tian
Department of Nursing Science, Second Military Medical University, Shanghai, China

Ze-Yu Zhang and Hui-Hui Deng
Department of Traditional Chinese Medicine, Third Clinical Medical College of Zhejiang Chinese Medical University, Hangzhou, Zhejiang, China

Zhe Liu
Department of of Neurobiology and Acupuncture Research, Third Clinical College of Zhejiang Chinese Medical University, Hangzhou, Zhejiang, China

Qin Chen
Department of Acupuncture, Zhejiang Chinese Medical University Affiliated Third Hospital, Hangzhou, Zhejiang, China

Index